Practical Clinical Electrophysiology

EDITORS

Peter J. Zimetbaum, MD

Associate Professor of Medicine
Harvard Medical School
Director, Clinical Cardiology
Cardiovascular Division
Beth Israel Deaconess Medical Center
Boston, Massachusetts

Mark E. Josephson, MD

Herman C. Dana Professor of Medicine
Harvard Medical School
Chief of the Cardiovascular Division
Chief Medical Officer and Chief Academic Officer of the Cardiovascular Institute
of the Beth Israel Deaconess Medical Center
Director, Harvard-Thorndike Electrophysiology Institute
and Arrhythmia Service
Beth Israel Deaconess Medical Center
Boston, Massachusetts

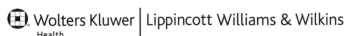
Wolters Kluwer | Lippincott Williams & Wilkins
Health

Philadelphia · Baltimore · New York · London
Buenos Aires · Hong Kong · Sydney · Tokyo

Acquisitions Editor: Frances R. DeStefano
Managing Editor: Chris Potash
Project Manager: Alicia Jackson
Manufacturing Coordinator: Kathleen Brown
Manufacturing Manager: Kimberly Schonberger
Design Coordinator: Holly McLaughlin
Cover Designer: Louis Fuiano
Production Services: Laserwords Private Limited, Chennai, India

© 2009 by LIPPINCOTT WILLIAMS & WILKINS, a WOLTERS KLUWER business
530 Walnut Street
Philadelphia, PA 19106 USA
LWW.com

Printed in the USA

Library of Congress Cataloging-in-Publication Data

Practical clinical electrophysiology/editors, Peter J. Zimetbaum, Mark E. Josephson.
  p.; cm.
  Includes bibliographical references and index.
  ISBN-13: 978-0-7817-6603-6
  ISBN-10: 0-7817-6603-6
  1. Arrhythmia. 2. Heart—Electric properties. 3. Electrophysiology. I. Zimetbaum, Peter J.
II. Josephson, Mark E.
  [DNLM: 1. Arrhythmias, Cardiac—physiopathology. 2. Cardiac Electrophysiology—methods.
3. Arrhythmias, Cardiac—diagnosis. 4. Arrhythmias, Cardiac—therapy. WG 330 P8954 2009]
  RC685.A65P693 2009
  616.1'28—dc22

                                                                    2008028374

Care has been taken to confirm the accuracy of the information presented and to describe generally accepted practices. However, the authors, editors, and publisher are not responsible for errors or omissions or for any consequences from application of the information in this book and make no warranty, expressed or implied, with respect to the currency, completeness, or accuracy of the contents of the publication. Application of the information in a particular situation remains the professional responsibility of the practitioner.

The authors, editors, and publisher have exerted every effort to ensure that drug selection and dosage set forth in this text are in accordance with current recommendations and practice at the time of publication. However, in view of ongoing research, changes in government regulations, and the constant flow of information relating to drug therapy and drug reactions, the reader is urged to check the package insert for each drug for any change in indications and dosage and for added warnings and precautions. This is particularly important when the recommended agent is a new or infrequently employed drug.

Some drugs and medical devices presented in this publication have Food and Drug Administration (FDA) clearance for limited use in restricted research settings. It is the responsibility of health care provider to ascertain the FDA status of each drug or device planned for use in their clinical practice.

To purchase additional copies of this book, call our customer service department at (800) 638-3030 or fax orders to (301) 223-2320. International customers should call (301) 223-2300.

Visit Lippincott Williams & Wilkins on the Internet: at LWW.com. Lippincott Williams & Wilkins customer service representatives are available from 8:30 am to 6 pm, EST.

                                                        10 9 8 7 6 5 4 3 2 1

To Ben, Molly, and Roberta—for your love, encouragement, and understanding

To Sylvie Tessa, Elan Robert, Joan, Rachel, Todd, Stephanie, and Jesse—for their love and support.

Contributing
Authors

David J. Callans, MD
Director, Electrophysiology Laboratory
Professor of Medicine
Cardiovascular Medicine Division
Hospital of The University of Pennsylvania
Philadelphia, Pennsylvania
Atrial Flutter

Daniel R. Frisch, MD
Assistant Professor of Medicine
Division of Cardiology
Electrophysiology Section
Thomas Jefferson University
Philadelphia, Pennsylvania
Supraventricular Tachycardia

William H. Maisel, MD, MPH
Assistant Professor of Medicine
Harvard Medical School
Director of the Pacemaker and ICD Service
Beth Israel Deaconess Medical Center
Boston, Massachusetts

Permanent Pacemakers
Clinical Management of Patients with Implantable Cardioverter Defibrillators

Michael McLaughlin, MD
Instructor in Medicine
Harvard Medical School
Division of Cardiology
Beth Israel Deaconess Medical Center
Boston, Massachusetts

Sudden Death Syndromes
Implantable Cardioverter Defibrillator Indications

Christopher Pickett, MD
Assistant Professor of Medicine
University of Connecticut
Division of Cardiology
University of Connecticut Health Center
Farmington, Connecticut

Clinical Management of Patients with Implantable Cardioverter Defibrillators

Heiko Schmitt, MD, PhD
Assistant Professor of Medicine
University of Connecticut
Division of Cardiology
University of Connecticut Health Center
Farmington, Connecticut

Permanent Pacemakers

John V. Wylie Jr., MD
Instructor in Medicine
Harvard Medical School,
Director, Arrhythmia Monitoring Laboratory
Division of Cardiology
Beth Israel Deaconess Medical Center
Boston, Massachusetts

Wolff-Parkinson-White Syndrome and Variants

Preface

The last decade has seen an explosion in the therapeutic options available for the management of cardiac arrhythmias. As a result, the focus of electrophysiology training has turned toward acquiring the technical skills necessary to perform catheter ablation and complex device implantation and away from the diagnostic skills required for arrhythmia management. Our goal in writing this book is to provide a succinct and practical clinical approach to the major arrhythmia disorders encountered in the clinic as well as the electrophysiology laboratory. We have focused on the clinical history, electrocardiogram and diagnostic electrophysiology study. More comprehensive texts are available, which delineate the details of diagnostic and therapeutic invasive electrophysiology studies. We hope it will prove equally useful to the internist evaluating syncope, the cardiologist deciding if a pacemaker is needed during a myocardial infarction complicated by complete heart block, and the electrophysiology fellow learning how to differentiate the various forms of supraventricular tachycardia in the electrophysiology laboratory.

As is true for most fields of medicine there is as much art as there is science in electrophysiology. We and the contributing authors to this book share a common "style" of arrhythmia management and passion for the clinical care of patients with arrhythmia disorders, which we hope will prove helpful to physicians caring for these fascinating patients.

Peter J. Zimetbaum, MD
Mark E. Josephson, MD

Acknowledgments

We would like to thank the current and past medical housestaff and cardiology fellows at the Beth Israel Deaconess Medical Center—it is their enthusiasm for learning and commitment to the care of our patients, which keeps us motivated to continue teaching electrophysiology. We would especially like to thank Karen Thomas, MD and Joseph Germano, DO for their assistance in proof reading selected chapters.

Contents

Contributing Authors   vii

Preface   ix

Acknowledgments   xi

1 Anatomy in Clinical Electrophysiology   1

2 Cellular Electrophysiology   13

3 Mechanism of Tachycardias   19

4 The Basic Electrophysiology Study   25

5 Basic Principles in Clinical Electrophysiology   41

6 Atrial Fibrillation   55

7 Atrial Flutter 73

8 Supraventricular Tachycardia 85

9 Wolff-Parkinson-White Syndrome and Variants 119

10 Ventricular Tachycardia 137

11 Bradycardias 163

12 Syncope 179

13 Sudden Death Syndromes 193

14 Implantable Cardioverter Defibrillator Indications 219

15 Permanent Pacemakers 231

16 Clinical Management of Patients with Implantable Cardioverter Defibrillators 251

17 Noninvasive Diagnostic Testing 269

18 Antiarrhythmic Drugs 279

Index 297

Anatomy in Clinical Electrophysiology

An understanding of cardiac anatomy is essential to the diagnosis and treatment of arrhythmias. This knowledge is required to allow recording of normal and abnormal electrical activity as well as anticipate electrophysiological consequences of various types of cardiac pathology.

RIGHT ATRIUM

Normal electrical activation of the heart begins in the sinus node complex located as a subepicardial structure at the junction of the high right atrium (RA) and the superior vena cava (see Fig. 1-1). The sinus node is a spindle-shaped complex of cells that generally lies in a superior and lateral location in the RA but occasionally extends posteromedially to the interatrial groove. The right phrenic nerve runs in close proximity to the sinus node on the epicardial surface of the RA. The sinus node is supplied by the right coronary artery (RCA) in 60% of patients and left circumflex artery (LCX) in 40% of patients (see Table 1-1). The sinus node is heavily innervated by parasympathetic and sympathetic inputs.

    Once the impulse leaves the sinus node it travels inferiorly toward the atrioventricular (AV) node located in the low septal aspect of the RA. Conduction to the left atrium occurs through activation of the coronary sinus (CS) and through a series of fibers called the *Bachmann bundle* that extend from the crest

1

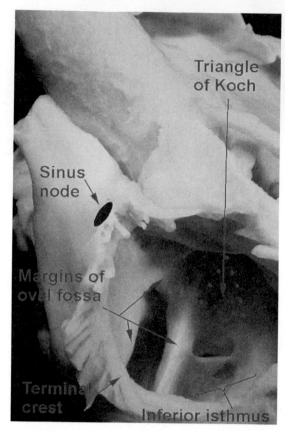

FIGURE 1-1. Right atrium opened, demonstrating the epicardial location of the sinus node in relation to the crista terminalis (terminal crest). The fossa ovalis and triangle of Koch are also demonstrated. (Courtesy Prof RH Anderson) (See color insert.)

TABLE 1-1 Vascular Supply of the Cardiac Conduction System

- Sinoatrial (SA) node: RCA (60%), LCX (40%)
- AV node: RCA (90%), LCX (10%)
- His bundle: RCA with small contribution from septal perforators of LAD
- Main and proximal left bundle branch block (LBBB): LAD (proximal), small collateral contribution from LCX or RCA
- Left anterior fascicle: anterior septal perforator, 50% of population has contribution from AV nodal artery
- Left posterior fascicle: proximal portion—AV nodal artery—distal portion—anterior and posterior septal perforators
- Right bundle branch block (RBBB): anterior septal perforators and collateral flow from RCA and LCX

RCA, right coronary artery; LCX, left circumflex artery, AV, atrioventricular node; LAD, left anterior descending coronary artery.

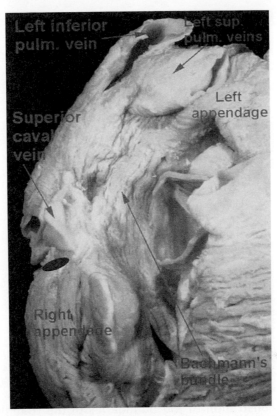

FIGURE 1-2. Right atrium demonstrating the location of the Bachmann bundle. The *blue oval* represents the sinus node. (Courtesy Prof RH Anderson) (See color insert.)

of the right atrial appendage through the transverse sinus behind the aorta and across the interatrial groove toward the left atrial appendage (LAA) (see Fig. 1-2). There is also some activation through the fossa ovalis.

The ostium of the CS lies in an inferior and posterior location in the RA. It forms the base of the triangle of Koch within which lies the compact AV node. The two sides of this triangle which emanate from this base include the septal leaflet of the tricuspid valve (TV) and the tendon of Todoro. The tendon of Todoro is a fibrous structure that forms as an extension of the Eustachian valve of the inferior vena cava and the Thebesian valve of the CS ostium (see Fig. 1-3). This tendon runs septally into the central fibrous body (CFB). The CFB is a confluence of fibrous tissue formed by the connection of the membranous septum with the fibrous trigones. The right and left fibrous trigones represent the areas of thickening at the edges of the connected or shared aspects of the aortic and mitral valves (*anterior* mitral leaflet). The right fibrous trigone connects with the membranous septum to form the CFB. The right coronary cusp of the aortic valve overlies and is continuous with the membranous septum. The noncoronary cusp overlies the right fibrous trigone and the left

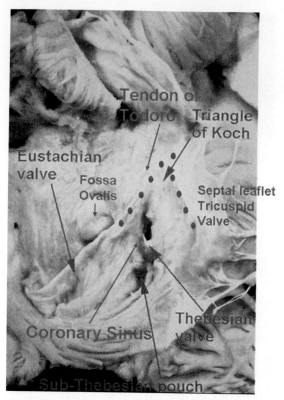

FIGURE 1-3. Demonstration of the boundaries of the triangle of Koch, right atrium, and fossa ovalis. (See color insert.)

coronary cusp overlies the left fibrous trigone. The aortic-mitral curtain is suspended between the trigones and forms the posterior aspect of the aortic outflow tract (see Fig. 1-4).

The fossa ovalis is the rim demarcating closure of the septum secundum and remnant of the septum primum. It is roughly at a 90-degree angle from but at the same level as the AV node/His bundle. The roof of the fossa ovale is formed by a muscular ridge called the *limbus*. Direct placement of a needle through the fossa will lead to the left atrium (Fig. 1-3). Penetration anterior to the fossa will enter the aorta. Penetration posterior and superior to the fossa will enter the invaginated groove or cleft between the right and left atria. This is the space commonly used by surgeons to access the left atrium and mitral valve.

The crista terminalis is a thick fibrous band of tissue that connects the inferior and superior vena cavae. It is located in the posterolateral aspect of the RA and can be identified by characteristic fractionated or split electrical recordings during electrophysiology study. This structure is a particularly common site for the development of atrial tachycardia.

The right atrial appendage is a relatively large structure which lies on the anterolateral surface of the left atrium. As is true of most of the RA it is full

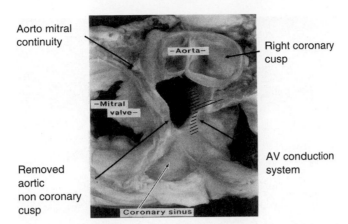

Aorto mitral
continuity

Right coronary
cusp

AV conduction
system

Removed
aortic
non coronary
cusp

FIGURE 1-4. Cross-section of the heart with the noncoronary cusp of the aortic valve removed. The relationship of the mitral valve, aortomitral continuity, aortic valve, and atrioventricular (AV) conduction system is shown.

of pectinate muscles. The shape of this structure facilitates stable pacemaker lead placement; however, its proximity to the TV sometimes results in "far field" sensing of ventricular electrical activity.

LEFT ATRIUM

The left atrium lies posterior to the RA. Four pulmonary veins (right and left superior and inferior) drain into the posterior aspect of the left atrium. The branching structure and size of these veins can vary greatly (see Fig. 1-5). A series of autonomic ganglia is present around the base of the pulmonary veins. The LAA lies just lateral to the left superior pulmonary vein and is separated from it on the endocardial surface by a thick muscular ridge of tissue. The appendage is composed of pectinate muscles and is the site of most thrombus formation associated with atrial fibrillation. The left phrenic nerve travels along the LAA and down along the obtuse margin of the left ventricle. The surgeon must carefully avoid this structure when placing a left ventricular pacing lead. The left main artery arises from the left coronary cusp between the pulmonary trunk and the LAA with the left circumflex running in close proximity to the LAA and CS.

The AV groove forms the posterior separation of the left atrium and ventricle. The LCX runs in this space, as does the CS. The anatomy of the CS is of particular importance to the electrophysiologist because it is utilized for pacing and recording of electrical activity involving the left side of the heart. Both the left atrium and the left ventricle can be recorded and paced through the CS. The CS runs in the AV groove along with the LCX. The body of the CS typically receives branches, which overlie the left ventricle (see Fig. 1-6). The great cardiac vein or anterior intraventricular vein is the branch which lies in

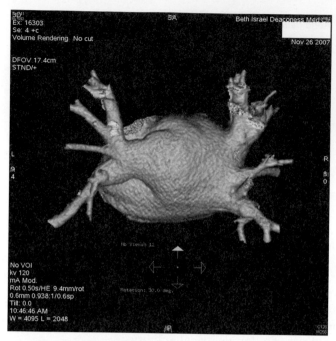

FIGURE 1-5. Computed tomographic (CT) angiogram of the posterior aspect of the left atrium. (See color insert.)

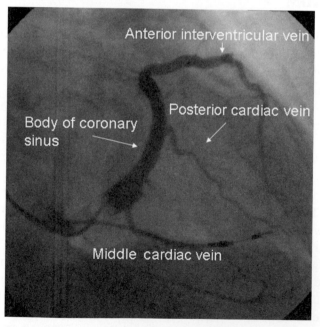

FIGURE 1-6. Right anterior oblique (RAO) coronary sinus venogram demonstrating the major branches of the coronary sinus. The posterior cardiac vein is the preferred target for coronary sinus lead placement.

the septum between the ventricles. It receives flow from the anterolateral branches and forms the posterior body of the CS. The posterolateral vein typically enters the mid portion of the CS and is the favored location for placement of pacing leads for ventricular resynchronization. The posterior branch enters more proximally in the CS and comes from the apex of the LV. This branch may enter the CS so proximally, that it forms a bifurcated ostium. As noted earlier, the Thebesian valve may be present at the CS ostium.

Ligament of Marshall

A remnant of the left superior vena cava, the ligament of Marshall, in most adults is a fold of pericardium which contains blood vessels, muscle fibers, and sympathetic nerve fibers (see Fig. 1-7). This structure lies above the LAA and lateral to the left superior pulmonary vein and drains into the CS through the oblique vein of the left atrium.

Atrioventricular Node

The AV node is a complex of cells, which, as noted earlier, lies within the confines of the triangle of Koch. The compact or dense AV node is present within atrial musculature above the septal leaflet of the TV. The AV node complex is composed of layers of transitional cells with varying electrical properties. The blood supply of the AV node derives from the AV nodal branch of the RCA in most patients. This AV nodal branch comes off the RCA at the crux of the heart (intersection of the AV and interventricular grooves).

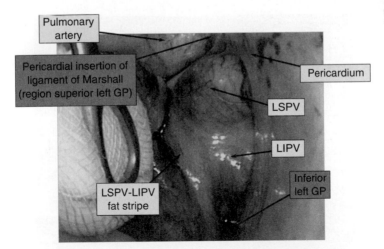

FIGURE 1-7. Epicardial exposure of the left atrium with the left superior pulmonary vein (LSPV), left inferior pulmonary vein (LIPV), ligament of Marshall, and ganglionic plexi (GP). (Courtesy Robert Hagberg, MD) (See color insert.)

His-Purkinje System

The proximal portion of the His bundle begins on the atrial aspect of the TV in the membranous atrial septum. The *AV junction* refers to the combination of the AV node and the proximal portion of the His bundle. The His bundle penetrates the septum between the CFB and the septal leaflet of the TV and splits into the left and right bundle branch systems. The left bundle branch begins in the membranous septum directly below the right and noncoronary aortic cusps (see Fig. 1-8). It is composed of a posteromedial or left posterior fascicle and the anterolateral or anterior fascicle. There usually is a septal branch of the left bundle. The right bundle branch runs in the septum as an insulated sheath until it reaches the base of the right ventricular papillary muscles. It then fans out into the myocardium at the apex of the right ventricle (RV).

After the impulse leaves the AV node it travels into the specialized infranodal conducting system, that is, through the His bundle, right and left bundle branches, and into the Purkinje network. The Purkinje network extends or fans out throughout the ventricular endocardium. The excellent insulation of the His-Purkinje system facilitates rapid conduction with near-simultaneous activation of the ventricles. Once out of the Purkinje network, the impulse proceeds relatively slowly through cell-to-cell contact through gap junctions from the endocardial to epicardial ventricular surface.

The normal pattern or sequence of activation occurs with early activation of the left ventricle in the septum and the anterior and posterior regions through the fascicles. The RV is activated shortly thereafter. The impulse next spreads to the subendocardial layer of the apical and free wall aspects of both ventricles through the Purkinje network. The last areas to be depolarized

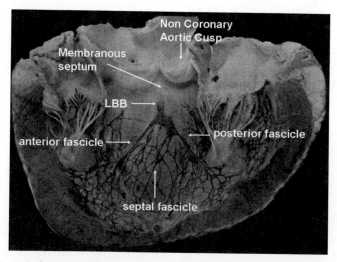

FIGURE 1-8. A left ventricle with the membranous septum and the left bundle branch delineated. LBB, left bundle branch. (See color insert.)

are the posterobasal portions of the ventricles. Repolarization occurs in the opposite direction from depolarization, that is, epicardium to endocardium.

The His bundle receives its blood supply from the septal perforating branches of the proximal left anterior descending (LAD) artery and the RCA. The right bundle branch and left anterior fascicle also receive their blood supply from the LAD artery. The left posterior fascicle has a dual blood supply from the RCA as well as the LAD.

RIGHT VENTRICLE

The RV is a particularly important structure from an electrophysiological standpoint. The right bundle branch travels in the interventricular septum to the apex of the RV and terminates at the base of the anterior papillary muscle. The RV, a highly trabeculated structure, is the standard site for temporary and permanent pacing. It is a relatively thin-walled structure, particularly at its apex and therefore prone to perforation. The inlet to the RV occurs through the TV. The TV contains septal, inferior, and anterosuperior leaflets. These leaflets are attached through chordae from anterior and medial papillary muscles. There are prominent fibrous trabeculations in the RV, the most notable of which is the moderator band. This structure runs from the septum to the anterior papillary muscle and is easily visualized by echocardiography.

The outlet or outflow tract of the RV is a musculature structure. The tissue separating the tricuspid and pulmonic valves is called the *supraventricular crest*, behind which lies the AV groove with the RCA. The supraventricular crest leads into the infundibular region of the right ventricular outflow tract (RVOT) in which the pulmonic valve sits. The RVOT is a common site for ventricular ectopic activity causing idiopathic ventricular tachycardia and is also the site of ventricular arrhythmias following repair of tetralogy of Fallot.

LEFT VENTRICLE

The surfaces of the left ventricle are described as inferior, septal, anterior, posterior, basal, and apical. Scar in these regions, often due to previous myocardial infarction, may form the substate for ventricular tachycardia. The mitral valve is a bileaflet structure with a posterior or mural leaflet and an anterior leaflet. The anterior leaflet is also called the *aortic leaflet* because it forms part of the left ventricular outflow tract. As noted earlier, this leaflet is continuous with a curtain of fibrous tissue (aortomitral curtain) which connects superiorly with the noncoronary and left coronary cusps of the aortic valve. This structure forms the posterior aspect of the aortic outflow tract while the membranous and muscular septum forms the septal surface.

The His bundle can be recorded on this septal side between the right coronary and noncoronary cusps before it continues on within the membranous septum to form the left bundle branch. The papillary muscles attach to the mitral valve leaflets through a complex "seaweed-like" network of chordae tendenae. The electrophysiologist must be careful to avoid entangling catheters in this network.

FLUOROSCOPIC ANATOMY

Most electrophysiology procedures continue to be performed under standard fluoroscopic guidance. The right anterior oblique (RAO) 30-degree and left anterior oblique (LAO) 45-degree views are most commonly employed (see Figs. 1-9 and 1-10).

Placement of the standard catheters for diagnostic and therapeutic electrophysiology studies are performed in the RAO projection as shown in Fig. 1-10. The RA is on the left with the AV groove/TV annulus lined up with the spine and the RV to the right of the spine. In this view, the right atrial catheter is placed in the right atrial appendage as shown. In real time, the catheter will move in a distinctive side-to-side motion. The His bundle catheter is placed across the TV annulus and the right ventricular catheter is placed in the apex.

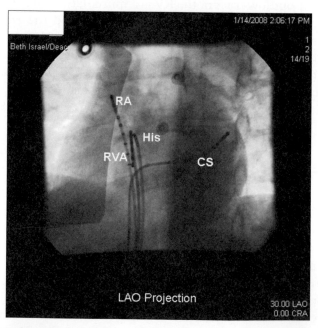

FIGURE 1-9. Left anterior oblique (LAO) fluoroscopic projection of catheter placement in a standard electrophysiology study. RA, right atrium; CS, coronary sinus; RVA, right ventricular apex.

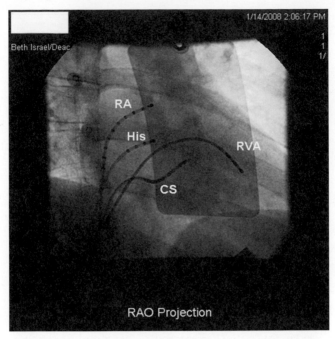

FIGURE 1-10. Right anterior oblique (RAO) fluoroscopic projection of catheter placement in a standard electrophysiology study. RA, right atrium; CS, coronary sinus; RVA, right ventricular apex.

The CS catheter enters the ostium in the low right posterior atrium and is seen extending over the course of the AV groove.

In the LAO projection the RA and ventricle are seen to the left, the septum is directly in the middle lined up with the spine, and the left atrium and ventricle are visualized to the right of the spine. This view is helpful to demonstrate that the CS catheter is in place and to direct catheters toward the septum when required. This is also the best view to image the lateral walls of the respective chambers. The LAO view is also critical for evaluation of CS lead placement for cardiac resynchronization. In this view the anterior interventricular vein can be distinguished from the lateral target veins.

Recently, laboratory systems have been developed to recreate anatomy based on the three-dimensional (3D) location of electrical signals. One system (CARTO-Biosense—Webster, Diamond Bar, California) uses a stable magnetic field placed under the patient and a sensor at the catheter tip in the heart to create an electroanatomic map. The catheter is maneuvered throughout the chamber of interest and a 3D reconstruction can be produced (see Fig. 1-11). As the catheter is manipulated around the chamber, a display of the local voltage of the myocardium is produced and the timing of electrical activation in that region (underneath the electrode) compared with a reference catheter is displayed (activation mapping).

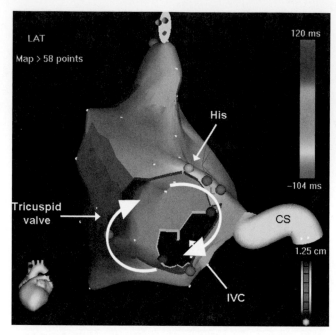

FIGURE 1-11. Electroanatomic (CARTO) image of the activation sequence during clockwise atrial flutter. The "head" and "tail" of the reentrant circuit meet where red meets purple/blue. LAT, local activation time; CS, coronary sinus; IVC, inferior vena cava. (See color insert.)

SELECTED BIBLIOGRAPHY

Anderson R, Hos S, Becker A. The surgical anatomy of the conduction tissues. *Thorax*. 1983;38:408–420.

Anderson R, Levy J. *Electrical anatomy of the atrial chambers*. 2000.

Josephson ME. *Clinical cardiac electrophysiology*, 4th ed. Philadelphia: Lippincott Williams and Wilkins; 2008.

Mazgalev T, Hos S, Anderson R. Anatomic-electrophysiological correlations concerning the pathways for atrioventricular conduction. *Circulation*. 2001;103:2660–2667.

Zimetbaum P, Josephson ME. Use of the electrocardiogram in acute myocardial infarction. *N Engl J Med*. 2003;348:933–940.

Cellular Electrophysiology

The action potential (AP) is the fundamental electrophysiologic event in cardiac cells. The coordinated flux of ions into and out of the cardiac cell forms the basis for cardiac depolarization and repolarization. These ions flow through a series of ion channels, which are the object of intensive and ongoing investigation. It is increasingly appreciated that alterations in the function of these channels through inherited abnormalities, metabolic alterations, or drug modulation can result both in arrhythmia suppression and life-threatening proarrhythmia.

The AP differs in fundamental ways between tissues responsible for slow impulse conduction (nodal tissue) and those responsible for rapid impulse propagation (His-Purkinje system [HPS], ventricular myocardium). Furthermore, important differences exist between the AP of ventricular tissues which appear to be dependent on the layer of cells that are examined (endo-, mid-, and epicardial tissue layers).

ACTION POTENTIAL

Action Potential of Sinus Node and Atrioventricular Node

The AP of nodal tissues differs from the AP of other myocytes by its absence of a resting membrane potential. The sinus and atrioventricular (AV) nodes

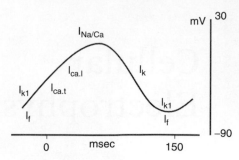

FIGURE 2-1. Calcium-dependent nodal action potentials.

rely largely on calcium-dependent APs which have a slow upstroke and an absence of a resting potential (see Fig. 2-1). These slow response tissues (sinus node and AV node) do not depend on voltage-sensitive sodium channels to initiate cardiac depolarization. During diastole (repolarization) the membrane potential drops to −50 to −60 and then slowly and spontaneously depolarizes again. This spontaneous "pacemaker" current is conducted through a nonselective inward current called I_f (allows Na and Ca in and K out). I_{k1} is also operative during this hyperpolarized potential and turns off as the cell is more depolarized. Depolarization is largely driven through slow voltage-gated inward calcium channels. There is a paucity of fast-activating sodium channels in nodal cells. Repolarization is achieved as the dominant current shifts to the outward (delayed rectifier) potassium current mediated by I_k.

Atrial, His-Purkinje System, and Ventricular Myocytes

In contrast to nodal tissue, conduction in atrial and ventricular muscle as well as the His-Purkinje network occurs rapidly due to sodium-dependent APs (see Fig. 2-2). These fast-response tissues (atria, bundle of His, fascicles/bundle branches, terminal Purkinje fibers, and ventricular tissue) depend on these sodium channels under normal circumstances.

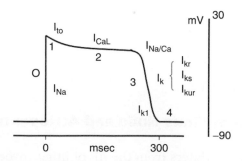

FIGURE 2-2. Sodium-dependent action potentials.

Phase 0: upstroke of AP due to rapid, transient influx of Na^+ (I_{Na})

Phase 1: Termination of upstroke of AP and early repolarization due to inactivation of Na channels and transient efflux of K^+ ($I_{to,f}$)

Phase 2: Plateau of AP—balance between influx of Ca^{2+} (I_{ca}) and outward repolarizing K^+ currents

Phase 3: Efflux of K^+ (I_{kr} and I_{ks})

Phase 4: Resting potential maintained by inward rectifier K^+ current (I_{k1})

Atrial and ventricular myocytes are stimulated or excited to begin the process of depolarization (opening of sodium channels) by current generated from the pacemaker tissues. The time it takes for the sodium channels to recover from inactivation is the time from the upstroke of the AP to the end of repolarization and defines the *refractory period* of normal ventricular tissues. The inward sodium channel is the dominant factor determining conduction velocity.

Selected Action Potential Alterations and Influence on Electrocardiogram

Deviation of the ST segment is likely due to the development of voltage gradients between the endocardium and epicardium (see Fig. 2-3). In the normal state, the AP of the epicardium has a distinct notch or "spike and dome." This notch is due to prominent I_{to} mediated outward potassium current during phase 1 of the AP. There is significantly more I_{to} in epicardial compared with endocardial layers and significantly more I_{to} in right ventricular compared with left ventricular epicardium. This difference between the epicardium and endocardium creates a transmural voltage gradient, which is represented typically by J point elevation. Factors that lead to a net *increase* in outward current during phase 1 will reduce the dome of the AP in the epicardial tissue compared with the endocardial tissue and cause a voltage gradient to develop. This voltage gradient is manifested in the electrocardiogram as ST elevation. Factors which increase outward current during phase 1 include potassium channel openers and sodium channel blockers.

A reduced I_{to}-mediated AP dome in the epicardial tissue compared with the endocardial tissue is likely responsible for the J point and ST elevation associated with early repolarization during slow heart rates. This typically produces an upward concave ST segment.

DEPOLARIZATION AND THE QRS INTERVAL

The QRS interval represents ventricular depolarization and is prolonged as a result of delay or block in conduction in the bundle branches. The QRS

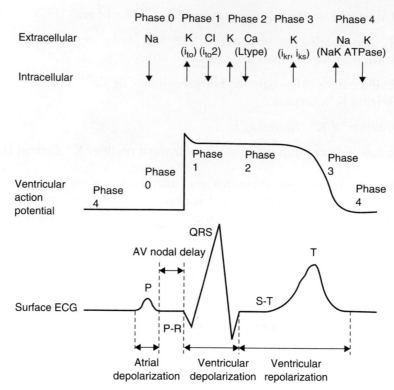

FIGURE 2-3. Ion channels and phases of the action potential and electrocardiogram (ECG). ATP, adenosine triphosphate.

complex can also be prolonged due to slow or abnormal conduction through the ventricular muscle. Drugs that block sodium channels can prolong the QRS complex. This occurs most often with type 1C antiarrhythmic drugs. These drugs block sodium channels in a use-dependent manner. In other words, although the QRS may be normal at resting heart rates, with increased heart rates there is increased binding (and less unbinding) of the medication and increased QRS prolongation. The class 1A drugs have a faster onset of binding and may produce QRS widening at rest.

REPOLARIZATION AND THE QT INTERVAL

The QT interval is the electrocardiographic representation of ventricular repolarization. Repolarization is determined by the balance between depolarizing (inward) current and repolarizing (outward) current. The predominant inward currents include the L-type Ca^{2+} current and the inward Na^+ current. The outward currents include the delayed rectifier potassium currents (slowly [I_{ks}] and rapidly [I_{kr}] acting). Any action that prolongs the AP duration will prolong the QT interval. Specifically any function that prolongs the inward current (e.g., potentiation of inward sodium current) or decreases the outward current (inhibition of outward potassium current) will prolong the QT interval. Most often the QT interval is prolonged due to drugs or congenital abnormalities of sodium or potassium channel function (see Chapter 18 and Chapter 13). Block of the inward calcium current during the plateau phase of atrial and ventricular tissues will shorten the AP duration.

SELECTED BIBLIOGRAPHY

Ackerman MJ, Clapham DE. Ion channels—basic science and clinical disease. *N Engl J Med*. 1997;336:1575–1586.

Arnsdorf MF. The cellular basis of cardiac arrhythmias: A matrical perspective. *Ann N Y Acad Sci*. 1990;601:263.

Josephson ME. *Clinical cardiac electrophysiology*, 4th ed. Philadelphia: Lippincott Williams and Wilkins; 2008.

Mechanism of Tachycardias

Most cardiac arrhythmias can be described as abnormalities of impulse formation, impulse conduction, or a combination of both. For example, the ventricular premature complex (VPC) which initiates monomorphic ventricular tachycardia in a patient with a prior anterior myocardial infarction represents an abnormality of impulse formation whereas the scar-mediated reentrant ventricular tachycardia is a manifestation of abnormal impulse conduction.

Triggered activity and abnormal automaticity, two common mechanisms of arrhythmia, are categorized as disorders of impulse formation.

TRIGGERED ACTIVITY

Triggered activity is the development of firing of a cluster of myocardial cells triggered by a series of preceding impulses. It is generated by a series of afterdepolarizations, which are spawned from a reduced level of membrane potential. These oscillations in membrane potential, if they reach threshold potential, can trigger the development of specific arrhythmias. Afterdepolarizations that develop before the completion of repolarization (during phase 2 or 3 of the action potential) are called *early afterdepolarizations* (EADs). Afterdepolarizations which occur following repolarization are called *delayed afterdepolarizations* (DADs) (see Fig. 3-1).

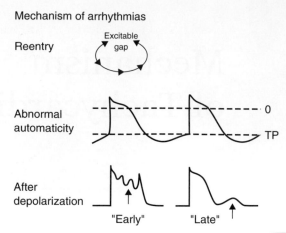

FIGURE 3-1. Different mechanisms of tachycardias.

EADs are believed to be responsible for arrhythmias associated with the acquired and congenital long QT syndromes. Slow heart rates and long coupled intervals promote the development of EADs, whereas faster heart rates and shorter coupled intervals suppress EADs. The administration of magnesium may suppress the development of EADs, explaining its effect in the management of polymorphic VT secondary to a prolonged QT interval (*torsades de pointes*).

DADs are felt to arise from transient inward currents which trigger membrane depolarizations. These transient inward currents occur in response to intracellular calcium overload and subsequent calcium release from the sarcoplasmic reticulum. DADs are due to an inward current produced by the Na/Ca exchanger. DADs have been demonstrated in tissue exposed to digitalis and many of the digoxin-associated arrhythmias are felt to be due to triggered activity. Accelerated idioventricular rhythms following myocardial infarction are also likely due to calcium loading and DADs resulting in triggered activity.

Clinical presentation (see Table 3-1): Clinical clues that an arrhythmia is due to triggered activity include the development of a tachycardia following an increase in sinus rate. The most common example is idiopathic right ventricular outflow tract tachycardia occurring in the setting of exercise or in response to a β-agonist and felt in many instances to be due to DADs.

Response to electrophysiologic study

- **Overdrive acceleration:** This refers to the observation that in rhythms due to triggered activity (due to DADs) when the heart is paced at a rate greater than the tachycardia rate the tachycardia rate increases following cessation of pacing (see Table 3-2).

TABLE 3-1 Mechanism of Common Clinical Arrhythmias

Reentry	*Triggered Activity*	*Automaticity*
Atrial tachycardia (initiates w/APD)	Atrial tachycardia (paroxysmal and associated with block e.g., digoxin toxicity due to DADs)	Atrial tachycardia (warms up, incessant younger patients)
AVNRT	RVOT VT	Reperfusion VT
AVRT	LQT (EADs)	Ischemic VT
Atrial flutter		
VT (scar mediated)		Fascicular VT
Idiopathic VT (verapamil sensitive)		

APD, atrial premature depolarization; DAD, delayed after depolarization;
AVNRT, atrioventricular nodal reentrant tachycardia; RVOT, right ventricular outflow tract;
VT, ventricular tachycardia; AVRT, atrioventricular reentrant tachycardia; LQT, long QT;
EAD, early after depolarization.

TABLE 3-2 Influence of Electrophysiologic Study (EPS) and Drugs on Different Mechanisms of Tachycardia

	Reentry	*Triggered Activity*	*Automaticity (Abnormal)*
Overdrive pacing	Entrain	Accelerate	Suppress
Premature stimuli	Initiate or terminate	Initiate or terminate	No
Afterdepolarizations recorded	Yes	Yes	No
Valsalva	Terminate	Terminate	No
Adenosine	Terminate	Terminate	No
Verapamil	Terminate	Terminate	No
Typical heart rates (AIVR, PV firing)	100–300	80–140	70–300

AIVR, accelerated idioventricular rhythm; PV, pulmonary vein.

- **Response to premature stimuli:** Premature stimuli can initiate or terminate triggered rhythms due to DADs but this is less reproducible than by overdrive pacing. Progressively premature stimuli result in a progressively shorter interval to first initiated tachycardia beat.

ABNORMAL AUTOMATICITY

Abnormal automaticity refers to the automatic rhythms which are felt to result from abnormal phase 4 depolarization of myocardial cells. These rhythms occur in atrial, junctional, or ventricular tissue. Idioventricular rhythms, parasystole, and incessant junctional tachycardia as is often seen following heart surgery are also felt to be automatic rhythms (Table 3-1).

Response to Electrophysiologic Study

- These rhythms exhibit either no overdrive suppression (depolarized tissue) or partial overdrive suppression of tissue (i.e., membrane potential of −70 to −80 mV). This is in contrast to normal automaticity such as in the sinus node or His-Purkinje system, which exhibits overdrive suppression (Table 3-2).

REENTRY

Reentry represents the most common mechanism of cardiac arrhythmias and is a disorder of impulse conduction. This mechanism requires two separate routes or pathways for electrical conduction (Fig. 3-1). These routes can be anatomically or functionally distinct. Arrhythmias develop with the introduction of a premature stimulus. The stimulus blocks in one pathway and conducts slowly in the other. The wave travels slowly enough to allow the blocked pathway to recover and conduct retrogradely through the originally blocked pathway. A single beat of re-entry is called an *echo beat*. The perpetuation of this reentry is tachycardia. The reentrant wavelength is equal to the conduction velocity of the impulse multiplied by the longest or most limiting refractory period of the circuit.

The anatomic substrate for reentry must be large enough to encompass the entire wavelength (the product of the refractory period and conduction velocity). If the length of the anatomic substrate is greater than the wavelength, there is a time interval or space between the tail of the circuit (end of refractoriness of preceding impulse) and the head (leading edge of depolarization) of the next impulse called the *excitable gap*. This excitable gap represents tissue, which is not refractory and therefore capable of being activated during the

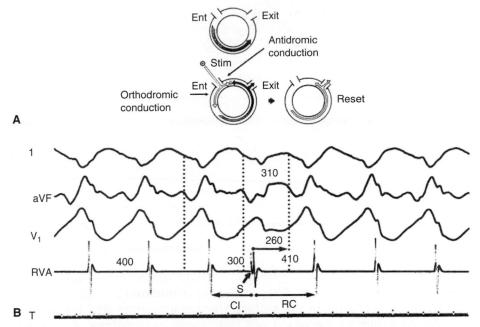

FIGURE 3-2. Schema of reentry with the introduction of a premature beat resulting in resetting of the tachycardia. **A:** The tachycardia wavefront is propagating in the circuit with the head represented by the black homogenous line representing absolutely refractory tissue and the gray stippled part representing partially refractory tissue. A stimulus is introduced into the circuit at the entrance (ENT). It conducts retrogradely (antidromic conduction) to collide with the head of the tachycardia and antegradely (orthodromic conduction). In **(B)** a ventricular premature depolarization (VPD) (*S*) is introduced at a coupling interval of 300 msec. It captures the ventricle with surface fusion and advances (reset) the next beat of the tachycardia. RVA; right ventricular apex; CI, coupling interval; RC, return cycle. (Adapted from Josephson ME. *Clinical Cardiac Electrophysiology*, 4th ed. 2008.)

tachycardia. The introduction of stimuli that penetrate the excitable gap can advance or reset the tachycardia or can terminate it (see Fig. 3-2). Resetting is the interaction of a premature wavefront with a tachycardia resulting in either advancement or delay of the subsequent tachycardia beat. In reentry the premature wavefront enters the excitable gap to collide retrogradely (antidromic) with the preceding tachycardia wavefront and to conduct antegradely (orthodromic) through excitable tissue in the circuit to produce an early complex. Resetting with fusion implies a reentrant mechanism with separate circuit entrance and exit sites. Fusion may be manifest on the electrocardiogram (ECG), or may be seen only on the local electrogram.

Continuous resetting of the tachycardia is called *entrainment,* another maneuver which proves reentry (see Fig. 3-3).

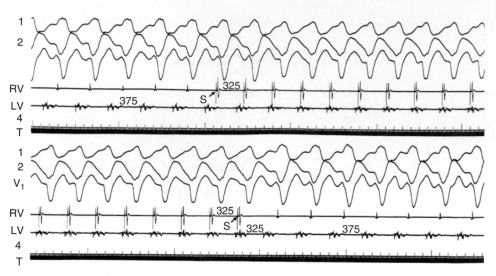

FIGURE 3-3. Entrainment of ventricular tachycardia. Ventricular tachycardia occurs at a cycle length of 375 msec. Pacing is initiated at a cycle length of 323 msec with a change in the surface electrocardiogram (ECG) morphology representing fusion of the paced and tachycardia morphology. Pacing is terminated in the bottom panel and the tachycardia resumes with the original morphology and cycle length. RV, right ventricle; LV, left ventricle. (Adapted from Josephson ME. *Clinical Cardiac Electrophysiology*, 4th ed. 2008.)

Response to Electrophysiologic Study

- Reproducible initiation and termination with premature stimulation

- Resetting (with single or double extrastimuli) or entrainment (with rapid pacing) (Table 3-2)

SELECTED BIBLIOGRAPHY

Josephson ME. *Clinical cardiac electrophysiology*, 3rd ed. Philadelphia: Lippincott Williams & Wilkins; 2002.

Josephson ME. *Clinical cardiac electrophysiology*, 4th ed. Philadelphia: Lippincott Williams & Wilkins; 2008.

The Basic Electrophysiology Study

The basic electrophysiologic (EP) investigation involves the placement of recording catheters in standard locations in the heart. Catheters with multiple (4 to 10) platinum electrodes through which electrical activity can be delivered and recorded are advanced through the venous system (inferior vena cava [IVC] or superior vena cava [SVC]) or retrogradely through the aorta. During a basic diagnostic EP study, catheters are placed in the right atrium (usually right atrial appendage [RAA]), across the tricuspid annulus, in the coronary sinus (CS) and in the right ventricular apex. The catheter in the RAA records a right atrial electrogram. The catheter placed across the tricuspid valve can record an atrial electrogram as well as a His bundle deflection and a ventricular electrogram (see Fig. 4-1).

The size of the atrial electrogram in reference to the ventricular electrogram defines whether the recording is a more proximal or distal His bundle tracing. In other words, if the atrial deflection is large or equal to the ventricular electrogram, the His electrogram represents a proximal His potential. Conversely, if the atrial deflection is small compared with the ventricular electrogram, the His deflection represents a distal His recording (see Fig. 4-2). The proximal portion of the His bundle can also be recorded from the left side of the heart by placement of a recording catheter in the noncoronary cusp or just below the aortic valve (see Fig. 4-3).

The CS is usually cannulated with a decapolar catheter. The proximal poles record activity near the CS and the distal poles record activity in the

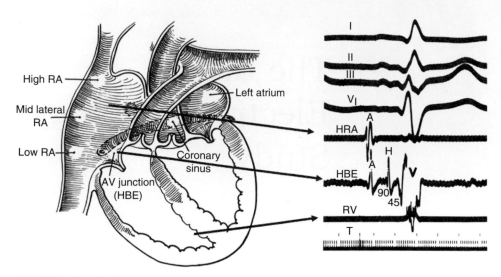

FIGURE 4-1. Schematic diagram of standard diagnostic catheters positioned to measure conduction intervals. RA, right atrium; HRA, high right atrium; AV, atrioventricular; HBE, His bundle electrogram; RV, right ventricle. (Adapted from Josephson ME. *Clinical Cardiac Electrophysiology*, 4th ed. 2008.)

anterolateral region of the atrioventricular (AV) groove. In general, normal atrial conduction will demonstrate activation of the CS from proximal to distal to the lateral wall of the left atrium indicating earliest activation from the right atrium at the region of the ostium of the CS. When the catheter is placed deep in the CS near the anterior interventricular vein, activation will occur earlier or simultaneously in the distal CS recording electrodes as the proximal CS. This indicates conduction over the Bachmann bundle (see Fig. 4-4).

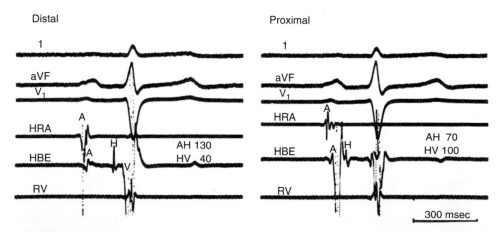

FIGURE 4-2. Demonstration of a distal and proximal recorded His electrogram. HRA, high right atrium; HBE, His bundle electrogram; RV, right ventricle. (Adapted from Josephson ME. *Clinical Cardiac Electrophysiology*, 4th ed. 2008.)

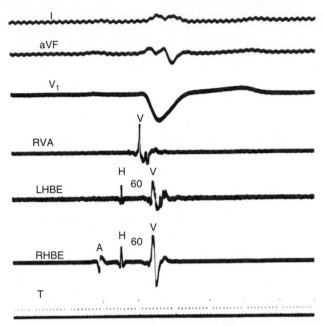

FIGURE 4-3. Demonstration of His bundle electrograms recorded from the right ventricle and left ventricle. RVA, right ventricular apex; LHBE, left His bundle electrogram; RHBE, right His bundle electrogram. (Adapted from Josephson ME. *Clinical Cardiac Electrophysiology*, 4th ed. 2008.)

The right ventricular catheter is placed at the apex and/or outflow tract and records a right ventricular electrogram. A potential representing the right bundle (RB) branch can be detected approximately 10 to 30 msec before the ventricular electrogram depending on catheter position (see Fig. 4-5). The most important feature of A, V, and CS catheters is position, stability, and good pacing thresholds.

NORMAL INTERVALS

The AH interval is measured in the His bundle tracing and represents conduction time from the low right atrium through the AV node to the His bundle (see Fig. 4-6). Most AH interval represents delay in conduction through the AV node which is engaged during the middle of the sinus P wave on the electrocardiogram and is significantly modulated by autonomic tone. The normal AH interval is 60 to 125 msec.

A long list of abnormalities can cause baseline prolongation in the AH interval including heightened vagal tone, infectious processes such as Lyme disease, infarction (inferior myocardial infarction [MI]), or fibrocalcific degeneration. An abnormally short AH interval is generally the result of accelerated AV nodal conduction, most often due to heightened sympathetic tone. This may occur

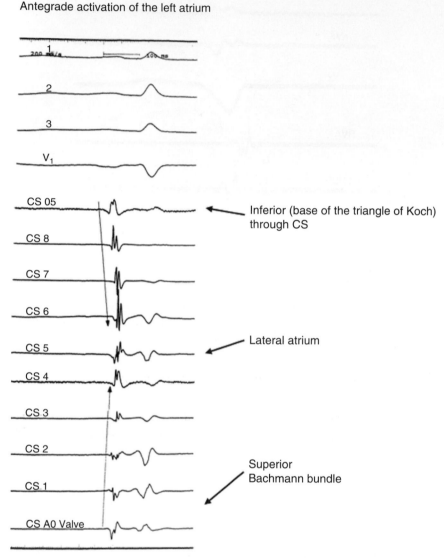

FIGURE 4-4. Demonstration of the Bachmann bundle conduction with simultaneous activation of the coronary sinus ostium (CS OS) and the distal coronary sinus (CS 1 and CS aortic valve).

due to conduction over a fast pathway in an individual with dual AV nodal pathways. Another rare cause of an abnormally short AH interval with normal ventricular activation (e.g., narrow QRS) is a bypass tract between the atrium and His bundle (i.e., atrio-His bypass tract).

The HV interval is the time from the earliest (most proximal) recorded His potential to the earliest recorded ventricular deflection (measured in the His tracing or surface QRS) (Fig. 4-6). The duration of the normal His deflection is at most 25 to 30 msec and the normal range for HV intervals is 35 to

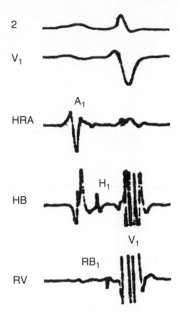

FIGURE 4-5. Demonstration of the timing of the His bundle (HB) and right bundle (RB) branch electrograms. HRA, high right atrium; RV, right ventricle.

55 msec. In the presence of left bundle branch block (LBBB), the HV can be up to 60 msec. Care must be taken to record the most proximal His potential (a His catheter recording which has an atrial signal on it as well). Occasionally a split His recording will be noted. In this case two potentials, each representing His activation, will be recorded after the atrial signal (see Fig. 4-7). This finding is

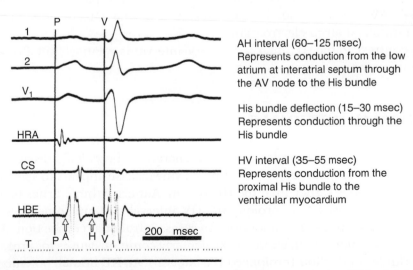

AH interval (60–125 msec)
Represents conduction from the low atrium at interatrial septum through the AV node to the His bundle

His bundle deflection (15–30 msec)
Represents conduction through the His bundle

HV interval (35–55 msec)
Represents conduction from the proximal His bundle to the ventricular myocardium

FIGURE 4-6. Determination of basic conduction intervals. HRA, high right atrium; CS, coronary sinus; HBE, His bundle electrogram; AV, atrioventricular.

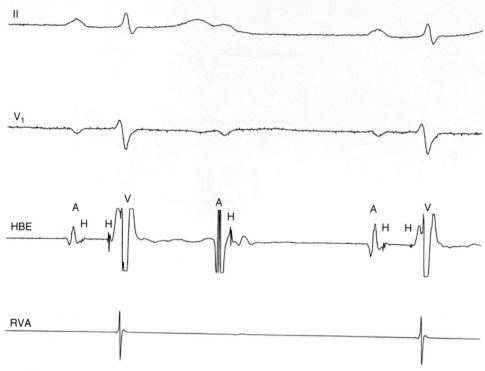

FIGURE 4-7. Two to one conduction with a split His bundle electrogram (HBE) on the conducted beats and block after the first component of the split His on the nonconducted beats. RVA, right ventricular apex.

indicative of His bundle disease. A multicomponent atrial electrogram can be confused for a His bundle potential. Incremental atrial pacing or maneuvers to delay AV nodal conduction will separate a true His potential from a multicomponent atrial electrogram.

In contrast to the AH interval, the HV interval is relatively unaffected by autonomic tone.

ABNORMAL INTERVALS

The HV interval can be prolonged by degenerative fibrocalcific disease, infiltrative processes, or surgery. Interestingly Lyme disease appears to specifically affect the AV node rather than the HP system. Antiarrhythmic drugs like procainamide can specifically prolong the HV interval and are sometimes used as a "stress test" in the EP laboratory to assess infranodal conduction. Aortic and mitral annular calcification are particularly common causes for prolonged His-Purkinje conduction (prolonged HV interval). An RB branch potential can often be identified and must be distinguished from the His electrogram. In general, the RB to ventricular electrogram is <30 msec.

Causes of an abnormally short HV interval include the following:

1. Conduction over an accessory pathway (AP). In this case, antegrade conduction occurs both over the AP and the AV node–His bundle routes. The ventricle is preexcited by conduction over the AP and causes the HV to appear shorter than normal.

2. A ventricular premature depolarization can result in a short HV interval through retrograde activation of the His bundle.

3. Inadvertent measurement of the RB-V interval instead of the HV interval. In this circumstance, the atrial electrogram is extremely small or absent.

The surface PR interval represents the surface manifestation of conduction through the atrium to the atrial electrogram on the recording catheter (PA interval), AH interval (largely conduction through the AV node), and infranodal conduction (HV interval) (Fig. 4-6). The vast majority of this time is attributable to AV nodal conduction.

Retrograde Atrial Activation

Retrograde activation of the atria can occur in association with ventricular premature complexes, as a manifestation of the retrograde limb of reentrant supraventricular tachycardias (e.g., AV nodal reentrant tachycardia, AV reentrant tachycardia) or as a consequence of ventricular pacing. *Concentric* retrograde activation refers to the midline activation of the atria through the AV node. This sequence generally reaches the AV node through the His-Purkinje network with earliest atrial activation noted at the His bundle or proximal CS electrogram (see Fig. 4-8). Retrograde conduction which is not midline is termed *eccentric conduction*. Eccentric conduction describes the pattern of activation observed during ectopic atrial tachycardia or with retrograde conduction over a free wall AP (Fig. 4-8).

PACING TECHNIQUES

Fixed cycle length pacing and pacing with the introduction of premature stimuli are typically performed in the EP laboratory to assess EP function and to induce arrhythmias. Fixed cycle length pacing refers to pacing at a fixed rate. The rate is called the *cycle length* and is determined by the following formula:

Pacing rate or heart rate (beats per minute) $= 60,000/$cycle length

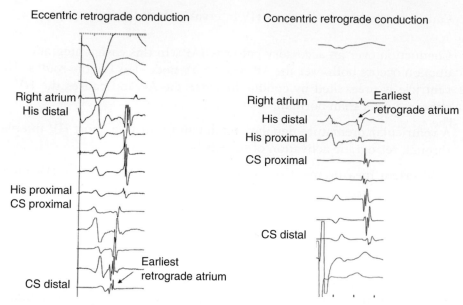

FIGURE 4-8. Eccentric and concentric retrograde conduction. Eccentric retrograde conduction is defined by earliest retrograde atrial activation recorded in the distal coronary sinus (CS) and latest atrial activation in the His bundle. Concentric retrograde activation is demonstrated by earliest atrial activation in the His bundle tracing and latest atrial activation in the distal CS recording.

Some basic cycle length/heart rate relationships include:

Heart Rate or Pacing Rate (bpm)	Cycle Length (msec)
100	600
120	500
150	400
200	300
300	200

Fixed rate pacing is performed with the introduction of stimuli (S_1) at a stable cycle length (e.g., 600 msec, 500 msec, etc.). This technique is used to assess the functional properties of the sinus, AV node, and His-Purkinje system (HPS) (see subsequent text). It is also used to induce certain types of tachyarrhythmias.

Pacing with the introduction of premature stimuli (incremental pacing) involves fixed cycle length pacing for a predefined number of beats followed by the introduction of premature stimuli. Typically 8 beats (S_1) at a cycle length of 600 or 400 msec are followed by a premature stimuli (S_2) beginning at 400 msec. S_2 is brought in by 10 to 20 msec increments until it fails to capture the myocardium. Failure to capture the myocardium defines the refractory period of the stimulated tissue. Premature stimuli are generally not introduced at coupling intervals shorter than 180 msec.

The introduction of multiple extrastimuli (e.g., S_2, S_3, S_4) is useful for the induction of certain mechanisms of tachyarrhythmias (e.g., reentrant and much less commonly triggered).

Refractory Periods

As noted, refractory periods of tissue in the EP laboratory are determined by incremental pacing. These are influenced by prior cycle lengths; therefore, standardized pacing protocols deliver a series of beats (8 to 10) at a fixed cycle length (to stabilize rate-related refractoriness) followed by progressively premature extrastimuli. Three types of refractory periods are determined.

Effective Refractory Period

The longest coupling interval (S_1-S_2) that fails to depolarize the stimulated tissue; for example, the AV nodal effective refractory period (ERP) is the longest A_1-A_2 (measured at the His bundle electrogram) which fails to conduct to the His bundle and ventricle (see Fig. 4-9).

Functional Refractory Period

The functional refractory period (FRP) is the *shortest* interval between two consecutively conducted beats out of a tissue resulting from any two consecutive paced beats. This is a measure of the *output* of a tissue; for example, the FRP of the HPS is the shortest V_1-V_2 in response to any H_1-H_2 interval (Fig. 4-9).

Relative Refractory Period

The relative refractory period (RRP) is the longest coupling interval (S_1-S_2) that results in prolonged conduction of the premature beat relative to that of the preceding basic drive cycle (S_1-S_1). The RRP is the end of the full recovery period—just before failure to conduct (ERP). The RRP represents the period of latency of the stimulated tissue (Fig. 4-9).

Effect of Heart Rate on Refractoriness in Different Tissues

The ERP of the atrium, HPS, and ventricles decreases with faster heart rates (shorter cycle lengths). This type of response is called *nondecremental*

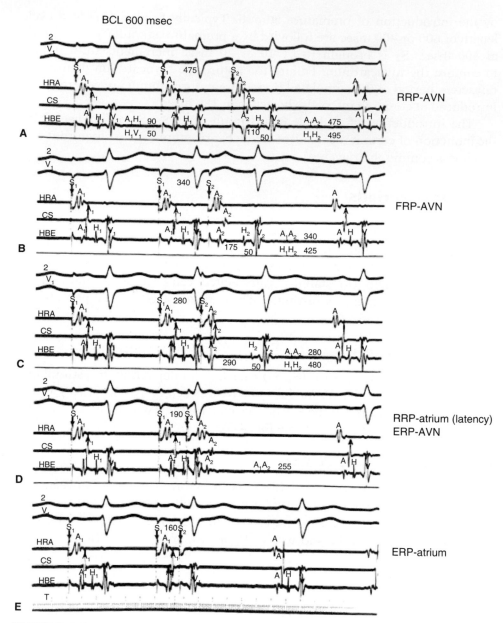

FIGURE 4-9. Demonstration of refractory periods. HRA, high right atrium electrogram; CS, coronary sinus; HBE, His bundle electrogram; RRP, relative refractory period; AVN, atrioventricular node; FRP, functional refractory period; ERP, effective refractory period.

and occurs because rapid pacing in these tissues shortens the action potentials, probably through an increase in the slow component of the delayed rectifier potassium channel (IKs). In contrast, the ERP of the AV node generally increases with faster rates. This is called *decremental conduction*.

The effect of abrupt changes in heart rate (basic drive cycles or premature impulses) have less predictable effects on the refractoriness of tissue—particularly in the HPS.

Effect of Abrupt Changes in Cycle Length on His-Purkinje System and Ventricular Refractoriness

Long-short change in cycle length (slow-paced cycle length followed by premature impulse) results in a *shortening* of the ERP and RRP of the HPS and the ventricular muscle refractory period. For example, an atrial premature impulse of 280 msec following a drive train of atrial pacing at a basic drive cycle of 600 msec (600/280) may not conduct through the HPS, whereas that same A_2 might very well conduct following a drive train of 400 msec (400/280) due to the shortening of HPS refractoriness associated with more rapid drive cycles. The same phenomena is observed with ventricular extrastimulation where an interval of 600/280 may not capture the ventricle but 400/280 will produce the ventricular capture).

Short-long change in cycle length (fast-paced cycle length followed by a long cycle and then premature impulse i.e., short-long-short) result in a *prolongation* of the ERP and RRP of the HPS.

RESPONSE TO ATRIAL PACING

The site of conduction delay and block can vary in response to atrial pacing. The most common response is the above-described decremental conduction in the AV node with eventual block. This introduction of progressively premature stimuli will result in ascertainment of the atrial ERP. Variations can occur in the site of conduction delay and block, which are likely due to differences in autonomic tone and sedation.

RESPONSE TO VENTRICULAR PACING

As noted, straight ventricular pacing is employed to determine the presence of retrograde conduction as well as the route of ventricle to atrial (VA) activation. Straight ventricular pacing with retrograde activation through the

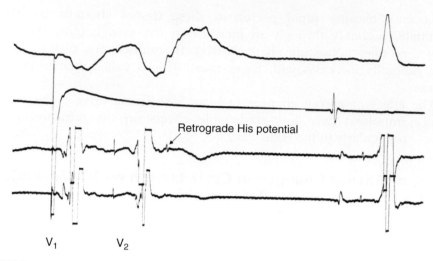

Retrograde His potential

V_1 V_2

FIGURE 4-10. Ventricular extrastimulation with demonstration of a retrograde His bundle potential.

AV node (concentric) results in progressive prolongation (decremental) of the VA interval until block occurs. This is in contradistinction to VA conduction through an AP, which is generally nondecremental and blocks without prior VA prolongation. Identifying the true site of retrograde block requires the recording of a retrograde His potential although this is often not possible (see Fig. 4-10).

The introduction of premature ventricular stimuli from the right ventricular apex allows determination of the ventricular effective refractory period (VERP). It also allows further assessment of retrograde conduction. Cycle length has a marked effect on the response to ventricular extrastimulation (i.e., faster cycle lengths result in decreases in the ERPs of the ventricular myocardium and HPS). At long coupling intervals, conduction typically occurs over the RB branch. Detailed mapping will demonstrate that the RB is activated followed by the His. In general, the His potential cannot be easily recorded because it is obscured within the ventricular electrogram. With progressively premature ventricular stimulation, the ERP of the RB is reached and conduction occurs solely across the septum and up the left bundle branch. In this case, the VA interval is prolonged and a retrograde H potential is noted after the ventricular electrogram in the His recording. The stimulus to H interval is generally >150 msec.

In general, retrograde conduction block in association with ventricular extrastimuli (VES) occurs most often in the HPS and much less commonly in the AV node. VES can also be used to identify the presence of an AP. In patients with AP(s) it is common to see fusion up both the AP and the normal midline activation route. With progressively premature VES, block can occur in the HPS and allow complete conduction over the AP (provided the ERP of the AP is less than that of the HPS).

Repetitive Ventricular Responses

Three types of repetitive responses may occur as a consequence of VES. They include the following:

1. Bundle branch reentry (BBR) beats (50% of healthy subjects)

2. AV nodal echo (15% of healthy subjects)

3. Intraventricular reentry (<15% of healthy persons)

Bundle Branch Reentry Beats

Premature stimulation of the right ventricle can result in retrograde block in the RB branch with transeptal conduction to the LBBB followed by retrograde activation of H. If this activation then proceeds around (reentry) to allow antegrade conduction of the RB and then the right ventricular myocardium it is called *BBR* (see Fig. 4-11). BBR occurs when progressively premature stimuli allow a critical amount of retrograde HPS delay (S_2-H_2) such that

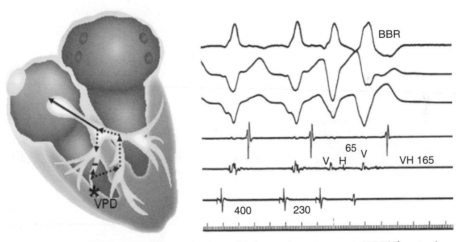

FIGURE 4-11. Demonstration of a bundle branch reentrant (BBR) beat. A ventricular extrastimulus blocks in the right bundle branch, conducts across the septum, and enters the left bundle branch. The impulse travels in a retrograde direction, activates the His bundle, and reenters the right bundle branch. The electrogram demonstrates the presence of a His bundle electrogram preceding activation of the right ventricle. VPD, ventricular premature depolarization. (See color insert.)

the antegrade limb (RB branch) has time to recover and allow reentry. BBR complexes typically have an LBBB morphology with left axis deviation because ventricular activation occurs from antegrade conduction over the RB branch. A similar phenomena can occur during left ventricular stimulation but then the BBR has a right bundle branch block (RBBB) pattern.

The HV interval generally approximates the HV during normal antegrade conduction (e.g., sinus rhythm).

Atrioventricular Nodal Echo Beat (Atrioventricular Nodal Reentry)

These extra beats stimulated by ventricular pacing result from reentry in the AV node. Retrograde conduction procedes over a slow AV nodal pathway and antegrade conduction over a fast AV nodal pathway. The antegrade conduction produces an extra beat with a normal or in some cases aberrant QRS conduction. The intracardiac recording of these extra beats will demonstrate retrograde activation of the atrium (surface P waves will be negative in 2, 3, and aVF). The atrial electrogram is followed by an H and V (see Fig. 4-12).

Ventricular Echo Beat

This type of response is intraventricular reentry occurring at a site distant from the pacing stimulus. This response is seen most often in patients with abnormal cardiac substrate, particularly MI. Multiple ventricular premature complexes may be induced and are considered nonsustained ventricular tachycardia if they do not exceed 30 consecutive complexes. Repetitive complexes may frequently be polymorphic.

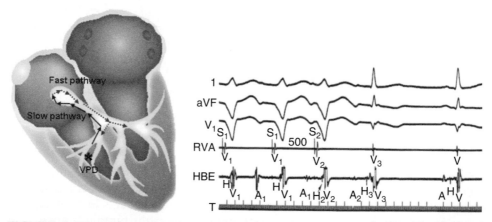

FIGURE 4-12. Ventricular pacing with ventricular extrastimulation resulting in an atypical atrioventricular (AV) nodal echo beat. VPD, ventricular premature depolarization; RVA, right ventricular apex; HBE, His bundle electrogram. (See color insert.)

SELECTED BIBLIOGRAPHY

Josephson ME. *Clinical cardiac electrophysiology*, 3rd ed. Philadelphia: Lippincott Williams & Wilkins; 2002.

Josephson ME. *Clinical cardiac electrophysiology*, 4th ed. Philadelphia: Lippincott Williams & Wilkins; 2008.

Basic Principles in Clinical Electrophysiology

WHAT IS NORMAL AND WHAT IS NOT

A thorough understanding of normal cardiac electrophysiology is necessary to accurately identify abnormalities. This chapter will define what is normal and how to identify what is abnormal.

Abnormalities in the electrical function of the heart can be identified through measurement of baseline intervals as well as patterns of conduction.

THE SINUS NODE AND ATRIAL CONDUCTION

The sinus node spontaneously depolarizes between 60 and 100 beats per minute (bpm). It is markedly influenced by parasympathetic and sympathetic tone. At rest, the sinus node is largely influenced by vagal tone. Sinus arrhythmia represents the normal manifestation of respiratory variation in heart rate. This occurs through a withdrawal of vagal tone (increased heart rate) associated with *inspiration*. The initial increase in heart rate associated with the onset of exertion is also caused first by the withdrawal of vagal tone followed by a sustained heart rate increase due to sympathetic tone. Complete blockade of both parasympathetic and sympathetic inputs to the sinus node (atropine and β-blocker administration) allows the determination of the intrinsic heart rate (IHR). The normal IHR is inversely related to the age of the patient and is calculated using the formula:

$$IHR = 117.2 - (0.52 \times age)$$

Testing sinus node function: The two tests used in the electrophysiology laboratory for assessment of sinus node function are called the *sinus node recovery time* (SNRT) and the *sinoatrial conduction time* (SACT).

Sinus Node Recovery Time

This is a measure of the recovery of sinus node *automaticity* following overdrive suppression. Unfortunately this test is not a pure assessment of automaticity alone, because conduction into and out of the sinus node is incorporated in its measurement. The test is performed by pacing the atrium for at least 1 minute at multiple cycle lengths above the intrinsic sinus rate. The sinus node is suppressed and once pacing is stopped the time required for sinus node automaticity to recover is measured. The corrected SNRT is used in clinical practice and is calculated by taking the longest interval from cessation of pacing to spontaneous sinus node activity (SNRT) and subtracting it from the baseline sinus cycle length (SCL). This is the most widely used electrophysiologic measure of sinus node function.

$$Corrected\ SNRT = SNRT - SCL$$

The normal corrected SNRT is 500 to 600 msec.

The SNRT may be falsely normal in patients with true sinus node dysfunction but slow sinus node cycle lengths.

Sinoatrial Conduction Time

SACT is a test of sinus node function, which is performed with the introduction of premature atrial stimuli during sinus rhythm following an 8- to 10-beat stable drive train at a cycle length just shorter than sinus. This test assumes that the time required to enter the sinus node is equal to the conduction time out of the sinus node and back to the recording/stimulating catheter (may not be true). It is calculated by subtracting the baseline SCL or A_1-A_1 from the time it takes for the sinus node to recover from the premature stimulus (A_2-A_3) divided by two for the time in and out of the sinus node.

$$SACT = [(A_2\text{-}A_3) - (A_1\text{-}A_1)]/2$$

A more accurate but rarely used measure of sinoatrial conduction is the recording of a sinus node electrogram. This signal is recorded with low pass filters and high gain. The time from phase 4 activity to the local atrial electrogram is the SCT.

Influences on Sinus Node Function

Enhanced: Catecholamines and withdrawal of vagal tone; denervation.

Inhibited: Drugs, trauma, fibrosis, ischemia, and congenital dysfunction.

ATRIOVENTRICULAR NODE FUNCTION

As noted, the atrioventricular (AV) node exhibits slower or decremental conduction in response to rapid atrial pacing or the introduction of premature stimuli to the AV node. Progressively rapid fixed cycle length pacing (A_1-A_1) is used to determine the AV Wenckebach (WB) cycle length. This critical cycle length is reached when there is atrial capture without capture of the His bundle or ventricle (see Fig. 5-1). The AV nodal WB cycle length is markedly influenced by the autonomic state. In general, antegrade AV nodal function is considered normal if there is conduction below a cycle length of 500 msec

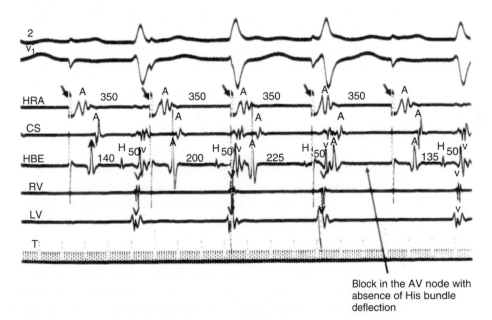

Block in the AV node with absence of His bundle deflection

FIGURE 5-1. Demonstration of normal atrioventricular (AV) Wenckebach physiology. Atrial pacing at 350 msec is associated with progressive prolongation in the AH interval. There is a block after the atrial electrogram and before the His bundle is activated. HRA, high right atrium; CS, coronary sinus; HBE, His bundle electrogram; RV, right ventricle; LV, left ventricle. (Adapted from Josephson ME. *Clinical Cardiac Electrophysiology*, 4th ed. 2008.)

(heart rate >120 bpm). AV nodal WB generally occurs below 500 msec and above 300 msec. If 1:1 conduction persists below 300 msec, this is considered enhanced AV nodal conduction. Conversely, AV nodal WB that occurs at rates slower than 600 msec (100 bpm) is considered abnormal. In patients with high vagal tone or on AV nodal blocking drugs, WB may occur at long cycle lengths. It is common and normal for well-trained athletes to exhibit WB while sleeping, particularly if during exercise AV conduction is normal.

The introduction of progressively premature stimuli is used to determine the refractory period of AV node. The atrioventricular nodal effective refractory period (AVNERP) is identified by a premature atrial stimuli, which captures the atrium without conduction to the His bundle or ventricle. It is measured in the His bundle electrogram. This must be distinguished from the atrial effective refractory period (AERP) that is reached by the longest A_1-A_2 interval, which fails to capture the atrium (see Chapter 4).

The physiological response to premature atrial stimuli is a progressive increase in A_2-H_2 interval as the A_1-A_2 interval becomes progressively shorter. This prolongation in the A_2-H_2 interval continues with progressively premature atrial stimuli until the refractory period of the atrium (AERP) or the AV node is reached (AVNERP).

In some patients, the introduction of progressively premature atrial stimuli will be associated with an abrupt (rather than the usual gradual) prolongation in the AH interval. This phenomenon is commonly referred to as *dual AV nodal pathways*. In this paradigm, there is conduction over two or, in some cases, multiple pathways. It is likely that these pathways represent different functional properties of the cells in the AV nodal region as opposed to distinct anatomic routes.

DUAL ATRIOVENTRICULAR NODAL PATHWAYS

Dual or multiple AV nodal pathways are present in 7% of the population representing a normal variation in human physiology. Most commonly there is a rapidly conducting (fast) and a slowly conducting (slow) pathway. Conduction over the fast pathway is associated with rapid (short AH interval) conduction and a long refractory period. In contrast, conduction over the slow pathway is associated with a long AH interval and a shorter refractory period. In patients with dual AV nodal pathways, conduction occurs over the fast pathway in most circumstances (short or normal PR interval). Conduction switches to the slow pathway when the refractory period of the fast pathway is reached and a "jump" to the slow pathway results (see Fig. 5-2). With the introduction of premature atrial stimuli a jump from the fast to the slow pathway is defined by a ≥50 msec increase in the A_2-H_2 interval in response to a 10 msec decrease in the A_1-A_2 coupling interval. This jump is most often elicited with the introduction of atrial premature stimuli but can occasionally be identified with straight fixed cycle length pacing.

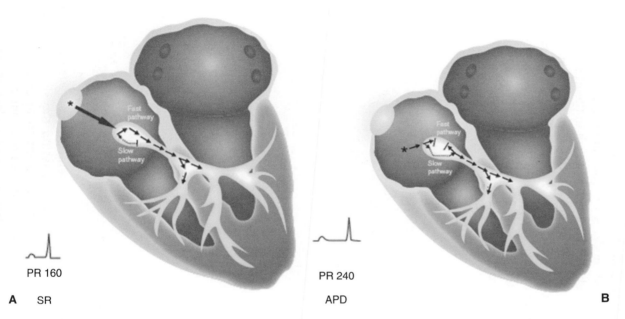

PR 160

A SR

PR 240

APD

B

FIGURE 5-2. Schema of dual atrioventricular (AV) nodal pathways. **A:** Demonstrates conduction down both the fast and slow pathways with a normal PR interval of 160 msec. **B:** Demonstrates an atrial premature depolarization (APD) with block in the fast pathway and conduction down the slow pathway yielding a longer PR interval of 240 msec. SR, sinus rhythm. (See color insert.)

Concealed Conduction

In electrophysiology, the term *concealed* refers to the inability to identify the electrophysiologic phenomenon on the surface electrocardiogram (ECG). Concealed conduction most commonly refers to the failure of propagation of impulses through the AV node as a result of previous penetration of that structure by atrial or ventricular rhythms. The result is delay or block of conduction of subsequent impulses. This phenomenon occurs during atrial fibrillation when in excess of 400 bpm bombard and result in concealed conduction delay in the AV node. A variable number of these impulses will ultimately conduct through the AV node and result in the irregular ventricular response associated with atrial fibrillation (AF). Another common example of concealed conduction is demonstrated by a prolonged PR interval following a ventricular premature depolarization (VPD). The VPD conducts to the AV node but fails to reach the atrium. The next sinus beat encounters delay in the AV node due to concealed activation of the AV node by the VPD (see Fig. 5-3).

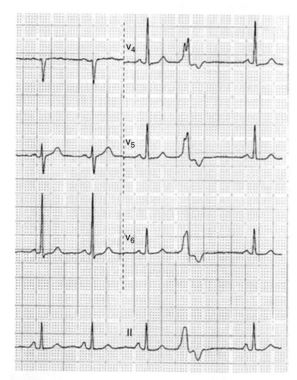

FIGURE 5-3. A wide complex beat consistent with a ventricular premature depolarization (VPD). The duration encompassing the sinus *p* wave before and after the wide complex beat is equivalent to three sinus complexes. A sinus *p* wave is seen after the VPD and does not conduct due to concealed conduction. HRA, high right atrium; HBE, His bundle electrogram.

Gap Phenomenon

This term describes the physiological delay or block in conduction with a premature stimulus followed by conduction without delay of a more premature stimulus. For example, atrial pacing at 600 msec with a premature stimulus at 320 msec (600/320) blocks before reaching the ventricle whereas a more premature stimuli (600/280) conducts. This seemingly paradoxical response to pacing is called the *gap phenomenon* and requires a site of distal block and proximal physiologic conduction delay. At the longer coupling interval there is block in the distal site. With progressively premature stimuli there is delay in the proximal site, which allows the distal site to recover and conduct. Therefore, the effective refractory period (ERP) of the distal tissue must be longer than the functional refractory period (FRP) of the proximal site of subsequent delay (see Fig. 5-4). This phenomenon commonly results from distal conduction block in the His-Purkinje system (HPS) with proximal delay in the AV node.

Supernormal Conduction

Conduction that is better than would be expected or occurs at a time when block or delay should occur is called *supernormal conduction*. The principle is that a short period of recovery of the transmembrane potential exists which corresponds to the end of the surface T wave and during which excitation is possible. This phenomenon occurs in the His-Purkinje tissue and is most commonly implied by the normalization of a wide QRS complex (bundle branch block [BBB]) when it would not be expected. For instance, supernormality may be implicated when acceleration-dependent aberration resolves despite continued heart rates at or above the rate at which aberration first developed.

Infranodal Conduction

Conduction through the His bundle, bundle branches, and ventricular myocardium is called *infranodal conduction*. Conduction through the His bundle is nondecremental. It is however strongly influenced by the preceding cycle lengths. For example, a premature stimulus delivered after a slow basic drive cycle (long H_1-H_1 intervals) may block in the HPS whereas the same coupling interval will conduct through the HPS if the preceding H_1-H_1 is shorter. This is a normal phenomenon and should not be considered an indication of HPS disease. In fact, in excess of 20% of individuals will demonstrate BBB or complete infranodal block in response to atrial premature beats delivered within the normal range of SCLs (800–1,000 msec). The longer the cycle length the more likely block or delay is to occur. This is due to the direct relationship of cycle length and refractory period of the HPS.

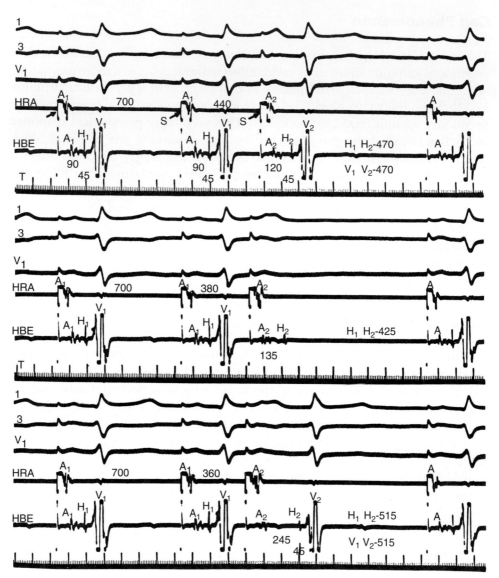

FIGURE 5-4. Three panels demonstrating the Gap phenomenon. The first atrial pacing drive at 700 msec with a premature impulse at 400 msec conducts with an H_1-H_2 interval of 470 msec. The second panel demonstrates a premature impulse delivered after 380 msec. This results in an H_1-H_2 interval of 425 msec, which blocks in the His bundle (after H_2). In the third panel, a premature atrial stimulus is delivered at 360 msec resulting in an H_1-H_2 interval of 515 msec, which results in conduction. (Adapted from Josephson ME. *Clinical Cardiac Electrophysiology*, 4th ed. 2008.)

Atrial pacing can be used to determine the conduction properties of the HPS.

The normal HPS should conduct at cycle lengths above 400 msec (heart rates of 150 or less). Block in the HPS at rates slower than 400 msec is indicative of a diseased HPS.

It may be difficult to fully evaluate the HPS because of block in the AV node with pacing. In this circumstance, atropine or isoproterenol should be administered to facilitate AV nodal conduction and allow input to the HPS.

Other important indicators of abnormal HPS conduction include an HV interval exceeding 55 msec. HV intervals of 100 msec or longer are considered an indication for pacemaker placement (see Chapter 11). Finally a split His potential (proximal and distal components) is indicative of intra His disease. Distinguishing a distal split His potential from a right bundle branch (RBB) potential is critical and can be confirmed by a potential to QRS duration of >30 msec.

MECHANISMS OF ABERRATION

The accurate differentiation of aberration from ventricular ectopy or tachycardia is a cornerstone of cardiac arrhythmia management. The differentiation of these entities requires a thorough understanding of the electrophysiological mechanisms, which promote aberration as well as the electrocardiographic patterns that favor a supraventricular or ventricular origin of tachycardia.

Atrial Premature Complex with Aberration or Ventricular Premature Complex?

Isolated wide complex beats may provide the clue to the mechanism of a wide complex tachycardia (WCT) if they are identical in morphology to the WCT. Ventricular premature beats can be identified by the presence of a compensatory pause. This physiology is based on the premise that a VPD blocks the conduction of a sinus impulse but does not actually reach the sinus node to reset or delay it. Therefore, the next sinus beat following the VPD comes on time and the interval preceding and following the premature complex comprise the duration of three normally timed sinus complexes (Fig. 5-3). A supraventricular beat will generally invade the sinus node and cause the next sinus beat to be reset so that the three intervals including the wide complex beat will not equal three normal sinus intervals. Unfortunately, VPDs can conduct retrogradely to the atrium and reset the sinus node as well.

Aberration/Transient Bundle Branch Block

Aberration results from the altered conduction of a supraventricular impulse, which encounters the refractory period of one of the bundle branches.

There are some basic principles of the conduction system that are helpful in understanding the mechanisms of aberration:

- The HPS has the longest refractory period in the heart at slow rates and is therefore most susceptible to conduction delay or block in response to premature atrial beats at slow sinus rates.

- Slow heart rates (long cycle lengths) prolong the refractory period and faster heart rates shorten the refractory period of the HPS.

- Abrupt changes in heart rate can result in corresponding changes in HP refractoriness (i.e., longer RR intervals lengthen HP refractoriness and promote BBB whereas short RR intervals shorten HP refractoriness).

- At relatively slow heart rates, the refractory period of the RBB exceeds that of the left bundle branch (LBB).

- At very rapid heart rates, the refractory period of the left bundle exceeds that of the right bundle.

- Preceding heart rates determine the degree of prematurity required to produce aberration (i.e., slow heart rates prolong HPS refractoriness and may lead to aberration of atrial premature depolarizations [APDs] with minimal prematurity whereas fast preceding heart rates will require a greater degree of prematurity to demonstrate aberration).

FORMS OF ABERRATION

There are four common forms of aberration: (a) associated with premature beats, (b) associated with an acceleration in heart rate, (c) associated with a deceleration in heart rate, and (d) retrograde invasion.

Aberration Associated with Premature Beats (Phase 3)

Phase 3 block refers to aberration resulting from encroachment on the refractory period during phase 3 of the action potential. Stimulation during phase 3 will result in excitation from a reduced (less negative) membrane potential. This reduced membrane potential is associated with a smaller number of open sodium channels and a resultant decreased conduction of the next action potential. As such, the refractory period is said to be voltage dependent. This results in aberration.

Phase 3 block is physiological and represents normal HPS behavior. This type of response is particularly common in the RBB because it has a relatively longer refractory period than the LBB. This type of aberrancy occurs frequently in association with atrial fibrillation and develops after a particularly long RR interval is followed by a shorter coupled interval (i.e., long–short sequence).

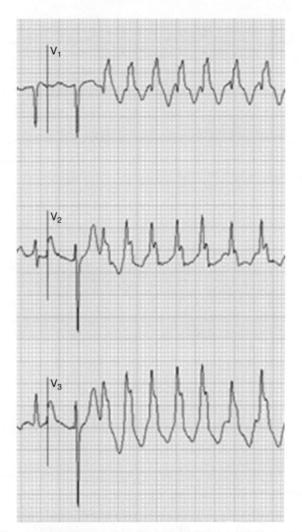

FIGURE 5-5. The development of right bundle branch block aberration during atrial fibrillation. Perpetuation of aberration is likely due to retrograde invasion.

Aberration following a premature atrial stimulus or a particularly long cycle during an irregular tachycardia such as atrial fibrillation most often occurs with right bundle branch block (RBBB). This is called an *Ashman phenomenon* and is due to the longer refractory period of the right bundle compared with the LBB (see Fig. 5-5). RBBB is more common because at slow heart rates the refractory period of the LBB is shorter than the RBB.

Acceleration-Dependent Block

This block often occurs at a critical increased heart rate. The heart rate need not be very rapid. In fact, acceleration-dependent aberration often occurs

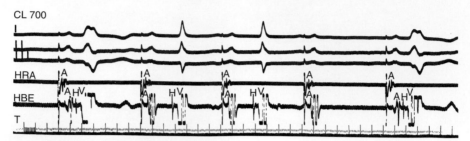

FIGURE 5-6. Atrial pacing at 700 msec results in atrioventricular (AV) Wenckebach. The sinus beat, which follows the pause conducts with left bundle branch block (LBBB) due to bradycardia-dependent or phase 4 block. HRA, high right atrium; HBE, His bundle electrogram. (Adapted from Josephson ME. *Clinical Cardiac Electrophysiology*, 4th ed. 2008.)

with relatively slow rates and with minimal (5 msec) increases in heart rate. This form of aberration occurs most often with an LBB morphology and is generally associated with underlying heart disease. The mechanism is related to abnormal excitability because the action potential duration is much shorter than the refractory period, which is time dependent not voltage dependent (i.e., phase 3).

Deceleration-Dependent Block (Phase 4)

Phase 4 block, also called *deceleration* or *bradycardic-dependent block*, describes aberration that occurs as a result of phase 4 depolarization (see Fig. 5-6). In this case, slower heart rates or pauses result in spontaneous diastolic phase 4 depolarization of the Purkinje fibers. An impulse arriving at these partially depolarized fibers will conduct with aberration or block. Stimulation of a cell, which has begun phase 4 depolarization, will result in an action potential with decreased conduction velocity and aberration on the ECG.

Although phase 4 depolarization can result in block or aberration, it can also result in spontaneous depolarization and the generation of automatic rhythms. This abnormal automaticity and conduction delay or block occur at sites of phase 4 activity.

Retrograde Invasion or Concealment

This aberration is produced by retrograde conduction into a bundle branch, which causes it to be refractory to the next conducted impulse. Retrograde invasion represents the most common cause of perpetuation of aberration. For example during RBBB, conduction occurs through the left bundle. The impulse then conducts transeptally and retrogradely invades the RBB to keep it in a state of refractoriness for subsequent impulses. Retrograde invasion of a bundle branch by a VPD can also initiate aberration (see Fig. 5-7).

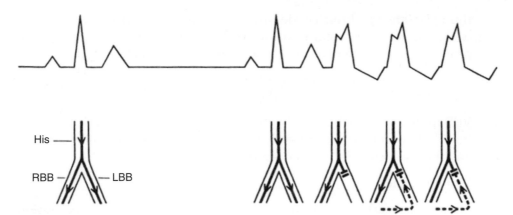

FIGURE 5-7. Schematic of pause-dependent aberration with perpetuation due to retrograde invasion of the left bundle branch (LBB). RBB, right bundle branch.

LOSS OF BUNDLE BRANCH BLOCK OR NORMALIZATION OF ABERRATION

There are multiple mechanisms through which aberration can be abolished. These include the following:

1. Interruption of retrograde invasion or "peeling back of refractoriness" (see Fig. 5-8)—As stated earlier, refractoriness is most often perpetuated

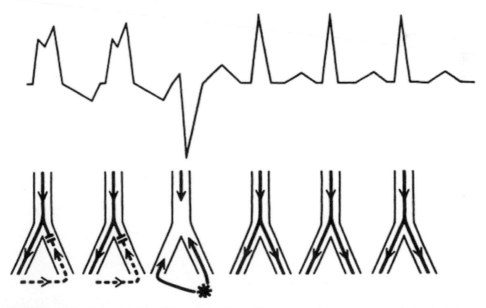

FIGURE 5-8. Schematic of interruption of retrograde invasion of the left bundle branch due to a ventricular premature depolarization.

through transseptal retrograde invasion of the distal RBB. A VPD, which occurs before transseptal invasion from the preceding tachycardia cycle can block retrograde invasion of the RBB and abolish aberration.

2. Equal delay in both bundle branches—This is very rare and must be accompanied by an increase in the PR interval.

3. VPD ipsilateral to BBB—If the VPD pre-excites the site of functional block, it will allow it time to recover before the next supraventricular impulse and therefore conduct without aberrancy.

4. Gap phenomenon.

5. Change in heart rate for rate dependent (acceleration or deceleration dependent block). In this form of loss of aberration as heart rate slows or speeds there is often a transition from wide to narrow over a few heartbeats.

SELECTED BIBLIOGRAPHY

Josephson ME. *Clinical cardiac electrophysiology*, 3rd ed. Philadelphia: Lippincott Williams & Wilkins; 2002.

Josephson ME. *Clinical cardiac electrophysiology*, 4th ed. Philadelphia: Lippincott Williams & Wilkins; 2008.

6 Atrial Fibrillation

Atrial fibrillation (AF) is the most common sustained arrhythmia encountered in clinical practice. It is both a disease of aging with a prevalence reaching 10% in patients older than 80 years as well as a disease of younger patients particularly when associated with autonomic triggers. These are probably underestimates due to asymptomatic and/or short-lived episodes that are never documented. The physician's current understanding of the pathogenesis of AF involves a theory of trigger and substrate. The trigger for arrhythmia initiation is an atrial premature depolarization, often originating from the left atrium in one or more of the pulmonary veins. The atrial tissue represents the substrate, which allows perpetuation of AF by reentry. Pulmonary vein firing may also be a perpetuating mechanism.

In some patients AF is paroxysmal, of short duration, and spontaneously terminating. In other patients, when AF develops it persists indefinitely unless a cardioversion is performed. Clinical factors including hypertension, aging, and congestive heart failure (CHF) as well as recurrent AF itself, result in atrial dilatation and fibrosis called *mechanical remodeling*. This type of mechanical remodeling promotes the development and perpetuation of AF. Electrical remodeling occurs in response to continuous and rapid electrical firing in the atria, which causes the loss of the normal adaptive shortening of atrial and pulmonary vein myocyte refractory periods in response to rapid heart rates (e.g., AF) (see Fig. 6-1).

Atrial remodeling = maintenance of AF
- Electrical (within hours) – rapid atrial activation →
  loss of nl shortening of atrial and PV myocyte
  refractory periods to rapid rates (decreases
  responsiveness to AADS
- Mechanical (within weeks) – fibrosis and dilatation

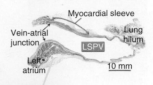

Inflammation
↑CRP
↑IL-6

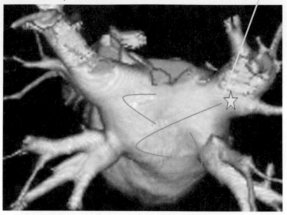

FIGURE 6-1. Current understanding of the mechanisms of atrial fibrillation. AF, atrial fibrillation; nl, normal; PV, pulmonary vein; AAD, antiarrhythmic drugs; LSPV, left superior pulmonary vein; CRP, C-reactive protein; IL-6, interkeukin 6. (See color insert.)

NOMENCLATURE

- The first episode of AF is classified as *new onset*.

- *Paroxysmal* AF is defined as recurrent AF that terminates spontaneously.

- *Persistent* AF is recurrent AF that does not terminate spontaneously and requires cardioversion for restoration of sinus rhythm.

- *Chronic* AF is persistent AF lasting for >6 months.

NATURAL HISTORY AND SUBTYPES OF ATRIAL FIBRILLATION

In almost all instances AF is a recurrent disease. Exceptions to this rule include AF associated with thyroid disease and AF which occurs in the postoperative state. The natural history of AF is difficult to predict. Paroxysmal AF generally lasts minutes to hours before spontaneous termination. This pattern may persist for decades or may progress to chronic AF. Other patients will develop persistent AF early in the course of their disease, which will become chronic if no attempts are made to restore sinus rhythm. A general principle accepted but not proven is the longer a patient is in AF the less likely sinus rhythm can be restored and maintained ("AF begets AF"). This is likely the consequence of electrical and mechanical remodeling.

Common conditions associated with the initial development and subsequent recurrence of AF include hypertension, aging, and structural heart disease (valve disease, cardiomyopathy, myocardial infarction [MI], pericardial disease, and CHF). Lung disease is also frequently complicated by AF and atrial flutter. Lone AF refers to patients younger than 65 years with AF in the absence of associated heart or lung disease. This group of patients often have autonomic triggers such as heightened adrenergic and vagal tone.

Age and Atrial Fibrillation

AF increases in frequency with aging, particularly in patients older than 65 years. At least 10% of the population older than 80 years will develop AF. The aging of a significant proportion of the population in the next 15 years will likely result in a significant increase in the number of patents with AF.

Autonomically Triggered Atrial Fibrillation

Adrenergically triggered AF generally occurs during exercise or in association with caffeine excess. This mechanism probably plays a role in AF associated with acute systemic illness or in the postoperative (noncardiac surgery) state. In the authors' experience, dietary caffeine is infrequently a consistent trigger for AF and they rarely limit caffeine intake in their patients. Vagally triggered AF is a relatively common form of AF. It is most often associated with sleep (particularly in the setting of obstructive sleep apnea), large meals, or the termination of significant exercise. A common scenario is the development of AF the evening or morning after an afternoon of significant exercise or activity. It may also occur in association with a vasovagal syncopal episode. This form of AF often develops during middle age and is most often paroxysmal and highly symptomatic. It may in fact be that some of what is believed to be vagal AF is really a combination of both enhanced sympathetic and vagal tone, particularly at the end of exercise and postoperatively.

Atrial Fibrillation Associated with Hyperthyroidism

AF is commonly associated with hyperthyroidism, whereas only 1% of cases of new-onset AF are due to hyperthyroidism. It is very difficult to maintain sinus rhythm in the presence of active hyperthyroidism and therefore rate control should be the strategy until a euthyroid state is achieved. β-Blockers are the first choice for rate control and combination therapy with a calcium channel blocker or digoxin may be required. There is some scant evidence that thromboembolic risk is increased in the presence of hyperthyroidism and therefore many practitioners choose to anticoagulate patients in this circumstance, even in the absence of other clinical risk factors for stroke.

Atrial Fibrillation Associated with Cardiovascular Surgery

There is a 50% to 60% risk of AF development post cardiovascular surgery. This risk is slightly higher with valvular disease compared with coronary artery bypass graft (CABG). The risk of AF development is greatest in the first week following surgery with a peak at days 2 to 3. It is important to realize that the likelihood of being in sinus rhythm 4 weeks following cardiac surgery is the same regardless of the strategy of rate or rhythm control employed. The authors choose to restore and maintain sinus rhythm in patients who are highly symptomatic in AF or difficult to rate control. Their preferred strategy is to load with amiodarone and continue therapy for a total of 6 weeks following surgery. Alternatives to amiodarone in this population include sotalol and dofetilide. Type 1A drugs are also useful particularly for patients with renal insufficiency.

Prophylactic therapy for AF prevention before cardiac surgery: It is well established that the discontinuation of previously prescribed β-blockers is associated with an increased risk of postoperative AF. It is therefore important to maintain β-blocker therapy through cardiovascular surgery. Amiodarone can be initiated in the week or weeks before electively scheduled cardiac surgery. This strategy will reduce the occurrence postoperative AF.

Atrial Fibrillation Post MAZE or Percutaneous Atrial Fibrillation Ablation Procedure

AF frequently occurs in the immediate period post MAZE or percutaneous AF ablation procedure. AF should be differentiated from atrial tachycardia, which also can occur as an arrhythmic complication of these procedures. In both circumstances, these arrhythmias often subside over a period of weeks. As a result, many practitioners choose to treat their postprocedure patients with an antiarrhythmic drug (AAD) for 4 to 12 weeks after the procedure.

Ischemia/Infarction as a Trigger for Atrial Fibrillation

AF is rarely, if ever, a manifestation of acute ischemia or infarction. When it does, it is usually in the setting of CHF with or without mitral regurgitation (MR) and is associated with a poor prognosis. It is common to develop AF with CHF or MR which develops in the setting of infarction. It is not common to develop AF in an uncomplicated MI or as a sole manifestation of ischemia or infarction. The authors do not recommend routine evaluation for coronary artery disease in patients with new onset AF unless there is other clinical evidence of ischemia.

Familial Atrial Fibrillation

There are likely multiple forms of familial AF. One phenotype which is easily identified is families with multiple members who develop AF at a young age (younger than 40 years). These patients often have significant atrial electrical dysfunction with sinus node dysfunction.

Alcohol and Atrial Fibrillation

Binge drinking is commonly associated with AF. Moderate alcohol consumption is probably not a risk for AF; however, excessive alcohol use does seem to predispose to AF.

Specific Electrocardiographic Patterns of Atrial Fibrillation

The term *coarse* as is often used when atrial activity in lead V_1 appears to be organized and is relatively high amplitude. If the remainder of the leads have low-amplitude fibrillatory waves and the ventricular response is irregularly irregular this rhythm should be characterized as typical AF.

A regular ventricular response during AF, particularly if slow, is indicative of heart block. This is shown in Figure 6-2.

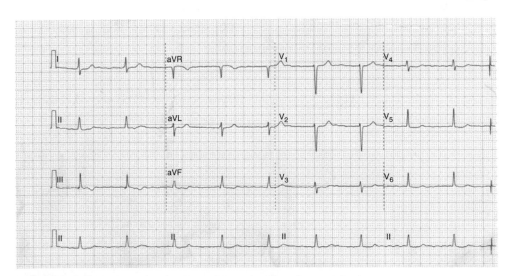

FIGURE 6-2. Atrial fibrillation with complete heart block.

Tachybrady Syndrome

Tachybrady syndrome refers to the presence of rapid and slow rhythms in the same patient (see Fig. 6-3). Most commonly this is AF with a rapid ventricular response and sinus bradycardia. This bradycardia often manifests as a prolonged sinus pause at the time of conversion from AF or flutter to sinus rhythm (Fig. 6-3).

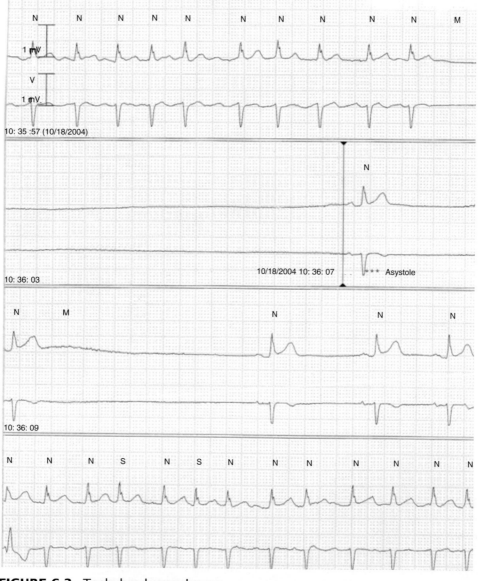

FIGURE 6-3. Tachybrady syndrome.

Symptoms and Hemodynamic Consequences Associated with Atrial Fibrillation

Most patients with new-onset AF have symptoms at the onset of their disease. With time and therapy many patients will report a significant reduction in their symptoms even with persistence of AF. The most commonly reported symptoms include dyspnea, palpitations, fatigue, and chest pain. Frequent urination may also be described as a consequence of atrial stretch-induced release of atrial natriuretic peptide. Patients with diastolic dysfunction, particularly those with hypertrophic cardiomyopathy and aortic stenosis, develop symptoms and hemodynamic compromise due to the loss of the atrial contribution to ventricular filling. Most other patients do not suffer significantly from the loss of atrial filling. Symptoms associated with AF result predominantly from a rapid ventricular response. This is particularly true if tachycardia-induced cardiomyopathy develops. Tachycardia-induced cardiomyopathy is characterized as a global cardiomyopathy which develops as a consequence of a rapid ventricular response. It is also believed that the ventricular irregularity associated with AF can be hemodynamically disadvantageous. Syncope or lightheadedness can also be associated with AF. This is almost always due to a sinus pause at the termination of AF, particularly in those with sinus node dysfunction. AF should be considered a proarrhythmic arrhythmia, particularly in the setting of old MI and CHF. AF can induce ventricular arrhythmias in this patient population.

Workup of New-Onset Atrial Fibrillation

History: All patients with a new diagnosis of AF should have a thorough history taken for common precipitants including alcohol, autonomic triggers, or evidence of a regular supraventricular tachycardia (SVT) (e.g., atrioventricular reentrant tachycardia [AVRT]) which initiates AF. The presence of family history should also be documented. Other associated conditions that will define the thromboembolic risk must also be documented.

Laboratory testing: The only critical laboratory test at the onset of AF is an assessment of thyroid function.

Exercise test: There is no need to perform an exercise test in patients with new-onset AF for the exclusion of coronary artery disease unless there is a strong clinical suspicion of ischemia. An exercise test may be helpful in assessing rate control or the presence of suspected exercise-induced AF or SVT.

Imaging: Transthoracic echocardiogram is indicated to define left atrial dimensions, left and right ventricular function, and identify occult valve disease or other forms of congenital heart disease.

Ambulatory electrocardiographic (ECG) monitoring: Ambulatory monitoring is useful to assess the symptom–rhythm correlation. It is clear from extensive monitoring data that in most patients with symptomatic AF there coexists frequent episodes of asymptomatic AF. It is also clear that symptoms felt to be AF will often prove to be associated with sinus rhythm. It may therefore be useful to perform a long-term continuous monitoring study to define the frequency and duration of recurrent AF events as well as the symptom–rhythm correlation between events in order to define the endpoint for therapy.

Atrial Fibrillation with Reduced Ventricular Function at Presentation

Occasionally patients will present with impaired ventricular function discovered on their initial echocardiogram after the diagnosis of AF. This may represent a cardiomyopathy with resultant AF or tachycardia-induced cardiomyopathy. Tachycardia-induced cardiomyopathy is a global left and often right ventricular myopathy, which can develop after a short period (weeks) of AF, generally with ventricular rates >110 beats per minute (bpm). These patients are frequently asymptomatic until they present with CHF. The authors' approach is to restore and maintain sinus rhythm, often with amiodarone, or to pursue aggressive rate control in these patients. The authors then perform another assessment of ejection fraction (EF) 2 to 3 months following the control of heart rate. If the EF is still impaired, they perform a standard evaluation for other causes of newly recognized cardiomyopathy.

STROKE RISK

The risk for stroke in patients with AF is based solely on their clinical risk factors and not on the frequency or duration of AF. The risk of stroke is the same for paroxysmal compared with chronic AF. Major risk factors for stroke include age older than 75 years particularly in women, hypertension, CHF, prior stroke, or transient ischemic attack (TIA). Valvular heart disease, in particular mitral stenosis, is also a significant risk factor for stroke. Diabetes mellitus and coronary artery disease are considered moderate risk factors. Age is an important risk factor for stroke with 25% of strokes attributed solely to AF in patients who are older than 80 years. Important transesophageal electroencephalogram (TEE)-based risk factors include dense spontaneous left atrial contrast ("smoke"), diminished left atrial appendage velocities (<20 m per second), and significant (>4 mm) aortic atheroma. The presence of any of these TEE characteristics is associated with a significant risk (>4%) of stroke even in the presence of therapeutic anticoagulation with warfarin.

The CHADS2 risk assessment score can be clinically useful to understand when counseling patients regarding the need for anticoagulation. This score uses pooled data on the clinical risk factors of congestive heart

TABLE 6-1 CHADS2-based Risk Rates	
CHADS2 Score	*Risk of Stroke Per Year*
CHADS2 of 0	0.5% per year
CHADS2 of 1–2	1.5%–2.5% per year
CHADS2 of 3	5.3%–6.9% per year

An important caveat to this risk-based assessment is that a CHADS2 score of 2 based on prior stroke should be viewed as an extremely high risk of recurrent stroke and mandates anticoagulation.

failure (C), hypertension (H), age older than 75 years (A), diabetes (D), and prior stroke/TIA (S). Each of these factors is assigned 1 point except for prior stroke which receives 2 points (see Tables 6-1 and 6-2).

Rhythm versus Rate Control

The decision to attempt to maintain sinus rhythm or accept rate control has now been thoroughly evaluated in a number of randomized controlled trials. These studies have all evaluated patients with at least one risk factor for stroke and an average age in the late 60s. These studies have shown that a strategy of rate control carried a similar associated mortality when compared with a strategy of rate control. Much of the mortality associated with the rhythm control strategy in these trials was due to AAD toxicity or stroke when warfarin was discontinued. The most important conclusion of these trials is that anticoagulation must be based on clinical risk factors for stroke and not the perception that sinus rhythm has been maintained and therefore stroke risk reduced by a rhythm control strategy. These studies did not evaluate patients with lone AF as well as the very elderly. It is likely that patients with highly symptomatic AF were also underrepresented in these trials. Moreover, those patients in either strategy who did best were those in sinus rhythm. The authors would suggest that sinus rhythm is best but it is difficult to achieve. Their general approach to AF management is shown in Figure 6-4.

Cardioversion

Cardioversion refers to restoration of sinus rhythm. Spontaneous cardioversion will occur in 50% of patients within the first 48 to 72 hours of AF. For those who do not convert spontaneously sinus rhythm can be restored with oral or intravenous (IV) medications or with electricity (direct current [DC]). Oral and IV pharmacotherapy restores sinus rhythm in 30% to

TABLE 6-2 Current Recommendations for Thromboembolic Prophylaxis Based on Risk Factors for Stroke	
No risk	Aspirin (81–325 mg daily) or nothing
One moderate risk factor (75 years or older, hypertension, heart failure LVEF ≤35%, diabetes mellitus)	Aspirin (81 or 325 mg) or warfarin (INR 2–3)
≥2 moderate risk factors or one high-risk factor (prior stroke/TIA, mitral stenosis, prosthetic valve)	Warfarin (INR 2–3, or 2.5–3.5 with prosthetic valve)

Cases where patients with one moderate risk factor should probably receive warfarin instead of only aspirin

Age 65–74 with DM or CAD

Age ≥65 with CHF

When to maintain aspirin (81 mg) with warfarin

In patients who need secondary prevention of CAD

Risks for bleeding on warfarin: The risk for significant bleeding (i.e., intracranial hemorrhage) on warfarin does not rise significantly until the INR is >5; if the INR can be maintained between 2 and 3, the risk for significant hemorrhage is <1%

Alternatives to warfarin: Clopidogrel and aspirin in combination are not equivalent to warfarin for thromboembolic prevention; a series of new medications including direct thrombin inhibitors and factor 10 A inhibitors are under investigation as alternatives to warfarin for stroke prevention in AF

LVEF, left ventricular ejection fraction; INR, international normalized ratio; TIA, transient ischemic attack; DM, diabetes mellitus; CAD, coronary artery disease; CHF, congestive heart failure; AF, atrial fibrillation.

50% of cases. The success of this approach is greatest early (within days) after the development of AF. DC cardioversion is highly effective particularly with the advent of biphasic waveforms. This approach restores sinus rhythm in >85% of cases. The definition of a successful cardioversion is a single beat of sinus rhythm even if it is rapidly succeeded by recurrent AF. Early recurrence of atrial fibrillation (ERAF) can occur immediately or in the first few minutes after cardioversion. There is no value to repeated attempts at cardioversion unless something is done differently (e.g., administration of an AAD). The authors' approach to patients with ERAF is to load them with an AAD for a minimum of 3 to 5 doses and repeat cardioversion. If the authors choose amiodarone, they will load this as an outpatient setting while in AF for at least 2 weeks and up to 1 month. In 50% of patients, sinus rhythm will be restored with this approach before return for repeat cardioversion.

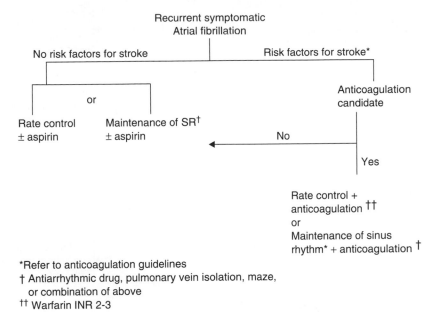

FIGURE 6-4. Algorithm for the management of patients with recurrent atrial fibrillation.

Anticoagulation Pericardioversion

The restoration of sinus rhythm is associated with a gradual recovery in atrial mechanical function over the first 2 to 3 weeks after cardioversion. Reduction in the risk of stroke associated with cardioversion is accomplished by assuring at least 3 weeks of therapeutic anticoagulation or a TEE without left atrial appendage thrombus at the time of cardioversion. Following cardioversion, anticoagulation should be continued for at least 3 to 4 weeks (see Fig. 6-5). After that period the continuation of warfarin is dependent on the clinical risk factors for stroke and/or the recurrence of AF. At present there is no data to support the use of Lovenox as a substitute for warfarin or heparin for stroke prevention in patients with AF.

Methods of Cardioversion

Intravenous antiarrhythmic drugs. Procainamide, ibutilide, and amiodarone are the only antiarrhythmic medications available in the United States for IV administration. IV procainamide is most successful at restoring sinus rhythm when administered at a dose of 10 to 15 mg per kg over 30 minutes. Patients must be monitored for hypotension and QT prolongation. Ibutilide is more effective for the conversion of atrial flutter than AF. It is also associated with QT prolongation and *torsades de pointes* (TDP) and patients must be monitored for approximately 4 hours after drug administration. IV amiodarone is modestly effective at restoring sinus rhythm. It may also be complicated by hypotension.

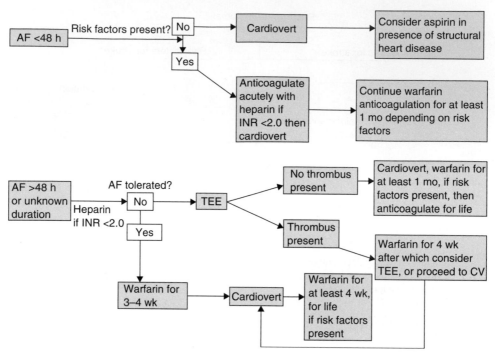

FIGURE 6-5. Guidelines for pericardioversion anticoagulation. AF, atrail fibrillation; TEE, transesophageal echocardiography; CV, cardioversion.

Oral therapy. "Pill in the pocket"—this approach is used mostly with type 1C drugs (flecainide and propafenone) in large dose (300 mg of flecainide or 600 mg of propafenone). It is restricted to patients with normal hearts, particularly in the absence of coronary artery disease. Patients should have this performed in a monitored setting at least once before recommending it as an outpatient management strategy.

Other oral therapies. Any oral antiarrhythmic medication can be used for cardioversion. Those with potassium channel blocking capability should be administered in a hospital setting due to the risk of TDP. Amiodarone is an exception which can be initiated in the outpatient setting during AF with a 50% rate of conversion to sinus rhythm over a month of drug loading.

Electrical cardioversion. DC or electrical cardioversion is routinely performed to restore sinus rhythm. It requires a short-acting anesthetic and when performed correctly is safe and highly effective. Most current defibrillators employ a biphasic waveform which results in >90% efficacy. Standard approaches to DC cardioversion employ an anterior and posterior (left scapular) paddle or patch orientation. Paddles can also be employed in an anterior and left axillary position. Pressure can be applied over the anterior patch to decrease chest wall impedance and improve efficacy. The anterior patch or paddle should be placed over or just to the right of the sternum (as opposed to over the left chest as is done when defibrillating the left ventricle) because the right atrium lies in front of the left atrium in the midchest. Causes for failure of DC cardioversion include increased anterior-posterior chest wall diameter and long-standing AF (particularly in association with enlarged left atrial dimension). Efficacy can be increased by the administration of ibutilide.

Complications of Cardioversion

Cardioversion is in general a safe procedure. It can be complicated by bradyarrhythmia if the sinus node is dysfunctional, particularly if large doses of rate controlling medications have been employed before cardioversion. It is the authors' practice to reduce the dose of these medications on the day or two before cardioversion if significant bradycardia is anticipated. Atropine can also be employed if marked bradycardia results after cardioversion. QT prolongation and TDP may also occur in the setting of prior treatment with potassium channel blocking drugs. A burn at the location of the patches or pads may occur. This is generally self-limited but can be treated when necessary with zinc oxide cream. Finally, postcardioversion pulmonary edema is a poorly characterized and rare but clinically important entity. In the authors' experience it presents in patients with prolonged periods of tachycardia before cardioversion. It need not be associated with left ventricular dysfunction and generally develops within 24 to 48 hours of cardioversion. It is managed with diuresis and may be a recurrent phenomena with subsequent cardioversions.

Maintenance of Sinus Rhythm

Antiarrhythmic Medications

The major issues to be considered when choosing an antiarrhythmic medication for maintenance of sinus rhythm include efficacy and antiarrhythmic toxicity. Amiodarone has uniformly been shown to be superior to all other antiarrhythmic medications for the maintenance of sinus rhythm. Specifically amiodarone is approximately 60% to 70% successful at suppressing symptomatic AF at 1 year compared with an efficacy of 40% to 50% for all other drugs. The realistic goal for AAD therapy is reduction in the frequency of symptomatic AF (also called *burden of AF*) rather than complete suppression of AF. A single recurrence of AF does not necessarily mean AAD failure. Patients who have done well for long periods on an AAD can be cardioverted and left on the previously successful AAD—often with long successive periods of sinus rhythm.

Choice of Antiarrhythmic Agents

Type 1C agents (propafenone and flecainide) are restricted to patients without structural heart disease, particularly coronary artery disease. They are well tolerated and often chosen as first-line agents for patients with lone AF or AF associated with hypertension. These agents should be used in association with an atrioventricular (AV) nodal slowing medication to avoid the development of atrial flutter with 1:1 conduction.

Sotalol and dofetilide are good choices for patients with coronary artery disease but should be avoided in the setting of significant renal dysfunction.

Amiodarone is an excellent choice for patients with significant structural heart disease, particularly CHF. Amiodarone should be avoided in patients with thyroid nodules that have the potential to become autonomous when exposed to the iodine moieties in amiodarone. It is also generally avoided in patients with significant liver disease. Amiodarone pulmonary toxicity occurs as an acute reaction after weeks of therapy or after large cumulative doses in the form of pulmonary fibrosis. Patients with significant pulmonary disease are not at greater risk of amiodarone lung toxicity but will tolerate it less well than patients without underlying lung disease.

Type 1A drugs are used less frequently than other agents due to concerns for toxicity. Disopyramide is used in patients without contraindications to the anticholinergic effects of this drug (i.e., avoid if prostatic hypertrophy or narrow angle glaucoma). It is a reasonable agent in patients with hypertrophy including hypertrophic obstructive cardiomyopathy.

The authors' approach to AAD selection is shown in Figure 6-6.

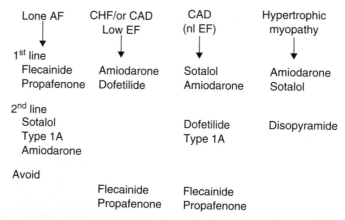

FIGURE 6-6. Antiarrhythmic drug selection based on clinical characteristics. Lone AF; absence of hypertension, coronary artery disease, diabetes mellitus, congestive heart failure, or valvular disease; CHF, congestive heart failure; CAD, coronary artery disease; EF, ejection fraction. Type 1A: quinidinene, procainamide, disopyramide.

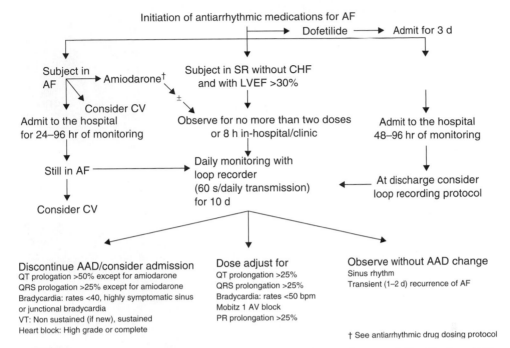

FIGURE 6-7. Initiation of antiarrhythmic medications for atrial fibrillation (AF). CHF, congestive heart failure; LVEF, left ventricular ejection fraction; CV, cardioversion; AAD, antiarrhythmic drug; VT, ventricular tachycardia; AV, atrioventricular.

Initiation of Antiarrhythmic Drugs for Atrial Fibrillation

Dofetilide is the only antiarrhythmic medication for which inpatient initiation is mandated. The authors favor a protocol of outpatient initiation of AADs for patients in sinus rhythm with close monitoring of heart rate, QRS interval (sodium channel blocking drugs), or QT interval (potassium channel blocking drugs) (see Fig. 6-7). Amiodarone is the one agent considered safe to load during AF in the ambulatory setting.

Nonpharmacologic Therapy

Nonpharmacologic therapies for the cure of AF comprise percutaneous catheter-based techniques and thoracotomy-based minimally invasive MAZE surgeries. Catheter techniques are based on the concept of electrical isolation of the pulmonary veins so that atrial premature depolarizations (APDs) cannot enter the left atrium from the pulmonary veins and trigger the initiation of AF (see Fig. 6-8). Variations of this procedure include additional ablation lines in the left and right atria. The surgical MAZE procedure is most often performed in conjunction with bypass or valve surgery. It comprises a series of ablation lines to isolate the pulmonary veins and create regions of conduction block

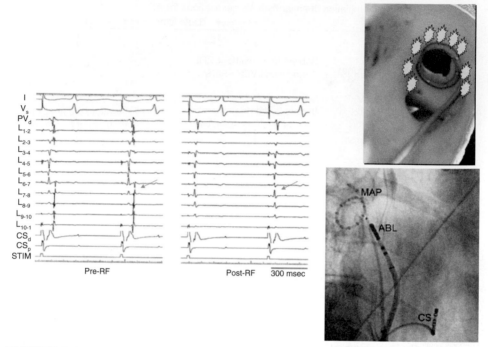

FIGURE 6-8. Percutaneous pulmonary vein isolation. The *arrows* point to pulmonary vein potentials present before ablation and absent following successful electrical isolation of the pulmonary vein. Channels labeled L represent the lasso or mapping catheter. STIM, stimulation channel; RF, radiofrequency; MAP, mapping catheter; ABL, ablation catheter; CS, coronary sinus.

throughout the left and right atria. The left atrial appendage is also resected or stapled shut as part of the surgical procedure. The minimally invasive MAZE procedure is a thoracoscopically guided epicardial isolation of the pulmonary veins combined with left atrial appendage stapling. Ablation of the parasympathetic ganglia in the region of the pulmonary vein ostia is also often performed as part of the MAZE procedure. The efficacy of these procedures requires careful evaluation and follow-up. The authors' experience with catheter-based pulmonary vein isolation is a 70% rate of significant decrease in AF frequency and symptoms. Approximately 15% of patients will require a second procedure for complete pulmonary vein isolation.

Principles of Rate Control

Control of the ventricular response is critical to mitigate symptoms associated with AF as well as the possibility of tachycardia-mediated cardiomyopathy.

First-line therapy for rate control is β-blockade. Calcium channel blockers (diltiazem, verapamil) are chosen in patients who are not good candidates for β-blockade (asthma, depression history) or do not tolerate them due to fatigue or other side effects (e.g., exacerbation of Raynaud phenomena). Digoxin is a relatively ineffective single agent for rate control but can be very useful in patients with cardiomyopathy particularly as a second agent with a β-blockers or calcium channel blockers.

The authors' target heart rate for rate control is a resting heart rate of ≤80 bpm and a rate with moderate exertion (e.g., 6-minute walk test) of ≤110 bpm. For patients who exercise at a higher level, the authors recommend keeping the rate at ≤160 to 170 bpm. Rate control in the conditioned athlete with resting bradycardia and exercise-induced tachycardia can be very challenging. An increased dose of β-blockade or calcium channel blockers before exercise is recommended in this group.

Atrioventricular junction (AVJ) ablation is an easily performed procedure to cause heart block and control of the heart rate. Patients who undergo AVJ ablation may have a junctional escape, but it should not be considered stable and a permanent ventricular pacemaker must be implanted. Patients who receive this therapy should be followed up with echocardiograms to make certain that they do not develop a pacing-induced cardiomyopathy. The physicians do not advocate the implantation of a coronary sinus lead for resynchronization at the time of AVJ ablation unless there is preexisting left ventricular dysfunction, particularly in the setting of chronic right ventricular pacing.

IMPORTANT PRINCIPLES IN ATRIAL FIBRILLATION MANAGEMENT AND CONSULTATION

- AF is almost never a one time event, it is a recurrent disease.

- For every symptomatic episode of AF, there are often multiple asymptomatic episodes.

- Stroke risk is dependent on clinical risk factors not the duration or frequency of AF.

- The elderly are at greatest risk of stroke with 25% of strokes attributed solely to AF in patients who are older than 80 years.

SELECTED BIBLIOGRAPHY

Allessie M, Ausma J, Schotten U. Electrical, contractile and structural remodeling during atrial fibrillation. *Cardiovasc Res.* 2002;54:230–246.

Falk R. Rate control is preferable to rhythm control in the majority of patients with atrial fibrillation. *Circulation.* 2005;111:3141–3150.

Fuster V, Ryden L, Cannom D, et al. ACC/AHA/ESC 2006 Guidelines for the management of patients with atrial fibrillation: A report of the American College of

Cardiology/American Heart Association Task Force on practice guidelines and the European Society of Cardiology Committee for practice guidelines. *Circulation*. 2006;114:e257–e354.

Haissaguerre M, Jais P, Shah D. Spontaneous initiation of atrial fibrillation by ectopic beats originating in the pulmonary veins. *N Engl J Med*. 1998;339:659–666.

Hauser T, Josephson ME, Zimetbaum P. Safety and feasibility of a clinical pathway for the outpatient initiation of antiarrhythmic medications in patients with atrial fibrillation and flutter. *Am J Cardiol*. 2003;91:1437–1441.

Josephson ME. *Clinical cardiac electrophysiology*, 4th ed. Philadelphia: Lippincott Williams & Wilkins; 2008.

Singh B, Singh S, Reda D, et al. Amiodarone versus sotalol for atrial fibrillation. *N Engl J Med*. 2005;352:1861–1872.

The Atrial Fibrillation Follow-up Investigation of Rhythm Management (AFFIRM) Investigators. A comparison of rate control and rhythm control in patients with atrial fibrillation. *N Engl J Med*. 2002;347:1825–1833.

Zimetbaum P. The argument for maintenance of sinus rhythm. *Circulation*. 2005; 111:3150–3155.

Atrial Flutter

CLINICAL CHARACTERISTICS

Atrial flutter is a regular, macro reentrant arrhythmia with an atrial rate of 250 to 320 beats per minute (bpm). The pathophysiology of atrial flutter is closely related to that of atrial fibrillation. The incidence of atrial flutter has been estimated at 0.88% of the general population, increasing to 5.87% in patients older than 80 years of age (see Table 7-1).

One of the difficulties in understanding atrial flutter is related to terminology. The term *atrial flutter* is used to describe several different macro reentrant arrhythmias, which differ in location and pathophysiology. These distinctions, although initially confusing, are particularly important with regard to ablative therapy for atrial flutter. The most frequent way of classifying atrial flutter is isthmus dependent (or typical) and non–isthmus dependent. Isthmus-dependent atrial flutter describes a right atrial circuit, bounded anteriorly by the tricuspid annulus and posteriorly by the caval veins, crista terminalis, and the Eustachian ridge (see Fig. 7-1). This circuit is most confined in the low atrium, as it passes around the inferior vena cava and the Eustachian ridge. These structures, with reference to the tricuspid valve, are the "isthmus" through which atrial flutter must pass and form the target for ablation therapy. Isthmus-dependent flutter has "sawtooth" flutter waves in the inferior leads (see Fig. 7-2). Viewing the atrium with the tricuspid valve turned up like a clockface, atrial flutter can traverse the same circuit in a clockwise (in which

TABLE 7-1   **Electrocardiographic (ECG) Characteristics of Atrial Flutter**
Be suspicious of any regular SVT with a ventricular rate of ≈150 bpm
1. Atrial rate from 250–310 bpm
2. Regular atrial activation in all leads, usually with a "sawtooth" pattern in the inferior leads
3. Regular ventricular response, with a consistent relationship between flutter waves and QRS complexes, usually in an even integral pattern (i.e., 2:1, 4:1, etc.)

SVT, supraventricular tachycardia.

case the inferior leads are positive) or a counterclockwise (in which the inferior leads are negative) direction (see Table 7-2).

Non–isthmus-dependent flutter refers to regular, macro reentrant atrial arrhythmias that occur outside of the isthmus, typically in regions of atrial scarring (see Fig. 7-3). This scarring may occur spontaneously, for reasons that are not well understood, or as the result of surgical incisions or extensive atrial

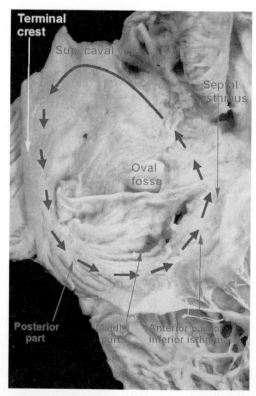

FIGURE 7-1. Anatomy of the right atrial flutter circuit. (See color insert.)

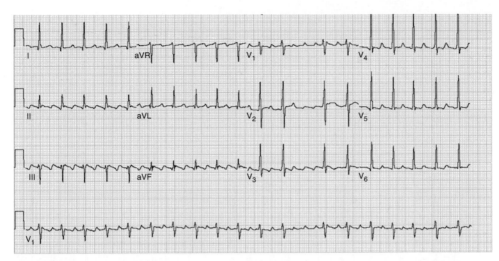

FIGURE 7-2. The electrocardiogram in isthmus-dependent, counterclockwise atrial flutter. The tracing shows a regular, narrow complex arrhythmia with an atrial rate of 240 bpm with 2:1 atrioventricular (AV) conduction resulting in an average ventricular rate of 120 bpm. The atrial rate is a little slower than typical because of marked atrial enlargement as well as antiarrhythmic drug effects. The flutter waves are negative in the inferior leads, positive in V_1 but negative in the remainder of the precordial leads.

ablation. In addition to natural barriers (such as the veins that enter the atria, or the valve annuli), scarring provides the boundaries for establishing atrial flutter circuits, as well as the requisite slow conduction. There is some overlap, both in atrial rate and electrocardiographic appearance between non–isthmus-dependent atrial flutter and pulmonary vein–related atrial tachycardia, which is probably due to reentry on a much smaller scale. Because of the wide

---

TABLE 7-2 Diagnosis of Isthmus-Dependent Atrial Flutter during Electrophysiologic (EP) Studies

1. Activation of the circular catheter progresses in a clockwise or counterclockwise manner
2. Right atrial activation requires the entire flutter cycle length
3. The onset of the surface flutter wave coincides with activation of a septal intracardiac electrogram (the His atrial recording in clockwise and the proximal CS in counterclockwise atrial flutter)
4. Entrainment pacing from the isthmus matches the activation during spontaneous atrial flutter
5. Following the cessation of entrainment pacing, activation occurs at the pacing site 1 atrial flutter cycle length from the last pacing stimulus

---

CS, coronary sinus.

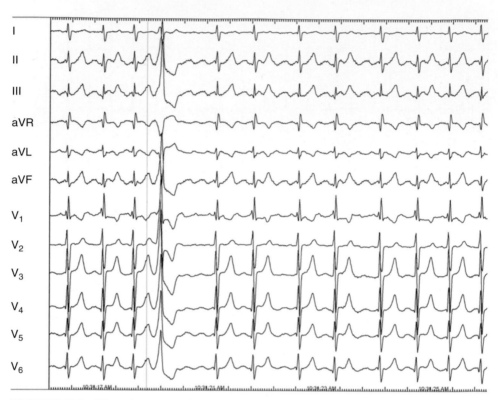

FIGURE 7-3. The electrocardiogram in non–isthmus-dependent atrial flutter. The atrial cycle length is 245 msec, and the flutter wave morphology is negative in the inferior leads, flat in lead I, but is positive in all of the precordial leads, indicating likely left atrial origin. This arrhythmia occurred in a patient who had undergone mitral valve replacement and represented complex reentry around the mitral annulus and in between the right and left pulmonary veins.

variability of this process and its relative rarity (at least before atrial fibrillation ablation procedures), this chapter will focus on isthmus-dependent atrial flutter.

Atrial flutter most often occurs in patients with structural heart disease, as some degree of right atrial enlargement and/or conduction slowing is required to make atrial flutter possible. One way of expressing this point is consideration of the wavelength, which is defined as the distance that the arrhythmia wave front travels in the average refractory period of the atrial tissue, or the conduction velocity × refractory period. In order for atrial flutter to occur, the wavelength must be shorter than the path length of the anatomic circuit or else the wave front would run into its refractory wake and extinguish. Anything that makes the wavelength shorter (fibrosis, antiarrhythmic drugs that block sodium channels) or the atrium larger (valvular heart disease, arrhythmia-induced remodeling, hypertension, cardiomyopathy) will facilitate atrial flutter.

There is a wide range of symptoms caused by atrial flutter, mostly dependent on ventricular rate, ranging from none to syncope. Characteristically, the ventricular rate has an even integral relationship with the atrial rate, usually 2:1. This results in a typical ventricular rate of 150 bpm, as the atrial rate is normally 300 bpm. Patients typically perceive this as rapid palpitations or as exercise intolerance because the rate is inappropriately high and does not change with increasing workload. Exercise intolerance and fatigue can occasionally occur because the ventricular rate is inappropriately slow, as would be observed in 8:1 flutter (ventricular rate ≈40 bpm). In other circumstances, there are no symptoms, perhaps owing to the fact that the atrial rhythm and more importantly the ventricular response, is regular. Atrial flutter may be paroxysmal, persistent, or may degenerate to atrial fibrillation.

Under unusual circumstances, the ventricular response to atrial flutter can be 1:1, a situation that has a high likelihood of causing syncope. The typical situation that leads to this is the use of sodium channel blocking antiarrhythmic drugs for atrial flutter or atrial fibrillation without atrioventricular (AV) nodal blocking agents. The antiarrhythmic drug slows the atrial rate during atrial flutter, and in some cases (classically with quinidine) facilitates AV conduction.

Atrial flutter and atrial fibrillation are interconnected on many levels. The pathophysiology of both are similar, and the two conditions coexist in many patients. Both arrhythmias are progressive, which is thought to be due to arrhythmia-related "remodeling" on structural (increased atrial size), electrical (shortening of the atrial refractory period), and ultrastructural (promoting atrial fibrosis) levels. Furthermore, the remodeling caused by one arrhythmia leads to progression of the other. Approximately 15% of patients treated with class IC antiarrhythmic agents or amiodarone for atrial fibrillation will develop atrial flutter, often exclusively. This observation led to the development of a "hybrid" management strategy of antiarrhythmic drugs to treat atrial fibrillation, and ablation to treat atrial flutter. On the other hand, approximately 50% of patients with "pure" atrial flutter will develop atrial fibrillation over 5 years. This progression occurs despite adequate treatment for atrial flutter and seems to be higher if episodes of atrial flutter continue.

ELECTROCARDIOGRAPHIC CLUES TO THE DIAGNOSIS

Isthmus-dependent atrial flutter is recognized on the electrocardiogram (ECG) by the following characteristics: (a) atrial rate from 250 to 310 bpm, (b) regular atrial activation in all leads, usually with a "sawtooth" pattern in the inferior leads, and (c) regular ventricular response, with a discernable and consistent relationship between flutter waves and QRS complexes, usually in an even integral relationship[1] (Fig. 7-2). The flutter waves in counterclockwise isthmus-dependent flutter are negative in the inferior leads, positive in V_1, and negative in the lateral precordial leads. The flutter waves in clockwise isthmus-dependent flutter are positive in the inferior leads, negative in V_1, and negative in the lateral precordial leads.

Non–isthmus-dependent atrial flutter follows the same "rules" described earlier, but the morphology of the flutter waves depends on the atrial site from which it arises (Fig. 7-3). When it originates from the left atrium, the flutter waves are not only more rightward in direction but also more likely to be positive in the precordial leads. This is owing to the fact that the left atrium is not only left but even more so posterior to the right atrium, allowing for more of the wave front to activate the anteriorly positioned precordial leads in a positive direction.

At first glance, identifying flutter waves can be difficult because they can be obscured by the T wave. A useful ECG pearl is to suspect atrial flutter whenever you see a supraventricular tachycardia (SVT) with a ventricular rate of approximately equal to 150 bpm. With this index of suspicion, it is easier to train the eye to start noticing the presence of two atrial activations for each QRS, and sorting out the flutter waves (particularly in the inferior leads) to confirm the diagnosis. When there is doubt on the initial ECG, infusion of adenosine may be helpful. This maneuver will not interrupt the arrhythmia, but will temporarily decrease AV conduction, allowing recognition of the flutter waves.

Atrial fibrillation is often confused with atrial flutter usually because of misinterpretation of organized atrial activity in lead V_1 (see Fig. 7-4). In this situation, apparently organized and repetitive atrial activation is observed in V_1, usually with a cycle length <200 msec. However, unlike the rules presented for atrial flutter earlier, (a) atrial activation is not organized in the frontal plane leads, (b) the ventricular response is irregular, and (c) even in V_1, there is no consistent relationship between the apparent "flutter waves" and QRS complexes. This is sometimes described as "coarse atrial fibrillation." Interestingly, V_1 in this instance seems to reflect uniform activation of the right atrium although the left atrium is fibrillating.

EVALUATION IN THE ELECTROPHYSIOLOGY LABORATORY

The primary indication for electrophysiologic study in patients with atrial flutter is to perform curative ablation. The diagnosis of atrial flutter is largely on the basis of preprocedural analysis of the ECG during tachycardia. There are some

---

[1]Atrial flutter with variable conduction (2:1 alternating with 4:1, or even multiple levels of AV block) can be confusing in this regard; however, there is always a consistent relationship between the flutter wave and the QRS, even if that relationship is more complex.

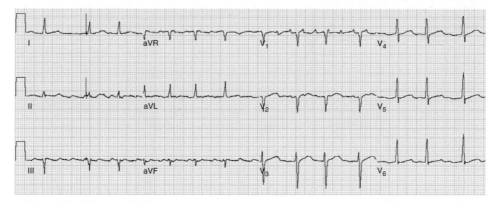

FIGURE 7-4. The electrocardiogram in "coarse" atrial fibrillation. Many mistake this arrhythmia for atrial flutter, owing to the apparent regular and uniform activation in lead V_1. Organized atrial activation is not apparent in any other electrocardiogram (ECG) lead, the ventricular response is irregular, and even in lead V_1, there is no consistent relationship between atrial and ventricular activation. These are all characteristic of atrial fibrillation.

difficulties in this, particularly distinguishing for certain isthmus-dependent and non–isthmus-dependent flutters after ablation or surgery. Because of this, it is useful to induce atrial flutter with atrial-programmed stimulation to confirm the diagnosis and establish the fact of isthmus dependency before ablation.

Isthmus-dependent atrial flutter provides a unique opportunity for understanding reentrant rhythms in general because the physicians can record from the entire circuit. This is typically done with a circular catheter, which is positioned close to the tricuspid annulus. Viewed from the perspective of intracardiac recordings, isthmus-dependent atrial flutter has the following characteristics: (a) activation of the circular catheter occurs in a clockwise or counterclockwise progression (see Fig. 7-5), (b) activation of the right atrium requires the entire atrial cycle length, (c) the onset of the surface flutter wave coincides with activation of a septal intracardiac electrogram (the His catheter atrial recording in clockwise and the proximal coronary sinus [CS] atrial recording in counterclockwise atrial flutter), and (d) a consistent response to overdrive pacing from the circuit during atrial flutter (entrainment). Entrainment is the most important laboratory technique in confirming the diagnosis. If the arrhythmia is actually isthmus dependent (as opposed to passive activation of the right atrium by a left atrial arrhythmia), then pacing from the isthmus during atrial flutter should result in the following: (a) the flutter waves and the intracardiac recordings should have the same activation patterns and timing during pacing and the spontaneous flutter and (b) after pacing is stopped, the electrogram recorded at the pacing site should occur one flutter cycle length (i.e., one revolution of the circle) from the pacing stimulus (Fig. 7-5). This second characteristic makes more sense when considering the opposite. If pacing was done outside of the tachycardia circuit, the amount of

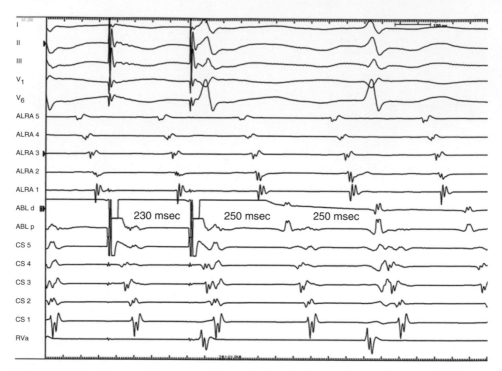

FIGURE 7-5. Intracardiac recordings during isthmus-dependent atrial flutter. Recordings from surface electrocardiogram (ECG) leads, coronary sinus (CS 1 is distal and CS 5 is proximal), and anterolateral right atrium (ALRA 1 is distal and ALRA 5 is proximal). Pacing at 230 milliseconds (msec) from the ablation catheter (ABL) is demonstrated on the left of the panel with entrainment of the tachycardia. The atrial activation is identical to that recorded during atrial flutter. When pacing is stopped, the wave front comes back around to the pacing site at a duration (250 msec) which is exactly equal to the atrial flutter cycle length. These findings confirm the diagnosis of isthmus-dependent atrial flutter.

time it would take for the next tachycardia wave front to return to the pacing site would be longer than the flutter cycle length (= flutter cycle length + the amount of time it takes to travel from the pacing site to the circuit and return back to the pacing site).

Once the diagnosis is confirmed with activation and entrainment mapping, ablation can be performed, either during atrial flutter or pacing from the CS. Ablation is targeted to the isthmus of tissue between the tricuspid valve to the inferior vena cava, taking advantage of the most anatomically constricted portion of the circuit. Block across the line of ablation lesions is confirmed by termination of the atrial flutter and by failure of conduction during pacing on both sides of the isthmus (see Fig. 7-6). When a perpendicular wave front is launched with pacing (as from the proximal CS) with the ablation catheter positioned on the ablation line, widely split double potentials are observed.

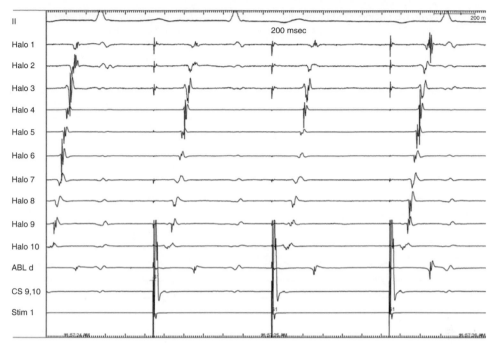

FIGURE 7-6. Intracardiac recordings after isthmus ablation. The ablation target was in the low medial right atrium, in between the coronary sinus and Halo 1. Pacing from the coronary sinus after ablation confirms the presence of block across the isthmus: the wave front cannot directly travel the short distance from the coronary sinus to Halo 1, but instead has to traverse the rest of the atrium to get there "the long way."

This represents initial early activation on the proximal side of the line, which blocks, and subsequent late activation at the same site after the impulse travels "the long way" around the tricuspid annulus (Fig. 7-6). During ablation in sinus rhythm conduction, block in the isthmus can be demonstrated with a change in the activation sequence of the lateral right atrium while pacing the CS or vice versa (see Fig. 7-7).

MANAGEMENT OF ATRIAL FLUTTER

Treatment of atrial flutter presents many of the same management considerations as atrial fibrillation. The issues include control of symptoms, which are usually due to inappropriately high ventricular rate, prevention of atrial remodeling, prevention of rate-related cardiomyopathy, and prevention of stroke (see Table 7-3). As mentioned earlier, rate control of atrial flutter is often difficult. Large doses and/or multiple AV nodal blocking drugs are typically required, often with the attendant side effect of producing bradyarrhythmias during sinus rhythm. Although only small amounts of data are available regarding the

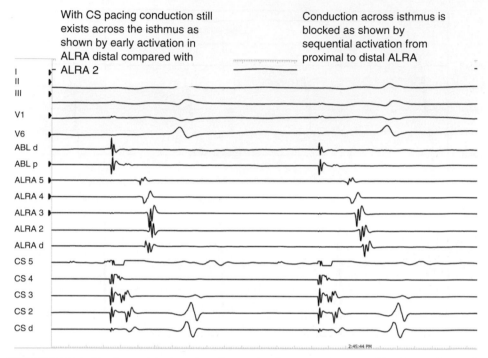

FIGURE 7-7. During ablation in sinus rhythm conduction block in the isthmus can be demonstrated with a change in the activation sequence of the lateral right atrium while pacing the coronary sinus (CS) or vice versa. ALRA, anterolateral right atrium.

efficacy of antiarrhythmic drugs for prevention of recurrent atrial flutter, it is thought that this strategy is largely frustrating. It is easy to understand, given consideration of the wavelength phenomenon, why sodium channel blocking agents are likely to be ineffective; however, it has not been demonstrated that class III agents are more successful. In a small study of patients randomized to antiarrhythmic drugs versus atrial flutter ablation, ablation was much more likely to prevent recurrence of atrial flutter as well as the progression to atrial fibrillation over short-term follow-up.

TABLE 7-3 Clinical "Pearls" Regarding the Management of Atrial Flutter

1. Rate control of atrial flutter is often difficult
2. Antiarrhythmic drugs can make atrial flutter more frequent and make episodes more persistent
3. The rules for anticoagulation of atrial flutter are the same as those for atrial fibrillation
4. Atrial flutter and atrial fibrillation frequently coexist

Because of its satisfactory safety profile and high efficacy, ablation therapy is the primary therapy in patients with isthmus-dependent atrial flutter, particularly in the absence of accompanying atrial fibrillation. In some patients with "mixed" atrial fibrillation and atrial flutter, ablation can also be helpful, either as part of a hybrid therapy approach or if atrial flutter but not atrial fibrillation is refractory to rhythm or rate control strategies. The acute success in contemporary series of ablation for isthmus-dependent atrial flutter is approximately >90%; the recurrence rate at 1 to 2 years of follow-up is 5% to 10%, and is associated with recovery of conduction in the sub-Eustachian isthmus.

Ablation is more complicated in non–isthmus-dependent atrial fibrillation, but should still be considered, particularly as alternative treatments (rate and rhythm control with antiarrhythmic drugs) may be even more limited in this condition compared to isthmus-dependent flutter. Successful ablation is not as uniform for non–isthmus-dependent flutter, but favorable series have been published from several highly accomplished laboratories.

Patients with atrial flutter are at a similar risk of stroke as patients with atrial fibrillation, and similar recommendations are in place regarding the use of warfarin anticoagulation. In general, these are based on clinical risk profiles (such as the congestive heart failure, hypertension, age, diabetes, and stroke [CHADS] score), except in preparation for and following cardioversion or ablation, in which cases uniform prescription of warfarin for 1 month before and after is recommended. As is the case for atrial fibrillation, the use of warfarin before cardioversion can be preempted by transesophageal echocardiography.

In the absence of concomitant atrial fibrillation, anticoagulation is typically discontinued after successful ablation of atrial flutter. As mentioned earlier, this can be tricky because of the high incidence of atrial fibrillation over time in these patients. The absence of potential complications of anticoagulation therapy during the interlude between flutter and fibrillation justifies this practice. Nonetheless, it is important for both patient and physician to be vigilant for the development of atrial fibrillation and reinstitution of anticoagulation.

SELECTED BIBLIOGRAPHY

Anselme F, Savoure A, Cribier A, et al. Catheter ablation of typical atrial flutter: A randomized comparison of 2 methods for determining complete bidirectional isthmus block. *Circulation*. 2001;103:1434–1439.

Chinitz JS, Gerstenfeld EP, Marchlinski FE, et al. Atrial fibrillation is common after ablation of isolated atrial flutter. *Heart Rhythm*. 2007; in press.

Fischer B, Jais P, Shah D, et al. Radiofrequency catheter ablation of common atrial flutter in 200 patients. *J Cardiovasc Electrophysiol*. 1996;7:1225–1233.

Granada J, Uribe W, Chyou PH, et al. Incidence and predictors of atrial flutter in the general population. *J Am Coll Cardiol*. 2000;36:2242–2246.

Huang DT, Monahan KM, Zimetbaum P, et al. Hybrid pharmacologic and ablative therapy: A novel and effective approach for the management of atrial fibrillation. *J Cardiovasc Electrophysiol*. 1998;9:462–469.

Jais P, Shah DC, Haissaguerre M, et al. Mapping and ablation of left atrial flutters. *Circulation*. 2000;101:2928–2934.

Josephson ME. *Clinical cardiac electrophysiology*, 4th ed. Philadelphia: Lippincott Williams & Wilkins; 2008.

Nakagawa H, Lazzara R, Khastgir T, et al. Role of the tricuspid annulus and the eustachian valve/ridge on atrial flutter. Relevance to catheter ablation of the septal isthmus and a new technique for rapid identification of ablation success. *Circulation*. 1996;94:407–424.

Nakagawa H, Shah N, Matsudaira K, et al. Characterization of reentrant circuit in macroreentrant right atrial tachycardia after surgical repair of congenital heart disease: Isolated channels between scars allow 'focal' ablation. *Circulation*. 2001;103:699–709.

Natale A, Newby KH, Pisano E, et al. Prospective randomized comparison of antiar-rhythmic therapy versus first-line radiofrequency ablation in patients with atrial flutter. *J Am Coll Cardiol*. 2000;35:1898–1904.

Poty H, Saoudi N, Abdel Aziz A, et al. Radiofrequency catheter ablation of type 1 atrial flutter: Prediction of late success by electrophysiological criteria. *Circulation*. 1995;92:1389–1392.

Saoudi N, Cosio F, Waldo A, et al. Classification of atrial flutter and regular atrial tachycardia according to electrophysiologic mechanism and anatomic bases: A state-ment from a joint expert group from the Working Group of Arrhythmias of the European Society of Cardiology and the North American Society of Pacing and Electrophysiology. *J Cardiovasc Electrophysiol*. 2001;12:852–866.

Schwartzman D, Callans DJ, Gottlieb CD, et al. Conduction block in the inferior vena caval-tricuspid valve isthmus: Association with outcome of radiofrequency ablation of type I atrial flutter. *J Am Coll Cardiol*. 1996;28:1519–1531.

Tai CT, Chen SA, Chiang CE, et al. Electrophysiologic characteristics and radiofre-quency catheter ablation in patients with clockwise atrial flutter. *J Cardiovasc Electrophysiol*. 1997;8:24–34.

Waldo AL, Mackall JA, Biblo LA. Mechanisms and medical management of patients with atrial flutter. *Cardiol Clin*. 1997;15:661–676.

Wood KA, Eisenberg SJ, Kalman JM, et al. Risk of thromboembolism in chronic atrial flutter. *Am J Cardiol*. 1997;79:1043–1047.

Supraventricular Tachycardia

INTRODUCTION AND MECHANISMS

Supraventricular tachycardia (SVT) refers to regular, narrow QRS complex rhythms typically in excess of 100 beats per minute (bpm). Atrial flutter and atrial fibrillation will be discussed separately. The prevalence of SVT in the general population is 2.25 per 1,000 persons with an incidence of 35 per 100,000 person-years. In the absence of preexcitation, these tachycardias are divided into three major categories: atrioventricular nodal reentrant tachycardia (AVNRT), atrioventricular reentrant tachycardia due to a concealed accessory pathway (AP) (circus movement tachycardia [CMT]), and atrial tachycardia (AT). Although these three categories encompass the vast majority of regular, narrow-complex tachycardias, other rare tachycardia mechanisms separate from these may exist such as junctional ectopic tachycardia (JET).

AVNRT is the most common form of SVT. It is a form of reentry involving two functional "dual" pathways in the AV node. Although the true circuit is functionally based rather than anatomically based, AVNRT has been described as following a protected circuit within the AV node or AV junctional region along so-called slow pathway (SP) and fast pathway (FP). The SP input has been localized to the inferior portion of the triangle of Koch between the ostium of the coronary sinus (CS) and the septal leaflet of the tricuspid valve.

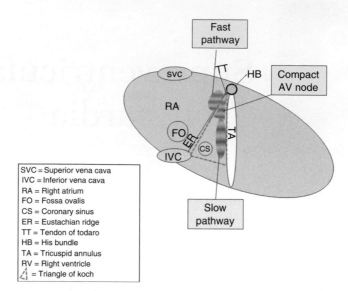

SVC = Superior vena cava
IVC = Inferior vena cava
RA = Right atrium
FO = Fossa ovalis
CS = Coronary sinus
ER = Eustachian ridge
TT = Tendon of todaro
HB = His bundle
TA = Tricuspid annulus
RV = Right ventricle
△ = Triangle of koch

FIGURE 8-1. Schematic of the functional anatomy of the atrioventricular (AV) node in the right anterior oblique (RAO) view. (See color insert.)

The FP input has been localized to the superior aspect of the tendon of Todaro at or just above this His bundle (see Fig. 8-1).

Dual pathways are required but not sufficient to have AVNRT. There must be block in one pathway and slow conduction in the other to allow reentry (echo beat) and this must be continuous to allow tachycardia (see Fig. 8-2). Linking of SP and FP is required for reentry to occur. Many patients will demonstrate dual pathways without being able to sustain tachycardia. In such cases there may be no linking, or more commonly a weak retrograde limb.

The typical or common form of AVNRT (97% of cases of AVNRT) involves antegrade conduction down the SP and retrograde conduction up the FP. The P wave is generated by the retrograde conduction from the AV node to the atrium. This generates a negative P wave, which is often buried in the QRS complex and invisible on the surface electrocardiogram (ECG). The P wave is seen within the QRS because retrograde conduction is rapid, occurs simultaneous with conduction to the ventricle, and the P wave is narrow. The uncommon or atypical form of AVNRT (3% of cases of AVNRT) conducts down the FP and back up the SP and is manifest as a long RP tachycardia with negative surface P waves in 2, 3, and aVF (see Fig. 8-3). P waves in this form of AVNRT tend to be broader and deeper than in typical AVNRT because earliest activation is near the CS ostium.

Atrioventricular Reentrant Tachycardia

Atrioventricular reentrant tachycardia (AVRT) refers to tachycardias which utilize an AP as at least one limb of the tachycardia (Fig. 8-3B). If there is

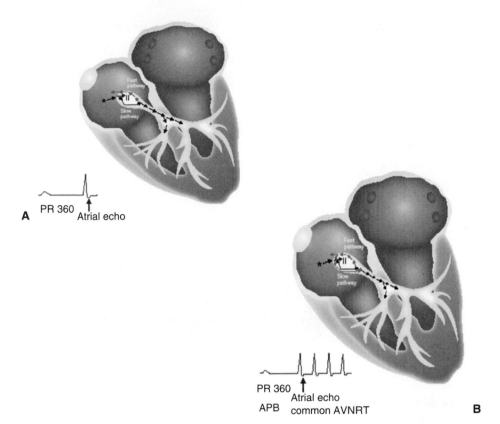

FIGURE 8-2. Diagrams of a typical atrioventricular (AV) nodal echo **(A)** and the initiation of atrioventricular nodal reentrant tachycardia (AVNRT) **(B)**. The *black arrow* represents initial conduction down the slow pathway. The *blue arrows* demonstrate retrograde conduction up the slow pathway (echo beat) with subsequent conduction back down the slow pathway with initiation of AVNRT. (See color insert.)

antegrade or manifest conduction over the AP in sinus rhythm and there is documented SVT it is called *Wolff-Parkinson-White syndrome* (see Chapter 9). If the pathway only conducts in the retrograde direction it is a "concealed" pathway. APs are considered congenital abnormalities. The locations of concealed APs are similar to manifest APs. Of all patients with SVT using a concealed AP, up to 10% have a second AP. Ninety percent of concealed APs are rapidly conducting. Of rapidly conducting concealed APs, 60% are left free wall, 27% are posteroseptal, 5% are anteroseptal, and 8% are right free wall. Because the circuit necessitates conduction through the His-Purkinje system (HPS) to the ventricles and then up an AP, the retrograde limb (represented by the VA interval) is longer than in AVNRT which does not need to reach the ventricle before activating the atrium. Unlike the AV node, which is characterized by decremental conduction, accessory atrioventricular connections tend to conduct in an "all-or-none" manner.

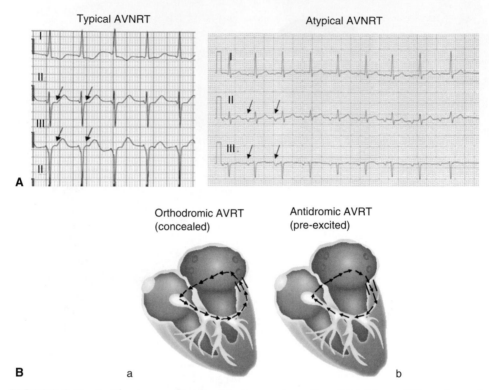

FIGURE 8-3. A: Electrocardiographic examples of typical (short RP) and atypical (long RP) atrioventricular nodal reentrant tachycardia (AVNRT). **B:** Atrioventricular reentrant tachycardia. (See color insert.)

During SVT with antegrade AV nodal conduction and retrograde conduction over an AP (orthodromic AVRT), retrograde conduction is said to conduct rapidly when the ECG RP interval is less than the PR interval. Although this is a good general rule, absolute RP intervals of up to 170 msec could be rapidly conducting. The RP interval is affected by the AV nodal conduction and the presence of bundle branch block (BBB). Tachycardias employing rapidly conducting APs tend to be paroxysmal. A small minority of SVTs using a concealed AP as the retrograde limb of circuit may demonstrate longer RP intervals (greater in duration than the PR interval) and are called *slowly conducting APs*. These APs frequently demonstrate decremental properties and can be incessant (PJRT or the permanent form of junctional reciprocating tachycardia). AVRT which conducts antegradely over the AP and retrogradely over the AV node or a second AP are called *antidromic tachycardias*.

Atrial Tachycardia

This is a form of SVT in which an atrial source drives the tachycardia independent of the route of AV conduction. The mechanism of this tachycardia may be automatic, triggered, or less commonly, reentrant. Reentrant forms of AT are generally considered macroreentrant if they can be entrained from sites over a distance of 1 or 2 cm whereas microreentrant circuits are more focal in nature. Large macroreentrant circuits are often related to atrial scarring. Frequently, AT is associated with structural heart disease and associated conditions such as myocardial infarction, chronic obstructive pulmonary disease (COPD), alcohol ingestion, hypoxia, hypokalemia, increased catecholamine states, and digoxin toxicity. Automatic atrial tachycardias (AATs) can be incessant and occasionally cause tachycardia-mediated cardiomyopathy.

Focal ATs generally develop in distinct anatomic locations. The crista terminalis is the most common site of AT in the right atrium and the pulmonary veins are the most common site of AT in the left atrium. Other important sites of AT include the lateral tricuspid annulus, CS ostium, para-Hisian region, mitral annulus, and atrial appendages. ATs coming from the superior crista terminalis may lie close to or originate within the sinus node complex. Reentry within the sinus node (sinus node reentry) can be considered a form of right AT. Rates in AT are often slower (100 to 180 bpm) than AVNRT or AVRT, but overlap exists.

Sinus tachycardia can be classified as appropriate in response to a stimulus such as anemia, volume depletion, or hyperthyroidism or inappropriate, indicating a rapid rate without a clear cause. Inappropriate sinus tachycardia may be due to reentry within the sinus node (sinus node reentry). Sinus node reentry tends to begin with a premature beat or rapid atrial rates and terminate spontaneously. Inappropriate sinus tachycardia may also occur as a syndrome in which the sinus rate increases in response to physical exertion, positional change, or emotional stimuli but remains rapid long after the stimulus is over. Postural orthostatic tachycardia syndrome (POTS) is a form of inappropriate sinus tachycardia in which movement from a supine to upright posture without associated orthostatic hypotension results in prolonged tachycardia. This is distinguished from orthostatic hypotension in which tachycardia occurs appropriately in response to a positional fall in blood pressure.

CLINICAL PRESENTATION

Demographics

The age of onset of tachycardia or palpitations and in some cases the gender of the patient, can help narrow down the differential diagnosis of SVT. Advanced age and the presence of structural heart disease increase the likelihood of AT. Conversely, palpitations since childhood favor AVRT. The onset of tachycardia during early adulthood, often with a period of quiescence and then recurrence in middle age is typical of AVNRT. However, AVNRT can present at any age. Male gender, particularly in a young person favors AVRT, whereas female gender, regardless of the age of onset, favors AVNRT.

Symptoms and Circumstances

Several signs and symptoms may suggest a particular type of SVT. For example, a pounding sensation in the neck may indicate atrial contraction against closed AV valves, which can be seen frequently in AVNRT due to near-simultaneous depolarization of the atria and ventricles. On physical examination, patients may display visible jugular venous pulsations ("frog sign") due to atrial contraction against a closed tricuspid valve.

The circumstances of initiation and termination may be suggestive of a particular diagnosis. Initiation after standing up from a bent-over position is common in patients with AVNRT, possibly from carotid sinus–driven changes in autonomic tone with change in posture. Similarly, termination by a vagal maneuver is common in AVNRT or AVRT. Although an abrupt onset and offset are classic manifestations of SVT (typically AVNRT or AVRT), increased sympathetic tone from tachycardia or related anxiety may blunt the sensation of an abrupt offset of tachycardia. Younger patients often have sinus tachycardia at the termination of an SVT episode, which may mask the feeling of an acute termination. Tachycardia that is incessant may lead to a cardiomyopathy. Such tachycardias are frequently due to AT or a slowly conducting AP (e.g., PJRT). The PJRT is characterized by an initiation with preceding sinus acceleration. It is often only slightly faster than the resting sinus rate and can start and stop throughout the day. Both AT and PJRT are sensitive to catecholamines, resulting in very rapid rates during daily exercise and slower rates at rest.

DIAGNOSIS

Electrocardiography

Because most SVTs can be diagnosed by ECG, great efforts should be made to document episodes of SVT on a 12-lead ECG before instituting empiric therapy. When a systematic approach is followed, diagnostic accuracy is improved.

P-Wave Axis and Morphology

The first step in analysis is to localize atrial activity. Because identification of the P wave may be difficult, perturbations in the tachycardia or comparison to a sinus rhythm tracing may provide assistance.

P waves that are identical to the sinus P wave suggest sinus node reentry or an AT coming from a site in the right atrium near the sinus node. P waves that are inverted in the inferior leads suggest retrograde activation of the atria as is characteristic of AVNRT or AVRT using a concealed AP in the posteroseptal region of the heart as the retrograde limb. A low right AT coming from the region of the CS can also produce a negative P wave in the inferior leads.

AT can usually be localized by P-wave morphology (see Table 8-1). Generally, an upright P-wave axis in the inferior limb leads favors AT over AVRT and rules out AVNRT. ATs originating in the left atrium most often have a positive (+) or occasionally a negative then positive (±) P wave in lead V_1 and frequently negative or biphasic P wave in aVL. Tachycardias arising from superior locations in either atrium (e.g., superior crista terminalis) have an inferior P-wave axis (+ II, III, and aVF), whereas ATs from inferior locations in the atria (e.g., CS ostium or inferolateral crista terminalis) have a superior (–II, III, and aVF) P-wave axis. A negative P wave in aVR suggests a site in the right atrium such as the sinus node or the crista terminalis but can be seen from the high right atrial septum or occasionally the right superior pulmonary vein. A characteristic "w-shaped" P wave is seen in AT arising from the lateral tricuspid valve (see Fig. 8-4).

ATs arising from the pulmonary veins are characterized by P waves that are positive across the precordial leads from V_1 to V_6, negative (–) or isoelectric in aVL, and negative in aVR. Notching is commonly seen in P waves produced by ATs from the left-sided veins in the inferior and precordial leads. P waves in V_1 are often wider in ATs from the left-sided veins compared with right-sided veins, and a positive P wave in lead I is highly suggestive of a right-sided focus. Additionally, the inferior leads are usually positive with a superior vein origin of AT.

When AVRT is considered, P-wave characteristics can localize the AP. During SVT using a septal AP as the retrograde limb, P waves are usually negative in II, III, aVF and positive in aVR and aVL, and biphasic or isoelectric in V_1. PJRT, which is a long RP tachycardia that is due to a concealed, slow decremental AP (>50 msec increase in VA with SVT or pacing) often reveals large inverted P waves in II, III, aVF (see Fig. 8-5). These pathways are located in the posteroseptal region. During SVT using a left free wall AP as the retrograde limb, P waves are usually negative in I whereas with right free wall pathways, the P wave is positive in I and negative in V_1.

P-Wave Relationship to the QRS

The relationship of the P wave to the QRS provides important insight into the tachycardia mechanism. The presence of AV dissociation or AV block excludes the possibility of AVRT because the atria and ventricles are obligate parts of the tachycardia circuit. In the presence of AV dissociation, AVNRT is less likely than AT, but not excluded because at least in some cases the atrium is not necessary to maintain AVNRT. A clue to the presence of AVNRT with 2:1 AV block is the finding that the blocked P wave is exactly halfway between each QRS (see Fig. 8-6). In typical AVNRT, because of simultaneous activation of the atria and ventricles, a retrograde P wave might not be observed when 2:1 AV conduction is present giving the appearance of a 1:1 (A:V) tachycardia with the P wave exactly halfway between the RR interval.

TABLE 8-1 Electrocardiographic Morphology of Atrial Tachycardia

Electrocardiographic Determination of Chamber of Origin of AT

	V_1 [a,b]	aVL
Right atrium	−	+
Left atrium	+	−

[a]Care must be taken to measure the initial deflection of the P wave in V1; an isoelectric segment may indicate origin from the coronary sinus ostium.

[b]V1(+) P wave during AT with V1(+/−) in SR is a better predictor of a left atrial (i.e. right superior pulmonary vein) focus than V1(+) during AT with V1(+) during SR, which may indicate a high crista terminalis focus.

Electrocardiographic Characteristics of Focal Atrial Tachycardias

Site	I	II	III	aVL	aVR	V_1	V_6	Comment
Right sided								
Sinus node	+	+	+	+	−	+/−	+	Tallest P in lead II
Crista terminalis (high)	+	+	+	+	−	+/−	+	Exclude SR and RSPV
Crista terminalis (low)	+	−	−	+	−	−	+	
Lateral tricuspid annulus	+	w	w	+	0	−	v	"W" shape in II, III, aVF
CS ostium	0	−	−	+	+	0/+	−/0	
Right atrial appendage	+	+	+	+	−	−	+	
Septum (superior)[b]	v	+	+	+	+	0	v	Narrower P than sinus
Septum (inferior)[b]	v	−	−	+	+	0	v	Narrower P than sinus
Left sided								
Left superior PV	−	+	+	−	−	+	+	Notch inferiorly and V_1-V_6
Left inferior PV	−	−	−	−	+/−	+	+	Notch inferiorly and V_1-V_6

TABLE 8-1 *Continued*

Electrocardiographic Characteristics of Focal Atrial Tachycardias

Right superior PV	+	+	+	$-^a$	−	+	+	Narrower P V_1 vs. LPV
Right inferior PV	+	−	−	$-^a$	−	+	+	Narrower P V_1 vs. LPV
Aortomitral continuity	v	+	+	−	v	−/+	v	
CS body	v	−	−	+	+	+	v	
Left atrial appendage	−	+	+	−	+	+	+	Deeply (−) in I

^{a}Right-sided PVs may have a P(+) in aVL.

^{b}Left-sided mapping is often performed as well.

CS, coronary sinus; SR, sinus rhythm; RSPV, right superior pulmonary vein; (+), positive polarity; (−), negative polarity; (0), isoelectric; (w), "W" shape; (v), variable

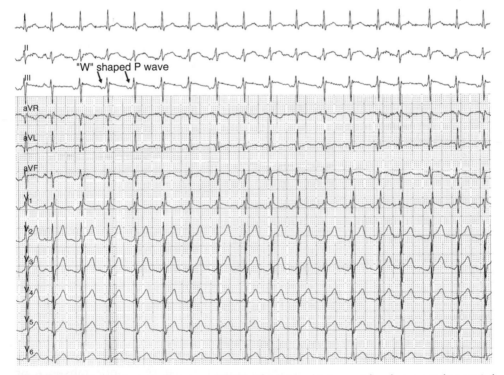

FIGURE 8-4. Electrocardiogram (ECG) of a lateral tricuspid valve annulus atrial tachycardia with the typical "W" P-wave morphology.

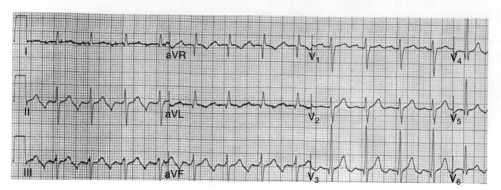

FIGURE 8-5. An electrocardiogram (ECG) of a long RP tachycardia due to the permanent form of junctional reciprocating tachycardia. The P waves are characteristically large and inverted in the inferior leads.

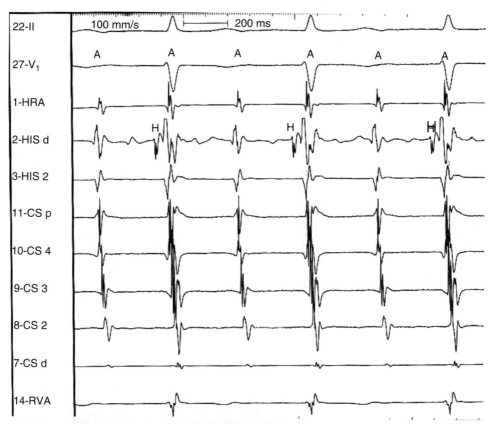

FIGURE 8-6. Intracardiac and surface electrocardiographic (ECG) recordings of atrioventricular nodal reentrant tachycardia (AVNRT) with 2:1 conduction to the ventricle. Block occurs in the atrioventricular (AV) node (absence of His electrogram after the blocked P waves). HRA, high right atrium; HIS, His bundle; CS, coronary sinus; RVA, right ventricular apex.

RP and PR Intervals

The RP interval should be measured and compared to the PR interval. In AT, the P wave drives the next QRS and is not mechanistically tied to the preceding QRS. As a result, spontaneous variations in the R to P (or V to A) interval frequently occur and favor AT over other forms of SVT. Less commonly (10%), extranodal AV connections demonstrate decremental conduction and gradual RP prolongation may occur. Although variable, this RP prolongation is predictively progressive. Most concealed APs have RP intervals shorter than PR intervals. A fixed RP interval with a 1:1 VA relationship regardless of the RR interval is compatible with the presence of a concealed AP. In AVNRT, the RP may be so short that it cannot be identified, and the P wave can appear as an R′ in V_1 or a pseudo S wave in the inferior leads (see Fig. 8-7).

The presence of a "negative RP" such that pseudo Q waves are present in the inferior leads is a specific finding in AVNRT. RP intervals >100 msec are less likely to represent the common form of AVNRT and may indicate the uncommon form of AVNRT or the presence of an AP. RP intervals that exceed

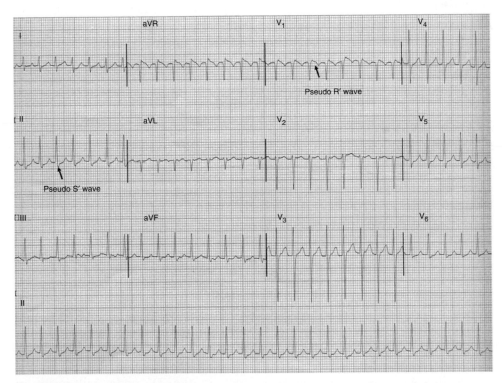

FIGURE 8-7. Electrocardiogram of typical atrioventricular nodal reentrant tachycardia (AVNRT) with pseudo R wave in lead V_1 and pseudo S wave in the inferior leads.

PR intervals are frequently due to AT, but may represent AVRT with a slowly conducting AP or the uncommon form of AVNRT. Theoretically, an AT can have a PR interval so long that the P wave is buried in the prior QRS mimicking AVNRT. Junctional tachycardia may also mimic AVNRT but is distinguished by its nonparoxysmal character.

QRS Alternans

Inspection for QRS alternans of >1 mV in multiple leads during SVT is a useful feature for determining tachycardia mechanism. Although insensitive, the presence of QRS alternans in an SVT that has been present for at least 10 seconds at a rate <180 bpm is specific for CMT.

Initiation and Termination of the Tachycardia

Documenting the onset of SVT with an atrial premature complex (APC) associated with a sudden increase in the initiating PR interval is characteristic of reentrant arrhythmias, typically AVNRT. Initiation with a ventricular premature depolarization (VPD) often occurs in AVRT. SVTs that initiate without a premature beat and a prolonged PR interval favor AT or AVRT using a slowly conducting AP. Furthermore, initiation without any AV delay is common with AT, and, in the case of automatic tachycardias, initiation may occur gradually ("warm up"). Similarly, AATs often terminate by "cooling down."

The initial P wave of the tachycardia is often the same as the subsequent P waves in AAT whereas the initial P wave will often be different in morphology to the subsequent P waves in AVRT or AVNRT.

Termination of the tachycardia after a P wave strongly suggests AVNRT or AVRT. AT is unlikely because termination of the tachycardia following a P wave requires the unlikely coincidence that at the moment the AT terminates spontaneous AV block occurs as well.

Ventricular Premature Depolarizations, Bundle Branch Block, and Atrioventricular Block

The development of a BBB during tachycardia that prolongs the tachycardia cycle length (TCL) or more specifically the RP interval suggests an AP ipsilateral (in the same ventricle) to the side of the BBB (e.g., prolongation of the TCL with a left bundle branch block [LBBB] is consistent with SVT mediated by a left-sided AP). ATs do not depend on conduction from the atria to the ventricles and therefore are not generally influenced by ventricular premature beats.

During AT, the development of block in the AV node will result in continuation of AT with a diminished ventricular response. This is in contradistinction to other forms of SVT (AVRT or AVNRT), which require conduction though the AV node and terminate when AV nodal conduction is blocked.

Vagal Maneuvers

For patients experiencing an episode of SVT, evaluation should include the response to vagal maneuvers. Effective vagal maneuvers include the Valsalva maneuver, carotid sinus massage, and coughing. These are most successful if done shortly after the onset of SVT. When performing these maneuvers, the patient should be placed in a supine position to avoid abrupt hemodynamic changes that may occur.

Enhancing vagal tone produces progressive slowing of AV conduction or block. If AV block occurs and SVT continues, AVRT can be excluded and P-wave morphology can be analyzed. When sinus tachycardia is a consideration, transient AV nodal slowing and sinus slowing may allow for P-wave morphology to be seen as distinct from preceding T waves. When termination occurs with vagal maneuvers, a diagnosis of AVNRT and AVRT is more likely than AT.

AT with 2:1 or higher degree conduction delay to the ventricles can be hard to differentiate from atrial flutter. ATs generally have a clear isoelectric interval between atrial waves whereas flutter is associated with more gradually sloping waves that merge into the next. Although less frequent than AVNRT or AVRT, AT may also be terminated with vagal maneuvers or AV nodal blocking drugs while these therapies will only slow but not terminate atrial flutter.

ELECTROPHYSIOLOGIC EVALUATION

Performance of an electrophysiologic study is the gold standard for diagnosis of SVT and affords the opportunity to perform catheter ablation. In order to obtain complete information catheters should record electrograms (EGMs) from the right atrium, left atrium (through the CS), His bundle, and right ventricular apex (RVA). In anticipation of ablation a fifth sheath is often placed that can accommodate an ablation catheter.

A complete evaluation of a clinical SVT includes initiation of the SVT, identification of the atrial activation sequence and AV relationship at onset and during SVT, effect of BBB on the SVT VA interval, requirement of atrium and ventricle to initiate and sustain the SVT, the effect of atrial and ventricular stimulation during tachycardia, and the effect of drugs and maneuvers on the tachycardia.

ATRIOVENTRICULAR NODAL REENTRANT TACHYCARDIA

Initiation

Initiation of the common form of AVNRT is typically due to an atrial premature depolarization (APD) that blocks antegradely in the FP, conducts down the SP (with pronounced AH prolongation), and then back up the FP (see Fig. 8-8). Dual AV nodal pathways are requisite in patients with AVNRT and are observed in most patients. Initiation of the common form of AVNRT is rare with single VPDs. This is primarily due to delay in the HPS, which limits the prematurity with which a VPD can reach the AV node. In contrast, single VPDs commonly initiate atypical AVNRT (antegrade conduction over the FP and retrograde conduction over the SP).

Atrial Activation Sequence and Atrioventricular Relationship

The atrial activation sequence during AVNRT is usually concentric: the earliest atrial depolarization is seen in the region of the His bundle. Earliest activation can be observed on the left side of the septum as well. Multiple, simultaneous atrial breakthroughs (along the CS catheter) are more consistent with AVNRT than an AP. In the common form of AVNRT, the minimum VA time (measured

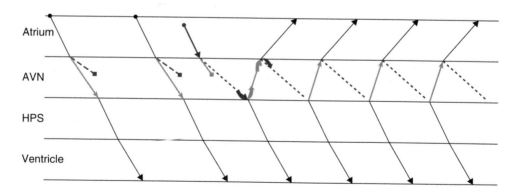

An APD blocks in the fast pathway, conducts antegrade over the slow pathway, and then retrograde over the fast pathway

→ Fast pathway
--► Slow pathway
↔ Atrial premature depolarization (APD)
-→ Block
↻ Indicates reentrant mechanism

FIGURE 8-8. Initiation of typical atrioventricular nodal reentrant tachycardia (AVNRT) with an atrial premature depolarization (APD). AVN, atrioventricular node; HPS, His-Purkinje system.

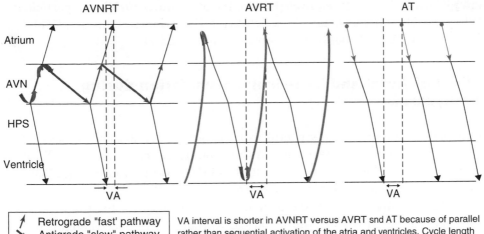

FIGURE 8-9. Ventriculoatrial (VA) intervals in atrioventricular nodal reentrant tachycardia (AVNRT), atrioventricular reentry tachycardia (AVRT), and atrial tachycardia (AT). AVN, atrioventricular node; HPS, His-Purkinje system; AP, accessory pathway.

from the earliest QRS, usually from the surface ECG to the earliest atrial EGM) is <60 to 70 msec (see Fig. 8-9). Negative VA times (atrial activation before the QRS, giving a pseudo Q appearance on ECG) is pathognomonic for AVNRT. The VA time measured from the earliest ventricular EGM to the high right atrial EGM is generally <90 msec in typical AVNRT. The AV relationship is usually 1:1, however, VA block is sometimes noted in AVNRT.

Effect of Bundle Branch Block on Ventriculoatrial Interval

BBB developing with AVNRT is uncommon in typical AVNRT because conduction over the SP provides ample time for recovery of conduction over the bundle branches as long as there is no change in the HV conduction. Significant prolongation of the HV can lead to retrograde activation of the atrium before ventricular activation leading to a P wave before the QRS.

Requirement of Atria and Ventricles to Initiate and Sustain Tachycardia

The AVNRT circuit is confined to the region of the AV node and consequently neither the atria nor the ventricles are required for perpetuation. Both AV and VA block can occur. The presence of AV or VA block excludes AVRT because a circuit involving an AP requires parts of the atria and ventricles to participate. When AV block does occur, block below the His is more common (75%) than block in the AV node below the reentrant circuit (25%).

Effect of Atrial and Ventricular Stimulation during Tachycardia

Delivery of APDs are rarely useful in making the diagnosis of AVNRT. Very short coupled VPDs can reset slow AVNRT but rarely can alter AVNRT with a cycle length (CL) of <375 msec. Multiple VPDs or ventricular pacing (VP) are more commonly needed to overdrive and reset AVNRT.

When pacing the ventricle at a CL 10 to 20 msec faster than the SVT, CL succeeds in advancing the atrial CL to that of the paced length; one of two responses upon cessation of pacing will be seen if the tachycardia continues. The first is atrial depolarization followed by ventricular depolarization, a so-called AV response, which is consistent with either AVNRT or AVRT (see Fig. 8-10). The second is two atrial depolarizations followed by a ventricular depolarization, a so-called A-A-V response, consistent with AT (See Fig. 8-11). In typical AVNRT, the last ventricular depolarization will conduct over the retrograde FP and return to the ventricle over the SP causing a V-A-V response. In the uncommon form of AVNRT, retrograde conduction goes up the

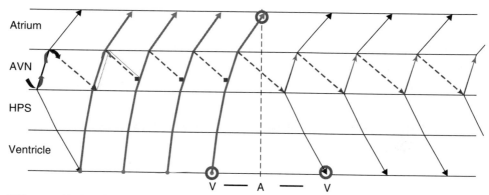

VAV response after cessation of ventricular pacing occurs beacuse of the presence of separate retrograde and antegrade tachycardia limbs. The same pattern would be expected in AVRT but not in atrial tachycardia.

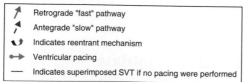

↗	Retrograde "fast" pathway
↗	Antegrade "slow" pathway
↻	Indicates reentrant mechanism
•→	Ventricular pacing
—	Indicates superimposed SVT if no pacing were performed

FIGURE 8-10. Ventricular pacing in atrioventricular nodal reentrant tachycardia (AVNRT) producing a V-A-V response. AVN, atrioventricular node; HPS, His-Purkinje system; AVRT, atrioventricular reentrant tachycardia; SVT, supraventricular tachycardia.

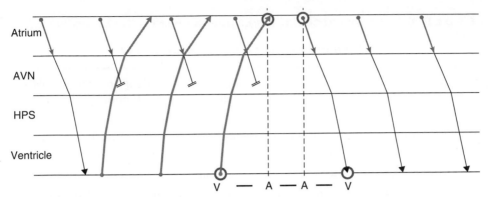

Atrium

AVN

HPS

Ventricle

V — A — A — V

VAAV response after cessation of ventricular pacing occurs beacuse of the presence of a single retrograde and antegrade tachycardia limb. The same pattern would not be expected in AVNRT or in AVRT.

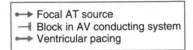

●→ Focal AT source
—⊣ Block in AV conducting system
●→ Ventricular pacing

FIGURE 8-11. Ventricular pacing in atrial tachycardia (AT) producing a V-A-A-V response. AVN, atrioventricular node; HPS, His-Purkinje system; AV, atrioventricular.

SP and antegrade conduction down the FP. Overdrive V pacing can make retrograde conduction so slow that it exceeds the paced CL giving rise to a pseudo V-A-A-V response. The fact that both As are at the paced CL makes the diagnosis of a pseudo V-A-A-V. The V-A-V response is assessed by measuring the postpacing interval (PPI) from the RVA channel. When used for SVTs with a concentric atrial activation sequence and normalized for TCL by subtracting the TCL from the PPI, a difference >115 msec has been shown to be highly specific for AVNRT (time from last RV paced complex to first return RV EGM minus the TCL).

Pharmacologic and Physiologic Maneuvers

During AVNRT, termination by vagal maneuvers often occurs with gradual slowing of the tachycardia followed by SP block. Atropine and isoproterenol often have the opposite effect in that each can improve retrograde fast and/or antegrade slow conduction particularly in patients with VA Wenckebach at relatively slow rates, dual retrograde pathways, and absent baseline VA conduction. These medications may sustain an otherwise nonsustained tachycardia. Calcium channel blockers, β-blockers, and digoxin tend to affect antegrade SP to a much greater degree than retrograde FP conduction. Class IA agents can produce block in the FP and may be effective in preventing or terminating AVNRT. Class IC antiarrhythmics can affect FP and SP as can amiodarone. Sotalol may render AVNRT noninducible in part due to its β-blocker effects.

Electrophysiologic observations for diagnosis of AVNRT are summarized in Table 8-2.

TABLE 8-2   Atrioventricular (AV) Nodal Reentrant Tachycardia

Diagnostic Criteria for Typical AVNRT

Initiation	Initiation dependent on a critical AH interval (dual AV nodal pathways present)
Atrial activation sequence and AV relationship at onset and during SVT	Earliest retrograde atrial activity in HBE ($VA_{min} \leq 60$ msec and $VA_{HRA} < 95$ msec)
Effect of BBB on VA interval	No change in VA interval
Requirement of A and V to initiate and sustain	AV dissociation during SVT possible
Effect of A and V stimulation during tachycardia	• V-A-V response upon cessation of RV pacing • PPI >115 msec of TCL after entrainment • $HA_{SVT}-HA_{Vpace@TCL} <0$ msec • $HA_{SVT}-VA_{Vpace@TCL} <-30$ msec • $VA_{Vpace@TCL}-VA_{SVT} >85$ msec • Longest V_1-V_2 from the RVA that advances the tachycardia subtracted from the TCL >100 msec (pre-excitation index)
Effect of drugs and maneuvers on tachycardia	Drugs that change conduction through AV node often terminate tachycardia

AVNRT, atrioventricular nodal reentrant tachycardia; AH, atrio-His; AV, atrioventricular; SVT, supraventricular tachycardia; HBE, His bundle electrogram; VA_{min}, minimal measured ventriculoatrial interval; VA_{HRA}, ventriculoatrial interval measured to the high right atrium; BBB, bundle branch block; RV, right ventricular; SVT, supraventricular tachycardia; PPI, postpacing interval; TCL, tachycardia cycle length; HA_{SVT}, His-atrial interval during supraventricular tachycardia; $HA_{Vpace@TCL}$, His-atrial interval during ventricular pacing at the tachycardia cycle length; $VA_{Vpace@TCL}$, ventriculoatrial interval during ventricular pacing at the tachycardia cycle length; VA_{SVT}, ventriculoatrial interval during supraventricular tachycardia.

ATRIOVENTRICULAR REENTRANT TACHYCARDIA

Initiation

Like AVNRT, initiation of orthodromic AVRT using a fast AP is often due to an APD with associated AV delay that allows enough time to exceed the retrograde refractory period of the AP. Unlike AVNRT, the critical AV delay may be due to delay not only in the AV node (AH delay) but also in the HPS

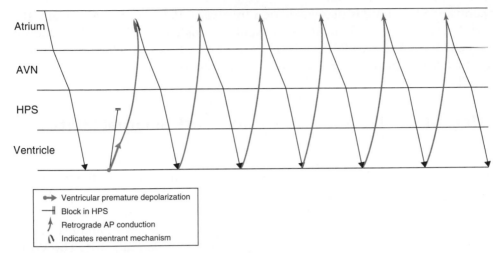

Atrium

AVN

HPS

Ventricle

➤ Ventricular premature depolarization
—⊣ Block in HPS
⌇ Retrograde AP conduction
(⅃ Indicates reentrant mechanism

FIGURE 8-12. Initiation of orthodromic atrioventricular reentrant tachycardia (AVRT) with a ventricular premature depolarization (VPD) which blocks in the His-Purkinje system (HPS) and conducts up the accessory pathway and back down the normal atrioventricular (AV) conducting system. AVN, atrioventricular node.

and ventricular myocardium. Programmed stimulation delivered near the site of the AP allows the most time for recovery of retrograde conduction.

VPDs commonly initiate AVRT (see Fig. 8-12). Unlike typical AVNRT, where delay occurs in the HPS and limits the prematurity with which the VPD can be delivered to the AV node, no such delay occurs with rapidly conducting APs. Approximately 60% of orthodromic AVRTs can be initiated with a single VPD (compared with a ~10% chance of initiating AVNRT by a VPD). Late coupled VPDs that initiate SVT are virtually diagnostic for SVT incorporating an AP. In such cases there is exclusive conduction up the AP, with block in the HPS.

Atrial Activation Sequence and Atrioventricular Relationship

Because the circuit in SVT incorporating an AP requires both the atria and ventricles, atrial activation must follow ventricular activation (unlike AVNRT). A hallmark of rapidly conducting APs is a fixed RP interval regardless of TCL, oscillations, or any PR interval change.

Although retrograde atrial activation can be assessed during right ventricular (RV) pacing or during SVT, activation is best evaluated during SVT because there may be fusion during RV pacing due to simultaneous conduction over the AP and the HPS/AVN. This is the rule with left-sided APs. Occasionally adenosine is needed to block AVN conduction. As a corollary, fusion during SVT suggests multiple APs. Eccentric atrial activation during reentrant SVT or VP is diagnostic of a free wall AP. For septal APs where the atrial activation is midline, there is usually a single breakthrough and the VA exceeds the VA in AVNRT (see Differentiating SVT Mechanisms in the subsequent text). Typically, the VA time ranges from 70 to 170 msec in concealed AVRT.

Effect of Bundle Branch Block on Ventriculoatrial Interval

The development of BBB may cause an increase in the SVT CL of a tachycardia using a free wall AP. However, diagnosis requires an increase in the measured VA interval compared with narrow-QRS conduction. An increase in VA by ≥35 msec with BBB is diagnostic of an AP on the same (ipsilateral) side as the site of BBB (or >45 msec with RVA pacing) (see Figs. 8-13 and 8-14). The VA will not change with BBB on the opposite (contralateral) side. The VA in posteroseptal APs may increase with LBBB (~10 msec) and anteroseptal APs may increase with right bundle branch block (RBBB) approximately 15 msec.

Requirement of Atria and Ventricles to Initiate and Sustain Tachycardia

In AVRT using a concealed AP, the reentrant circuit requires the atria and ventricles; therefore if AV (or VA) block occurs, then an AP-dependent tachycardia

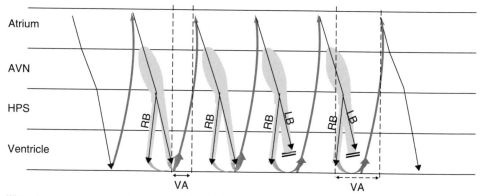

When a bundle branch block develops ipsilateral to the site of an accessory pathway (in this case a left bundle [LB] branch block in the presence of a left-sided AP) the VA interval increases with or without an increase in the tachycardia cycle length.

LB = left bundle
RB = right bundle

FIGURE 8-13. Ventriculoatrial (VA) intervals during orthodromic atrioventricular reentry tachycardia (AVRT) without and with ipsilateral bundle branch block. The VA interval prolongs with bundle branch block on the same side as the accessory pathway. AVN, atrioventricular node; HPS, His-Purkinje system.

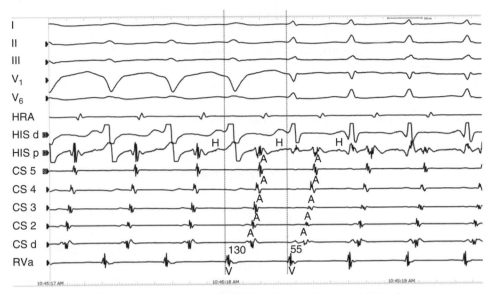

Spontaneous relief of left bundle branch block during supraventricular tachycardia with decrease in VA time from 130 to 55 msec indicating the participation of left-lateral accessory pathway in the tachycardia. Lines demonstrate onset of the surface QRS. Shown are surface leads I, II, III, V$_1$, and V$_6$ as well as electrograms from the high right atrium (HRA), His bundle (His d and His p) coronary sinus from proximal to distal (CS 5 to CS d), and right ventricular apex (RVA).

FIGURE 8-14. Left bundle branch block during orthodromic atrioventricular reentry tachycardia (AVRT) utilizing a left free wall accessory pathway.

is excluded. The failure to initiate the SVT with an APD that blocks in the AVN or HPS may be an early clue that the SVT employs an AP.

Effect of Atrial and Ventricular Stimulation during Tachycardia

The ability to alter a tachycardia is related to the proximity of the stimulation site to the circuit (see Table 8-3). Because both the atrium and ventricles are part of the tachycardia circuit, stimulating either chamber can affect the tachycardia. Programmed APDs can advance AVRT using a concealed AP with or without atrial fusion and can terminate AVRT often by producing block in the AVN or HPS.

Response to overdrive VP:

1. VP at 10 to 20 msec faster than the TCL (or single VPDs) would be expected to demonstrate a V-A-V response after cessation of pacing when the atrial activation is advanced and the SVT persists.

2. During overdrive V pacing, it is possible to see an antegrade His (i.e., fusion) proving CMT.

TABLE 8-3 Atrioventricular Reentrant Tachycardia (AVRT)

Diagnostic Criteria for Orthodromic AVRT

Initiation	Initiation dependent on a critical AV interval (dual AV nodal pathways not necessary)
Atrial activation sequence and AV relationship at onset and during SVT	Earliest retrograde atrial activity variable (VA ≥60 msec)
Effect of BBB on VA interval	Ipsilateral bundle branch block, prolongs VA by ≥35 msec
Requirement of A and V to initiate and sustain	Obligatory 1:1 AV relationship with constant VA despite TCL variations
Effect of A and V stimulation during tachycardia	• V-A-V response upon cessation of RV pacing • Longest V_1-V_2 from the RVA that advances the tachycardia subtracted from the TCL <100 msec (pre-excitation index) • VPD during His refractoriness advances atrial activation or terminates SVT without conduction to atrium
Effect of drugs and maneuvers on tachycardia	Drugs that change conduction through AV node often terminate tachycardia

AV, atrioventricular; SVT, supraventricular tachycardia; VA, ventriculoatrial; BBB, bundle branch block; TCL, tachycardia cycle length; RV, right ventricular; RVA, right ventricular apex; VPD, ventricular premature depolarization.

The responses to VPDs that demonstrate the presence of an AP include the following:

1. Capture of the atrium at the VPD coupling interval ("exact capture phenomenon")

2. Atrial capture during His refractoriness, with resetting of the SVT

3. Increase in VA time when stimulating from the contralateral ventricle

4. Delaying or terminating SVT with VPDs delivered during His refractoriness

5. A pre-excitation index, which quantifies the coupling interval of the longest RV VPD that can influence an SVT can be used to localize APs (see later section for details)

The response of slowly conducting APs to ventricular stimulation differ from fast APs. Because of decremental properties, ventricular stimulation often increases the VA interval. As stated earlier, a VPD introduced during His refractoriness that causes delay of the subsequent atrial depolarization and retards the SVT is diagnostic of participation of an AP in an SVT.

Pharmacologic and Physiologic Maneuvers

During AVRT, termination by vagal maneuvers often occurs with AVN block. Most often there is a nonconducted atrial potential which is the last echo beat. Calcium channel blockers, β-blockers, digoxin, and adenosine prolong AVN conduction and cause block in the AV node. Class IA and IC drugs exert their effect and may produce block in the AP. Class III agents prolong antegrade conduction and refractoriness of manifest APs. Infra-His block caused by a drug resulting in termination of the arrhythmia implies the necessity of the ventricles.

ATRIAL TACHYCARDIA

Initiation

Initiation of AAT is not associated with significant AV delay and typically "warms up" (progressive CL shortening as tachycardia proceeds) (see Table 8-4). Isoproterenol may be required to initiate such tachycardias.

TABLE 8-4   Atrial Tachycardia (AT)

Diagnostic Criteria for AT	
Initiation	Initiation not dependent on a critical AV interval (dual AV nodal pathways not necessary). Typically "warms up."
Atrial activation sequence and AV relationship at onset and during SVT	Earliest atrial activity variable. Initiating AV interval of tachycardia usually same as first beat of tachycardia. Varying AV and VA intervals
Effect of BBB on VA interval	No change in VA interval
Requirement of A and V to initiate and sustain	AV dissociation during SVT common
Effect of A and V stimulation during tachycardia	V-A-A-V response upon cessation of RV pacing
Effect of drugs and maneuvers on tachycardia	Drugs that change conduction through AV node may cause AV block with continuation of tachycardia

AV, atrioventricular; SVT, supraventricular tachycardia; VA, ventriculoatrial; BBB, bundle branch block; RV, right ventricular.

Programmed stimulation can initiate reentrant ATs and triggered ATs, such as those due to digitalis intoxication or catecholamines, but not AAT.

Atrial Activation Sequence and Atrioventricular Relationship

Because both AAT and triggered AT are focal, the first and subsequent atrial activation sequences (and P waves) are identical. This is in contrast to reentrant SVTs where the initiating P wave is often an APD with a different atrial activation sequence than the subsequent tachycardia. The same is true with intracardiac atrial activation. The atrial activation sequence of the initiating beat will be the same as the subsequent activation sequence during SVT (see Fig. 8-15).

Effect of Bundle Branch Block on Ventriculoatrial Interval

Because the specialized conduction system and ventricles are not required to maintain an SVT due to AT, BBB only transiently increases the RR and PR if the HV prolongs. Dual AV nodal pathways maybe present during AT and produce changes in the PR interval without affecting the RP interval.

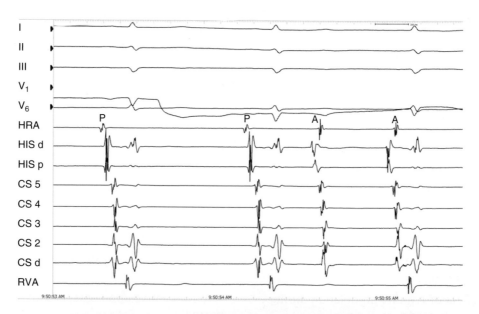

Spontaneous intiation of atrial tachycardia (A) during sinus rhythm (S). The atrial activation sequence of the initiating beat is the same as subsequent activation sequence.

FIGURE 8-15. Initiation of atrial tachycardia. HRA, high right atrium; HIS, His bundle; CS, coronary sinus; RVA, right ventricular apex.

Requirement of Atria and Ventricles to Initiate and Sustain Tachycardia

As mentioned, the specialized conduction system and ventricles are not required for maintenance of AATs. The presence of varying AV and VA intervals as well as AV block during an SVT is highly suggestive of AT. Furthermore, AT will continue following the development of block in the AV node.

Effect of Atrial and Ventricular Stimulation during Tachycardia

Because ATs do not depend on conduction from the atria to the ventricles, these SVTs are not generally influenced by VPDs. This property can be exploited during SVT by rapid VP. If the ventricles can be dissociated from the atria during ongoing tachycardia then a diagnosis can be made. If retrograde conduction occurs, a V-A-A-V response results following cessation of pacing if the AT continues. Occasionally, triggered AT may be terminated by VP with VA conduction.

Like other automatic tissues (e.g., the sinus node), long coupled APDs will not affect the focus and compensatory pauses will occur. Burst atrial pacing may produce overdrive suppression of the focus. Overdrive acceleration and shortening of the interval to the first beat of the tachycardia after overdrive atrial pacing are characteristic of a triggered mechanism, and may be useful to make a diagnosis of a triggered AT.

Rapid overdrive atrial pacing from different sites in the atria and observation of the delay between cessation of pacing and resumption of tachycardia may provide evidence for the location of the tachycardia. Pacing from the right atrium will result in a short return CL from right ATs and a longer return CL from left ATs, whereas left atrial pacing will produce an opposite response. This technique may be used to achieve a rough localization of a tachycardia early in a study although it has significant limitations involving differing degrees of tachycardia suppression and possible entrainment of macroreentrant tachycardias.

Pharmacologic and Physiologic Maneuvers

Vagal maneuvers may produce AV block but do not generally affect the AT (although transient slowing is possible). However, vagal maneuvers, adenosine, β-blockers, and calcium channel blockers can terminate ATs due to a triggered or reentrant mechanism. Incessant tachycardias respond poorly to antiarrhythmic therapy, although β-blockers may be useful in occasional cases to slow or terminate the tachycardia.

Tachycardias that terminate with a P wave favor a mechanism other than AT because the probability that the last beat of an AT will also fortuitously block before reaching the ventricles is unlikely.

DISTINGUISHING NARROW-COMPLEX, REGULAR TACHYCARDIAS WITH PACING MANEUVERS

Determining the tachycardia mechanism can sometimes prove difficult because there is overlap in the ECG and intracardiac EGM manifestations of AVNRT, AVRT, and AT. Various pacing maneuvers can be used to make a diagnosis (see Table 8-5).

TABLE 8-5 Distinguishing Narrow-Complex, Regular Tachycardias with Pacing Maneuvers

Septal Accessory Pathway versus AVNRT

Maneuver	Septal Accessory Pathway	AVNRT
VPD during His refractoriness	Advances atrial activation	No advancement of atrial activation
	Terminates SVT without conduction to atrium	
PPI–TCL after ventricular pacing	<115 msec	>115 msec
$VA_{Vpace@TCL} - VA_{SVT}$	<85 msec	>85 msec
Retrograde VA conduction	Nondecremental	Decremental
Atrial or ventricular pacing at TCL	Obligate 1:1 conduction	Wenckebach may occur
VA dissociation during SVT	Incompatible	Possible
VA interval in SVT	Often >60 msec	Often <60 msec
HA interval in SVT	Fixed	May vary
Basal vs. apical ventricular pacing	VA shorter with basal pacing	VA shorter with apical pacing
Para-Hisian Pacing	No change in stimulus-A with loss of His capture	Increased stimulus-A with loss of His capture

AVNRT, atrioventricular nodal reentrant tachycardia; VA, ventriculoatrial; VPD, ventricular premature depolarization; SVT, supraventricular tachycardia; PPI, postpacing interval; TCL, tachycardia cycle length; $VA_{Vpace@TCL}$, ventriculoatrial interval during ventricular pacing at the tachycardia cycle length; VA_{SVT}, ventriculoatrial interval during supraventricular tachycardia.

Response to Ventricular Pacing

Ventricular Premature Depolarizations

When the HPS is refractory that depolarizes the atrium with the same activation sequence as during the SVT indicates the presence of an AP.

Termination of SVT with a His-refractory pulmonary vascular congestion (PVC) without depolarization of the atria is proof of AVRT.

Pre-excitation index. This is based on the concept that the further a pacing impulse is from the anatomic tachycardia circuit it is trying to excite, the more premature it must be delivered to enter the retrograde limb of the circuit and preexcite the atria. It is determined by the following:

Tachycardia CL—longest-coupled VPD that preexcites the atrium

A coupling interval >90% of the TCL from the RVA indicates a right-sided or septal AP (with AVNRT it is >100 msec)

Anteroseptal or posteroseptal AP <45 msec

Because VPDs are usually delivered from the RVA, there may be considerable distance to a left free wall AP and therefore there is overlap in the values derived for AVNRT and left free wall APs.

Rapid VP (with capture of the atrium with *concentric* retrograde activation):

V-A-V response → PPI – TCL ⟶ ≥115 msec = AVNRT

↘ <115 msec = AVRT

V-A-A-V response → AT or "pseudo" V-A-A-V (see Fig. 8-16)

Exceptions and limitations to overdrive VP for discrimination of AT from AVNRT or AVRT include the following:

It can only be assessed if VA conduction occurs at a shorter CL than the tachycardia (i.e., without terminating it)

If 2:1 AV block during AVNRT occurs at the end of the entrainment

AT in patients with dual AV nodal physiology or concealed AT in which VP initiates a second arrhythmia (e.g., AVNRT)

AT coincident with AVNRT

"Pseudo V-A-A-V response" in atypical AVNRT or slowly conducting AP

1:2 response to the last paced beat (retrograde conduction up both the FP and SP)

His-Atrial and Ventriculoatrial Intervals

VA intervals are longer in AP-mediated tachycardias compared with AVNRT because the AVRT circuit involves both the ventricle and the atrium and these chambers are activated sequentially.

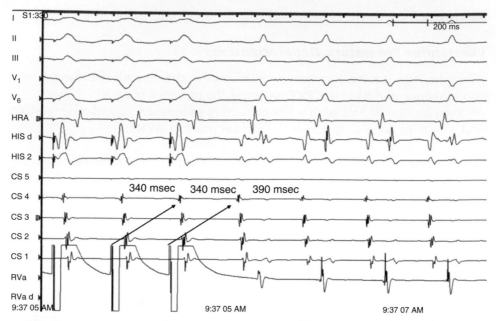

FIGURE 8-16. Example of a pseudo V-A-A-V during atypical atrioventricular nodal reentrant tachycardia (AVNRT). Ventricular pacing is demonstrated at 340 msec with conduction up a slow atrioventricular (AV) nodal pathway. The two atrial electrograms occur at the same rate as the preceding pacing rate (340 msec) indicating that they were produced by the ventricular pacing up a slowly conducting retrograde route (slow pathways) rather than atrial tachycardia. HRA, high right atrium; HIS, His bundle; CS, coronary sinus; RVA, right ventricular apex.

AVNRT: VA_{min}(V to earliest atrial electrogram) = -40 to $+75$

$$VA_{\text{high right atrium}} = <90 \text{ msec}$$

AVRT: 70 and 170 msec on average.

During VP, H and A are activated in series in AVNRT and in parallel in AVRT. During SVT, the H and A are activated in parallel in AVNRT but are activated in series in AVRT. Other measurements that can be used to discriminate AVNRT from AVRT include:

HA_{SVT}–$HA_{\text{ventricular pacing}} <+10$ msec

HA_{SVT}–$VA_{\text{ventricular pacing}} <-30$ msec   all suggest AVNRT

$VA_{\text{ventricular pacing}} - VA_{SVT} >+85$ msec

Differential Pacing

Basal right ventricular versus right ventricular Apical Pacing

In an SVT that relies exclusively on the specialized conduction system, the septal VA time would be expected to be longer with RV basal pacing compared with pacing at the RVA. This is because the time from impulse delivery until the time the HPS is engaged is longer at basal sites.

Para-Hisian Pacing

When pacing at a low current near the His bundle only the local myocardium would be expected to be stimulated (as evidenced by a wide QRS on ECG). The impulse would then have to propagate apically to the HPS before retrogradely activating the atria. If a septal AP were present the VA would be short. When pacing with higher current, the His bundle will be stimulated directly (as evidenced by a narrower QRS on ECG) and the impulse will conduct retrogradely from the His and the VA will be shorter. Several caveats to para-Hisian pacing have been stipulated for its results to be valid. These include the necessity of capturing the His bundle and local ventricular myocardium together (as opposed to the His bundle alone), the necessity of observing the same atrial activation sequence during capture at both current levels, and avoidance of direct atrial capture.

Atrial Premature Depolarizations

Although rare in adults, junctional tachycardia must sometimes be differentiated from AVNRT, both of which have similar ECG and intracardiac EGM appearances.

Scanning diastole with APDs can be used to clarify the mechanism. When the APD engages the HPS the AH should be measured. In AVNRT, the APD would have to enter the anterograde limb of the tachycardia circuit (i.e., the AV nodal SP) and would be expected to conduct to the His with an AH that is similar to or longer than the AH during SVT. In junctional tachycardia, both AV nodal pathways would be expected to be available for antegrade conduction and the resultant AH would be much shorter (if similar to the AH of the FP). A theoretic concern would be a 1:2 response in the AV node where the APD would conduct antegradely over the FP and then the SP both stopping and then reinitiating AVNRT.

TREATMENT

The most recent American College of Cardiology/American Heart Association/European Society of Cardiology guidelines give a class I recommendation to catheter ablation of AVNRT even after a single episode in patients who desire complete control of arrhythmia. These guidelines also give a class I recommendation to catheter ablation of symptomatic AVRT and a class IIa recommendation to ablation for single or infrequent episodes in patients who desire complete control of arrhythmia.

Ablation of Atrioventricular Nodal Reentrant Tachycardia

Ablation of the "SP" is directed anatomically at fibers between the tricuspid annulus and anterior lip of the CS. The initial ablation target is slightly superior to the ostium of the CS at the tricuspid annulus.

When positioning the ablation catheter (typically a 4- to 5-mm tip), attention should be paid to the A:V ratio, which should be approximately 1:3 with the atrial EGM having a multicomponent shape. The local A should be inscribed well after the A in the His bundle electrogram (HBE). To avoid complete AV block, the interval from atrial signal recorded on the HBE should be >20 msec later than the atrial signal on the ABL catheter (<20 msec is predictive of AV block) (see Fig. 8-17).

During effective ablation, junctional rhythm with 1:1 atrial conduction is frequently seen in the absence of SVT, rapid atrial pacing (>600 msec), or sinus tachycardia. The presence of AV or VA block should prompt immediate cessation of ablation and withdrawal of the ablation catheter. If junctional rhythm is absent after 10 to 15 seconds of ablation, radiofrequency delivery should be discontinued and a new spot chosen. Generally, target temperatures are 55°C to 60°C. Catheter position should be continuously monitored. After each ablation attempt, repeat stimulation should be performed. Success rate is generally >95% acutely with a 2% long-term recurrence rate.

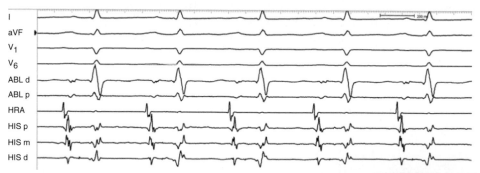

Ablation site for slow pathway. Note the fractionated appearance of the atrial signal on the distal pole of the ablation catheter (ABLD) and the timing of the atrial depolarization on ABLD relative to that on the His bundle cathwters (HBE) shown proximal (p), middle (m), and distal (d). Shown also are surface leads I, aVF, V₁, and V₆ as well as electrograms from the high right atrium (HRA).

FIGURE 8-17. Slow pathway ablation site for atrioventricular nodal reentrant tachycardia (AVNRT).

The principal endpoint for AVNRT ablation is noninducibility of the tachycardia even after isoproterenol and atropine. Ideally there should also be an increase in the AV Wenckebach cycle, no evidence of "SP" conduction, an increase in the AVN effective refractory period, no change (from baseline) of the AH during sinus rhythm, and maintenance of VA conduction. The persistence of an SP or even single echo beats (particularly, in a zone <30 msec) are also acceptable endpoint.

Although rare (~1%), the most important potential complication of SP ablation is inducing AV block necessitating pacemaker implantation. Other potential complications include cardiac tamponade, groin hematoma, and deep vein thrombosis.

Ablation of Concealed Posteroseptal Accessory Pathways

Although details about ablation are beyond the scope of this chapter, a few notes about posteroseptal APs are relevant. A major technical consideration is the decision to limit ablation to the right heart or to proceed with left heart mapping (through a transseptal or a retrograde aortic approach). Features that suggest ablation success from the right atrial approach include a difference in VA from the His and the VA at the earliest CS <25 msec, and a long RP tachycardia. Features that suggest the need for left atrial mapping include earliest retrograde atrial activity during SVT in the mid CS (>1.5 cm from CS ostium), a difference in VA time in His to VA in the earliest CS >25 msec, an increase in VA by 10 to 30 msec with LBBB, and R > S in V_1. Tachycardia features that suggest an epicardial AP may be present and include the presence of a CS diverticulum by venography, a negative delta wave in II, a steep positive delta wave in aVR, and a deep S wave in V_6.

Treatment of Atrial Tachycardia

Nonsustained or paroxysmal ATs are often asymptomatic and do not require treatment. Incessant tachycardias are more often symptomatic and may result in tachycardia-mediated cardiomyopathy. For this reason, patients who present with AT and cardiomyopathy of unclear etiology should be treated aggressively to suppress or cure the tachycardia and allow the cardiomyopathy to resolve. ATs due to automatic or triggered mechanisms are often unresponsive to medications and are best treated with ablation. Conversely, microreentrant ATs frequently respond well to β-blockers or calcium channel blockers. In general, it is reasonable to attempt a trial of β-blocker or calcium channel blocker as the first line of therapy. Antiarrhythmic drugs including sodium channel and potassium channel blockers are also quite effective for suppressing ATs.

If medications are unsuccessful or not tolerated electrophysiologic study with mapping and ablation is highly successful for AT and increasingly chosen as a first-line strategy. The site of origin of the tachycardia can be localized with a reasonable degree of certainty from the surface ECG as already described. Activation mapping can further identify the earliest site of activation and ablation is performed at that site. In general, successful sites of ablation are >20 msec earlier than the surface P wave.

Advanced mapping systems allow further characterization of arrhythmia mechanisms through mapping of the chamber of origin. Activation mapping allows the establishment of the earliest to latest points of arrhythmia activation. If the earliest point meets the latest in a large circuit involving the entire atrium, the diagnosis is a macroreentrant rhythm such as atrial flutter. If the rhythm emanates from a point in the atrium with the latest point distant from the earliest point, the diagnosis is consistent with a focal AT. The earliest mapped site of activation is the origin of the tachycardia.

Complications related to ablation of ATs usually develop from damage to structures in proximity to the site of ablation (e.g., sinus node damage or phrenic nerve paralysis when ablation tachycardias at the top of the crista terminalis, AV block with para-Hisian tachycardias, etc.).

SELECTED BIBLIOGRAPHY

Blomstrom-Lundqvist C, Scheinman MM, Aliot EM, et al. ACC/AHA/ESC guidelines for the management of patients with supraventricular arrhythmias – executive summary. *J Am Coll Cardiol*. 2003;42(8):1493–1531.

Field ME, Miyazaki H, Epstein LM, et al. Narrow complex tachycardia after slow pathway ablation: Continue ablating? *J Cardiovasc Electrophysiol*. 2006;17:557–559.

Frisch D, Zimetbaum P. *Vagal maneuvers in uptodate*, 2008.

Josephson ME. *Clinical cardiac electrophysiology*, 4th ed. Philadelphia: Lippincott Williams & Wilkins; 2008.

Josephson ME, Wellens HJJ. Differential diagnosis of supraventricular tachycardia. *Cardiol Clin*. 1990;8(3).

Katritsis DG, Ellenbogen KA, Becker AE. Atrial activation during atrioventricular nodal reentrant tachycardia: Studies on retrograde fast pathway conduction. *Heart Rythm*. 2006;3:993–1000.

Kistler PM, Robert-Thomson KC, Haqqani HM, et al. P-Wave morphology in focal atrial tachycardia. *J Am Coll Cardiol*. 2006;48:1010–1017.

Kistler PM, Sanders P, Fynn SP, et al. Electrophysiological and electrocardiographic characteristics of focal atrial tachycardia originating from the pulmonary veins. *Circulation*. 2003;108:1968–1975.

Kwaku KF, Josephson ME. Typical AVNRT – an update on mechanisms and therapy. *Card Electrophysiol Rev*. 2002;6:414–421.

Michaud GF, Tada H, Chough S, et al. Differentiation of atypical atrioventricular node re-entrant tachycardia from orthodromic reciprocating tachycardia using a septal accessory pathway by the response to ventricular pacing. *J Am Coll Cardiol.* 2001;38:1163–1167.

Miles WM, Yee R, Klein GJ, et al. The preexcitation index: An aid in determining the mechanism of supraventricular tachycardia and localizing accessory pathways. *Circluation.* 1986;74(3):493–500.

Orejarena LA. Paroxysmal supraventricular tachycardia in the general population. *J Am Coll Cardiol.* 1998;31:150–157.

Roberts-Thompson KC, Kistler PM, Kalman JM. Atrial tachycardia: mechanisms, diagnosis, and management. *Curr Probl Cardiol.* 2005;30:529–573.

Wolff-Parkinson-White Syndrome and Variants

Ventricular preexcitation occurs in 0.1 to 3.1 out of 1,000 people, and is defined as activation of the ventricular myocardium by an atrial impulse earlier than would be expected with normal atrioventricular (AV) conduction. A delta wave is often seen on the surface electrocardiogram (ECG), which represents activation of the ventricle by an "accessory" pathway (AP) before activation by the conducting system (see Fig. 9-1). Wolff-Parkinson-White (WPW) syndrome is defined as an AP-mediated tachycardia occurring in patients with ventricular preexcitation on a 12-lead ECG.

APs occur when there is an incomplete segmentation of the embryologic cardiac tube and formation of the fibrotic AV ring during fetal cardiac development. The most common type of pathway is AV, formed by myocardial tissue connecting the atrium and ventricle, and most pathways are epicardial. AV pathways may be "manifest," which means that they conduct antegradely from the atrium to the ventricle and result in preexcitation which can be seen on the surface ECG, or "inapparent," which means that preexcitation is not seen on the surface ECG, or concealed because normal AV conduction activates the ventricle faster than the AP or because the AP does not conduct in an antegrade manner. These latter APs conduct only "retrograde" from the ventricle to the atrium, and are clinically relevant only when they participate in a tachycardia. In fact a minority of APs only conduct in the antegrade manner (preexcitation) whereas the majority conduct in a retrograde direction. Pathways exhibiting antegrade conduction do so in an "all or none" manner

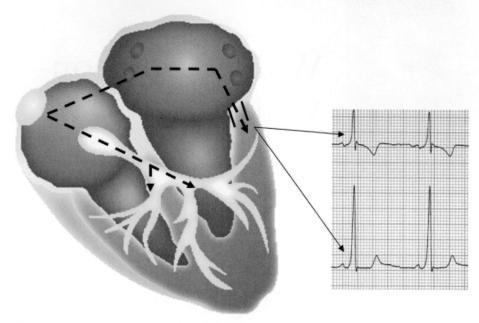

FIGURE 9-1. Diagram of antegrade conduction over both the normal atrioventricular (AV) conducting system and a left-sided accessory pathway. The amount of conduction over the accessory pathway corresponds to the degree of ventricular preexcitation or delta wave. (See color insert.)

99% of the time. Approximately 1% of antegradely conducting AV pathways exhibit decremental conduction, the vast majority of which are right sided.

APs can be located anywhere around the A-V ring except at the portion of the aortomitral continuity where there is no ventricular myocardium below the atrium. They are often slanted, with the ventricular insertion point located closer to the septum and the atrial insertion more lateral in inferior APs and the ventricular insertion site lateral and atrial insertion site septal in anterior and posterior APs. Less common variants of typical AV APs are atriofascicular, nodofascicular, nodoventricular, and fasciculoventricular pathways, representing AP conduction between combinations of the atrium, AV node, conducting system, and ventricle. These variants are quite rare, but all except fasciculoventricular pathways may participate in tachycardias.

CLINICAL EVALUATION

The first step in evaluating a patient who presents with preexcitation on an ECG is to take a thorough clinical history. The presence of symptoms associated with preexcitation often determines the course of the clinical evaluation. Symptoms may include sustained palpitations or syncope. A history of syncope must be taken carefully to differentiate neurocardiogenic or vasovagal syncope from

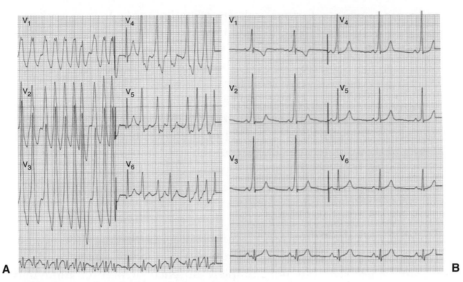

FIGURE 9-2. Precordial leads V_1-V_6 and a rhythm strip of lead 2 are shown for a patient with preexcitation through a left-sided accessory pathway. **A:** During atrial fibrillation (AF), overt preexcitation is seen with R-R intervals as short as 200 msec are seen, which may provoke hemodynamic instability and cardiac arrest. **B:** After restoration of sinus rhythm, the same preexcitation pattern seen during AF can be seen on the electrocardiogram (ECG).

syncope related to an AP-mediated tachycardia (see Chapter 12). Syncope due to an AP will often be preceded by palpitations and may even require urgent cardioversion or defibrillation if rapidly conducted atrial fibrillation (AF) is present (see Fig. 9-2). Many patients will never have symptoms related to an AP, and the management of these patients is controversial (see discussion in the subsequent text). A family history of preexcitation or sudden cardiac death is important, as a familial association has been described. In addition, the presence of congenital heart disease should be ascertained. Ebstein anomaly is associated with right-sided APs, and when present the APs are often multiple and slowly conducting. Ebstein anomaly may be seen in "corrected" or L-type transposition of the great arteries in which the tricuspid valve (TV) is the left AV valve.

Asymptomatic Patients

The evaluation of patients presenting without identifiable symptoms or history of syncope and preexcitation on an ECG is controversial. The two risks to such patients are the development of an AP-mediated supraventricular tachycardia (SVT) and the occurrence of AF with rapid conduction over the AP leading to ventricular fibrillation and/or cardiovascular collapse. The incidence of the latter is extremely low (<0.02% per year), and while the magnitude of this outcome warrants further risk stratification, this low risk should be stressed to the patient. The first step in risk stratification is noninvasive determination of the ability of the AP to conduct impulses rapidly from the atrium to the ventricle. If an AP is unable to conduct rapidly from the atrium to the ventricle, the risk of extremely rapid ventricular rates and ventricular fibrillation resulting from preexcited AF is low.

It should be noted that APs have properties similar to myocardium (see subsequent text), and that in a setting of high adrenergic tone their ability to conduct rapidly increases. Therefore, the first step in noninvasive testing is often exercise treadmill testing because it induces a rapid heart rate in a setting of high adrenergic tone. If preexcitation is noted to disappear suddenly during exercise testing, the AP refractory period is likely long, and therefore it should be unable to conduct rapidly to the ventricle during AF. Care must be taken in reviewing the ECGs during stress testing; however, as the heightened adrenergic tone also increases AV conduction down the normal conduction system, and a *decrease* but not complete absence of preexcitation may be observed. The abrupt loss of the delta wave must be recognized to confirm that the refractory period of the AP is reached during routine exercise and is therefore unlikely to ever conduct AF at a potentially lethal rate.

Another noninvasive test that may be used to risk-stratify patients with asymptomatic preexcitation is a 24-hour Holter monitor. If preexcitation is noted to be intermittent on ambulatory monitoring, the AP refractory period is probably long and it is unlikely to be able to sustain rapid conduction during AF. Intravenous (IV) administration of procainamide (10 mg per kg over 5 minutes) has been used in the past to risk-stratify patients—disappearance of preexcitation with drug administration is associated with longer AP refractory periods. However, this test is rarely used in current clinical practice. The downside of these two tests is that neither evaluates the function of the AP in the setting of high catecholamines, and therefore may underestimate the capacity of an AP to conduct rapidly.

Patients who do not exhibit low-risk characteristics on noninvasive evaluation as described earlier may be offered invasive electrophysiologic testing. A frank discussion about the low risk of sudden death in patients with asymptomatic preexcitation and the comparably low risks of electrophysiology study is warranted at this point in the clinical evaluation. Factors that often determine whether invasive evaluation is pursued include high-risk occupations such as commercial drivers and pilots and, more commonly, patient preference. Some authors argue that patients who are asymptomatic and in the age-group of 35 to 40 years represent a low-risk group and do not warrant electrophysiologic (EP) testing, but because AF may develop later in life and is the presenting arrhythmia in up to 20% of patients presenting with WPW syndrome, this recommendation may not be justified. However, in the authors' experience, they have not seen sudden death in this older age-group with preexcited AF, suggesting that the AP does not conduct at a rate conducive to the development of ventricular arrhythmia in this population. It should also be noted that these same authors discount the utility of noninvasive testing and recommend EP testing in all patients with asymptomatic preexcitation who are younger than 35 years. The goals of EP testing are to evaluate the refractory period of the AP and to assess for inducible AP-mediated tachyarrhythmias. Specific methods are discussed in subsequent text.

Symptomatic Patients

Patients presenting with symptomatic palpitations or syncope suggestive of a cardiac origin and preexcitation on an ECG should be offered an electrophysiology study for further characterization and often ablation of the AP (see subsequent text). This strategy is cost-effective and may allow a patient to avoid long-term medical therapy. For patients who do not wish to undergo invasive testing, drug therapy can be employed as a secondary approach. For patients with overt preexcitation, calcium channel blockers and digoxin should be avoided. Digoxin may shorten the refractory period of the AP, thereby allowing more rapid ventricular activation during AF and increasing the risk of ventricular fibrillation. Calcium channel blockers do not affect the refractory period of the AP in the baseline state, but have been shown to allow more rapid ventricular activation during AF when given intravenously, probably due to an increase in sympathetic tone secondary to hypotension induced by the medication or decreased retrograde concealment in the AP resulting from AV nodal slowing. The use of β-blocker is controversial, as these agents either do not affect or may even prolong AP refractoriness and slow the ventricular response in most patients with preexcited AF, but isolated reports of increased ventricular rates after their administration suggest that caution should be exercised in their use. Class IA and IC agents or amiodarone are the most effective at blocking conduction in the AP and preventing recurrences of documented tachycardia. Given the potential toxicities and proarrhythmic effects of these medications, symptomatic patients should be encouraged to undergo definitive treatment with ablation of the AP. Patients with tachycardia utilizing a concealed AP may be treated with β-blockers, calcium channel blockers, or digitalis. These medications slow conduction in the AV node and may suppress AV reentry. Figure 9-3 presents an algorithm for managing patients with known or suspected preexcitation who present with a tachycardia.

Electrocardiographic Interpretation

Evaluation of the 12-lead ECG of a patient with suspected preexcitation can provide significant information about the AP location. Algorithms have been proposed for the localization of APs, but none are >90% accurate and all have limitations. When interpreting a preexcited ECG, the duration of the PR interval and the vector of the delta wave are examined. In general, preexcitation caused by right-sided APs result in a shorter PR interval due to proximity to the

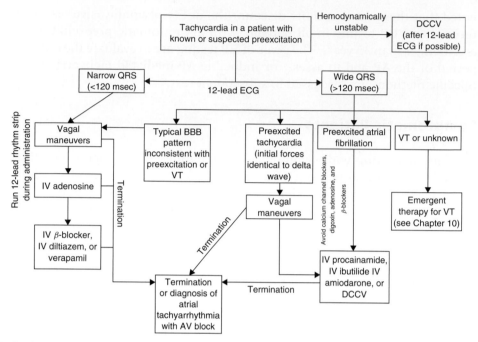

FIGURE 9-3. An algorithm for the management of tachycardia in a patient with known or suspected preexcitation. DCCV, direct current cardioversion; ECG, electrocardiogram; BBB, bundle branch block; VT, ventricular tachycardia; IV, intravenous; AV, atrioventricular.

sinus node, with the terminal portion of the P wave often interrupted by the onset of the delta wave (see Fig. 9-4). APs excite the ventricular myocardium from the site of insertion at the base of the ventricle and activation spreads from this point. Therefore, the vector of the delta wave is determined by the site of ventricular insertion. As an example, a posterior (previously described as left lateral, see subsequent text) AP activates the posterior and lateral portion of the ventricle first and activation spreads anteriorly and to the right, resulting in a rightward axis of the delta wave and positive delta wave in the precordial leads (see Fig. 9-5).

The traditional nomenclature describing APs was developed in the pathologic and surgical literature, and did not accurately locate the pathways as the heart sits in the chest cavity. Revised nomenclature has been developed which more accurately reflects the anatomic location of APs around the AV ring. Figure 9-6 depicts the location of APs using the revised nomenclature along with traditional designations. A synthesis of algorithms for localization of APs is presented in this figure, which can only be used as a general guide for localization. Factors which may affect ECG interpretation are multiple bypass tracts, rapid AV nodal conduction, intra-atrial conduction defects, hypertrophy, congenital heart disease, and prior myocardial infarction. More

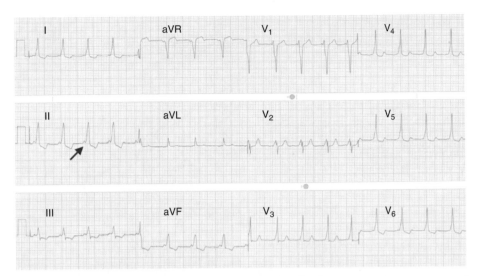

FIGURE 9-4. A 12-lead electrocardiogram (ECG) demonstrating an anterior (right free wall) accessory pathway is shown. Note the left inferior axis of the delta wave and the short PR interval. The delta wave interrupts the P wave (*arrow*), characteristic of right-sided accessory pathways.

accurate localization and characterization of APs requires an electrophysiologic study.

Fully preexcited tachycardias often present a diagnostic dilemma, as it may be difficult to differentiate the ECG from ventricular tachycardia (VT). Algorithms have been developed in an attempt to differentiate a preexcited tachycardia from VT. Absence of initial RS complexes across the precordium and other factors have been cited as morphologic criteria for VT (see Chapter 10). This criterion is useful, as negative initial forces suggest

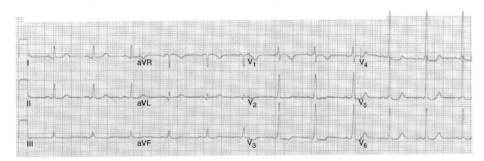

FIGURE 9-5. A 12-lead electrocardiogram (ECG) demonstrating a posterior (left free wall) accessory pathway is shown. Note the longer PR interval and vector of the delta wave consistent with the posterior location of the accessory pathway. There is a lesser degree of preexcitation due to the relative distance from the sinus node, which allows a greater degree of activation through the native conduction system.

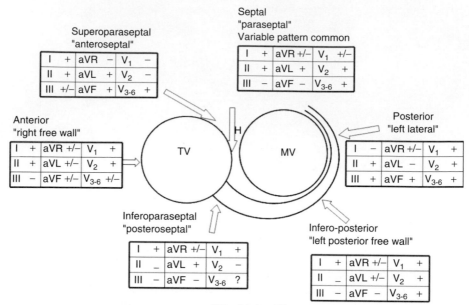

Superoparaseptal
"anteroseptal"

I	+	aVR	−	V$_1$	−
II	+	aVL	+	V$_2$	−
III	+/−	aVF	+	V$_{3-6}$	+

Septal
"paraseptal"
Variable pattern common

I	+	aVR	+/−	V$_1$	+/−
II	+	aVL	+	V$_2$	+
III	−	aVF	−	V$_{3-6}$	+

Anterior
"right free wall"

I	+	aVR	+/−	V$_1$	+
II	+	aVL	+/−	V$_2$	+
III	−	aVF	+/−	V$_{3-6}$	+/−

Posterior
"left lateral"

I	−	aVR	+/−	V$_1$	+
II	+	aVL	−	V$_2$	+
III	+	aVF	+	V$_{3-6}$	+

Inferoparaseptal
"posteroseptal"

I	+	aVR	+/−	V$_1$	+
II	−	aVL	+	V$_2$	−
III	−	aVF	−	V$_{3-6}$	?

Infero-posterior
"left posterior free wall"

I	+	aVR	+/−	V$_1$	+
II	−	aVL	+/−	V$_2$	+
III	−	aVF	−	V$_{3-6}$	+

TV   H   MV

R/S <1 in lead V$_1$
Left- sided: more negative in lead II, positive or isoelectric V$_1$
Right- sided: more negative in lead III, negative or isoelectric in
V$_1$ with abrupt transition in V$_2$

FIGURE 9-6. A schematic for localizing an accessory pathway (AP) from the surface electrocardiogram (ECG) is shown. The triscuspid valve (TV) and mitral valve (MV) annuli and the His bundle (H) are shown from a left anterior oblique view. The coronary sinus is depicted below the MV. The revised nomenclature for each AP location is given along with the traditional nomenclature in italics. The expected morphology of the delta wave in each surface lead is shown in the table associated with each location. A "+" sign indicated a positive delta wave deflection and "−" indicated a negative deflection. Note that the surface vector of the delta wave can be variable for many AP locations, and the "+/−" designation reflects that a positive, isoelectric, or negative delta wave may be seen in that lead.

an apical origin of the tachycardia which is incompatible with preexcitation. However, a fully preexcited ECG cannot be definitively distinguished from VT because ventricular activation in both tachycardias originates in the ventricular myocardium rather than using the native conducting system.

ELECTROPHYSIOLOGIC STUDY

The goals of an electrophysiologic study of a patient with preexcitation are to confirm the diagnosis of preexcitation, determine the location and the conduction properties of the AP, and evaluate any tachycardias which may involve the AP.

Characterizing the Accessory Pathway

The electrophysiologic properties of APs differ significantly from the AV node. APs generally conduct in an all-or-none manner, with stable conduction time at progressively shorter coupling intervals until sudden block is observed. This is consistent with the histologic finding that APs tend to resemble myocardium more than specialized conduction tissue. APs usually respond to administration of catecholamines (e.g., isoproterenol) with a decrease in refractory period. There are exceptions to this feature of APs, as rare right-sided AV APs may exhibit decremental conduction as well as preexcitation variants such as atriofascicular (Mahaim), nodofascicular, or nodoventricular APs. In addition, intermittent conduction over an AP may be observed, which usually suggests a long AP refractory period.

An initial step in the electrophysiologic study is to slow conduction down the AV node to maximize the portion of the ventricle activated by the AP. Carotid sinus massage or adenosine may be used to slow conduction down the AV node, although caution must be taken when administering adenosine, as it may induce AF resulting in a rapid ventricular response. During an intracardiac catheter study, introduction of premature atrial depolarizations or rapid atrial pacing may be used to prolong conduction down the AV node and maximize preexcitation. Pacing the atrium close to the suspected site of the AP is an important tool for localizing the atrial insertion site of the AP. Activation of the atrium close to the AP will cause a greater amount of ventricular myocardium to be activated by the AP rather than the conducting system. A hallmark of preexcitation is demonstration of an apparent short conduction time from the His bundle to ventricle. In sinus rhythm, the HV interval is generally short (shorter than normal, i.e., <30 msec) and may even be negative. Care must be taken to measure ventricular activation from the earliest deflection seen on the surface ECG or intracardiac recordings.

Localization of the atrial insertion of an AP may also be achieved by pacing the ventricle and noting the earliest recorded atrial electrogram. An estimate of the earliest site of atrial activation can be obtained from a standard decapolar catheter placed in the coronary sinus (CS) and a multipolar or halo catheter placed around the tricuspid annulus. More precise localization of the atrial insertion requires manipulation of a deflectable tip catheter in the right and/or left atrium. Mapping may be performed during ventricular pacing or, preferably, during orthodromic atrioventricular reentrant tachycardia (AVRT) (if inducible), because simultaneous conduction over the AV node during ventricular pacing may be confusing. It should be stressed that the shortest local V-A interval recorded does not always coincide with the site of earliest atrial activation due to the presence of slanted APs, as described in the preceding text. For APs near the septum, differentiation of the atrial insertion of the AP from retrograde conduction up the AV node may at times be difficult if localization is performed during ventricular pacing. Application of ventricular extrastimuli can demonstrate conduction up the AP and simultaneous block in the AV node. Mapping during this maneuver will then allow differentiation of ventriculoatrial (VA) conduction up the AP. Another method for determining the presence of an AP is pacing the ventricle from both the apex and the base. Pacing from the base of the right ventricle, closer to the ventricular insertion of the AP, will result in a shorter VA interval and earlier atrial activation in patients with an AP. This may allow differentiation of the atrial insertion of the AP from the AV node in patients with septal and anteroseptal APs.

Determination of the refractory period of antegrade conduction over an AP may help stratify a patient's risk for extremely rapid AV conduction during AF. Patients with long refractory periods are thought to be at low risk of sudden death due to a rapid preexcited atrial arrhythmia, whereas patients with refractory periods <220 msec, multiple APs, and septal APs may be at somewhat higher risk. As noted earlier, it must be stressed that the overall risk of sudden death in a patient with preexcitation is extremely low.

Patients with intermittent preexcitation are at low risk for rapid AV conduction over the AP, as this is usually a marker of longer refractory periods. Administration of procainamide, ibutilide, or amiodarone may produce block in the AP, which has been considered to be a marker for a longer AP refractory period and thereby lower risk for sudden death. This response can be reversed by catecholamines and as such is less helpful than other noninvasive tests. Direct determination of the refractory period of the AP using atrial extrastimuli is a more effective method once a patient has been committed to an electrophysiologic study. Owing to the catecholamine-sensitive nature of most APs, isoproterenol is routinely administered after assessment of the properties of the AP in the baseline state. After enough isoproterenol has been administered (the IV drip is titrated to a dose high enough to increase the sinus rate to >100 or be limited by hypotension), the AP is again assessed using atrial extrastimuli administered in decremental manner until refractoriness is reached. In addition, burst pacing is performed to evaluate the fastest rate at which an AP will conduct. Some advocate purposeful induction of AF using extremely fast atrial stimulation to assess the shortest conducted R-R interval to determine a patient's risk for developing ventricular fibrillation in the setting of AF. This technique often does not add much additional information to a diagnostic electrophysiologic study, however, and may add risk by necessitating anesthesia for direct-current cardioversion if the AF does not spontaneously terminate.

Fasciculoventricular pathways represent the rarest form of ventricular preexcitation. In this variant, conduction occurs in a normal fashion through the AV node and His bundle. The ventricle is then preexcited via a pathway from a fascicle to the ventricular tissue. These pathways do not participate in tachyarrhythmias. These pathways are easily identified with atrial pacing which will prolong the PR interval (and AH interval) due to AV nodal delay but not change the degree of preexcitation (because the pathway begins distal to the AV node)

Induction and Evaluation of Tachycardia

In patients who have had palpitations or in whom there is a suspicion for an AP-mediated tachycardia, programmed electrical stimulation is performed in an attempt to induce a tachycardia. Both ventricular and atrial extrastimuli can induce orthodromic tachycardia and both pacing maneuvers should be performed. In particular, atrial stimulation near the site of the AP is often successful in inducing a tachycardia. A premature atrial depolarization administered near the AP site can block in the AP and conduct down the AV node to the ventricle and then back up the AP, which is no longer refractory.

Once a tachycardia is induced, pacing maneuvers should be performed to determine the mechanism of tachycardia (see Chapter 8 for details) and document the involvement of the AP in the tachycardia (see Table 9-1). Insertion

---

TABLE 9-1 **Differentiation of an Accessory Pathway Conduction during Supraventricular Tachycardia (SVT) and Sinus Rhythm from Normal Retrograde Conduction up the Atrioventricular Node during Atrioventricular Nodal Reentry Tachycardia (AVNRT) and Sinus Rhythm**

During SVT

Eccentric atrial activation during SVT with atrial activation identical to atrial activation during ventricular pacing

Advance the atrium during SVT with a ventricular depolarization when the His bundle is refractory

Termination or delay of the tachycardia by a ventricular depolarization during His refractoriness

Prolongation of the VA interval >35 msec associated with ipsilateral bundle branch block

Inability to sustain SVT in presence of AV block

(for wide-complex tachycardia suspected to be antidromic AVRT): Advance the ventricle with an atrial depolarization when the atrium near the His bundle is refractory.

During NSR

VA interval shorter during basal ventricular pacing than apical pacing

HA during SVT less than HA or VA interval during ventricular pacing

Parahisian pacing with a change in HA interval with capture and no capture

Parahisian pacing with a change in V-A with capture and no capture (if atrial activation sequence identical)

AV, atrioventricular; AVRT, atrioventricular reciprocating tachycardia; NSR, normal sinus rhythm.

of ventricular premature beats (VPB) when the His bundle is refractory is the most important maneuver in the diagnosis of an AP-mediated tachycardia. If a His-refractory VPB is able to preexcite the atrium, the presence of an AP is demonstrated, and if this maneuver advances or delays the tachycardia, its participation in the tachycardia is proved.

For wide-complex tachycardias in which the diagnosis of antidromic tachycardia (utilizing the AP for AV conduction and the AV node for ventriculoatrial conduction) is suspected, pacing maneuvers may also confirm the diagnosis (Table 9-1). The most important maneuver in this situation is insertion of an atrial premature beat (APB) when the atrium recorded near the His bundle is refractory (see Fig. 9-7). The APB should be applied near the site of the AP and if it is able to preexcite the ventricles and affect the tachycardia, the AP participation in the tachycardia is proved. During antidromic tachycardia, QRS morphology represents fully preexcited ventricular activation and is suspected that the initial forces are identical to the delta wave pattern seen on the baseline ECG.

Tachycardias Involving Preexcitation Variants

The Lown-Ganong-Levine syndrome comprises patients with a short PR interval (<120 msec) and documented tachycardia. Most of these patients have a short PR due to enhanced AV nodal conduction, although some may be found to have atrio-His bypass tracts. During electrophysiology study, patients with enhanced AV nodal conduction will have decremental AH intervals with administration of atrial premature depolarizations (APDs), whereas patients with atrio-His APs will demonstrate a lack of AV delay during administration of APDs and a short HV interval. These APs have not been shown to participate in reentrant arrhythmias. However, patients with this syndrome may demonstrate extremely rapid conduction during atrial tachyarrhthmias and put a patient at risk for ventricular arrhythmias. Electrophysiologic testing should therefore include assessment of the AV refractory period. If this is very short and may allow extremely rapid conduction, therapy with a class I or III agent may be considered. More commonly, the tachycardias seen in patients with this syndrome are atrioventricular nodal reentry tachycardia (AVNRT) or AVRT using a separate concealed AP for retrograde conduction. These tachycardias are treated the same as in patients with a normal baseline PR interval.

APs with decremental conduction properties may by atriofascicular, AV, nodofascicular, or nodoventricular, and are commonly referred to as *Mahaim fibers* (see Fig. 9-8). The ventricular insertion sites of these APs tend to be in either the right ventricle or the right bundle branch. Reentrant tachycardias that utilize these APs as the antegrade limb of a circuit therefore have a left bundle branch block (BBB) with left axis ECG morphology. The degree of preexcitation seen with these APs is quite variable. During electrophysiology

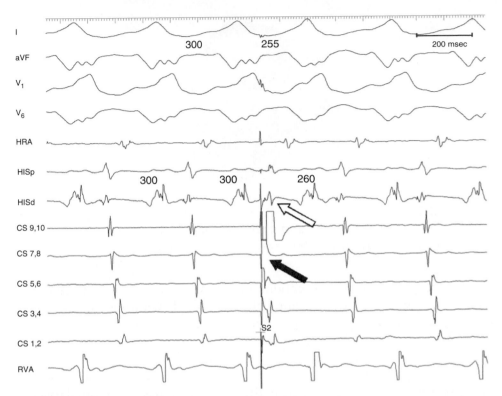

FIGURE 9-7. Demonstration of the mechanism of antidromic tachycardia. A wide-complex tachycardia with intracardiac electrograms is shown. An atrial premature beat (*closed arrow*) is delivered from the coronary sinus (CS) catheter when the atrium in the His bundle region is refractory (*open arrow*). The action potential duration (APD) does not affect the timing of the atrial depolarization but the next ventricular beat is advanced and the tachycardia is reset. This maneuver proves that the His bundle could not be used for atrioventricular conduction and that the mechanism of the wide-complex tachycardia is an antidromic tachycardia utilizing a left inferoposterior accessory pathway. Four surface leads (I, aVF, V₁, V₆) are shown, and intracardiac electrograms from the high right atrium (HRA), His bundle region (HISp and HISd), five bipolar pairs in the coronary sinus (CS 1,2 through 9,10), and the right ventricle atrium (RVA). Paper speed is 100 mm/sec, and numbers reflect timing in milliseconds between electrograms.

study, pacing near the atrial insertion site of atriofascicular or AV pathways (usually along the anterolateral tricuspid annulus) may increase the degree of preexcitation. These pathways are unique in that their histologic structure is similar to the specialized conduction tissue seen in the AV node and His bundle. AV and atriofascicular pathways can be traced along the right ventricle to their insertion sites in the apical right ventricle or right bundle. Detailed catheter mapping along their course is often able to identify a discrete potential similar to a His bundle potential.

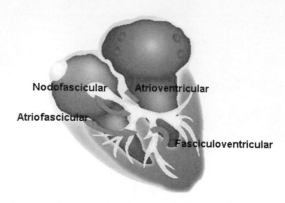

FIGURE 9-8. Variants of preexcitation: atriofascicular, atrioventricular, nodofascicular, nodoventricular, and fasciculoventricular pathways connecting the respective structures are depicted. (See color insert.)

Atriofascicular and slowly conducting AV APs generally do not participate as the retrograde limb of reentrant tachycardias. When a wide-complex tachycardia with left BBB, left axis morphology is seen, AV reentry using a slowly conduction AV or atriofascicular AP must be considered. Atrial activation sequence is usually consistent with retrograde conduction up the AV node. Insertion of an APB near the origin of the AP (usually in the anterolateral right atrium) after the atrium near the His bundle has been depolarized is able to advance the tachycardia and proves the mechanism of antidromic AV reentry. Nodoventricular and nodofascicular pathways are less common but may participate in reentrant tachycardias. When they serve as the retrograde limb of a reentrant circuit, they may be extremely difficult to differentiate from AV nodal reentry. Only the appearance of A-V dissociation or the ability to affect the timing of atrial activation while the His bundle is refractory may allow discrimination from AV nodal reentry.

Ablation Strategies

If an AP is shown to participate in a reentrant tachycardia or if a patient has documented evidence that a rapidly conducting pathway may allow extremely fast ventricular rates during atrial tachyarrhythmia, then ablation is usually indicated. Ablation is performed using a deflectable mapping catheter capable of applying radiofrequency energy. Generally a smaller tip 4 mm catheter is used to avoid excessive myocardial damage. Ablation of right-sided APs is usually performed from the atrial side, whereas left-sided APs can be approached from the ventricular side using a retrograde aortic approach or from the atrial side using a transseptal approach. Occasionally, epicardial inferoparaseptal APs may involve CS diverticula and require ablation within the CS.

Careful mapping must be performed to locate the insertion site of the AP. Mapping on the ventricular side of the AV ring in a patient with preexcitation should be performed during sinus rhythm or during atrial pacing. Pacing near the origin of the AP allows maximum preexcitation and the mapping catheter is manipulated until the earliest site of ventricular activation is found (usually 10 to 30 msec before the onset of the delta wave). Recording of unipolar signals is important, as this allows determination of whether the site of earliest activation is closer to the distal ablation pole or a more proximal recording pole of the catheter. At the ideal site, a QS pattern is seen in the unipolar recording from the distal tip of the ablation catheter. When ablating from the atrial aspect, a similar approach is used, but ventricular pacing is performed and the site of earliest atrial activation is sought. Ablation guided by the site of ventricular preexcitation (delta wave) in the author's opinion, is more accurate. Occasionally, a small electrogram spike between the atrial and ventricular signal may be seen, which may represent a direct recording of the AP potential. Careful atrial and ventricular pacing often reveals that what is thought to be an AP potential is actually a component of the atrial or ventricular signal. A true AP potential recording is rare, but when observed may predict a successful ablation site. When there is uncertainty regarding the optimal location using the method described earlier, pacing from the ablation catheter may provide further diagnostic information. Pacing from the atrial aspect will result in the shortest AV interval at the appropriate site, whereas pacing from the ventricular insertion site will result in the shortest VA interval.

Use of the local bipolar ventricular and atrial electrograms is also useful, but it should be noted that the shortest local VA or AV time during catheter mapping does not necessarily represent the optimal ablation site if a slant is present. In addition, although mapping during reentrant tachycardia may remove the uncertainty of fusion from mapping, ablation during tachycardia is not recommended. Abrupt termination of tachycardia during ablation may result in dislodgement of the catheter and inadequate ablation of the AP. Ablation during pacing as described earlier is preferred. When the optimal site is achieved, loss of preexcitation is usually seen within 10 to 15 seconds of the onset of application of radiofrequency energy. Absence of effect with longer periods of ablation suggests that the ablation site is inadequate and further mapping should be performed.

Ablation of decremental AV and atriofascicular APs is performed after mapping of the pathway. A Mahaim potential analogous to the His bundle potential can be recorded along the anterolateral tricuspid annulus and often traced down the free wall of the right ventricle. Ablation at the annulus where this potential is recorded is performed to achieve a durable result.

CONCLUSION

Patients presenting with ventricular preexcitation require a thorough clinical evaluation. A careful history is important to determine which patients may have symptoms related to the presence of an AP. Symptomatic patients merit a thorough electrophysiologic study and ablation of the AP if it can be demonstrated to participate in a clinical tachycardia. Given the extremely low incidence of sudden death in patients who are truly asymptomatic, the physicians recommend a conservative approach in such patients. However, a great deal of controversy exists over the management of such patients, and the recommendation for empiric electrophysiologic study in younger patients is an accepted strategy in many centers. An open discussion with each patient about the risks and benefits of these strategies is necessary in all cases.

SELECTED BIBLIOGRAPHY

Brugada P, Brugada J, Mont L, et al. A new approach to the differential diagnosis of a regular tachycardia with a wide QRS complex. *Circulation*. 1991;83(5):1649–1659.

Cosio FG, Anderson RH, Kuck K, et al. Living anatomy of the atrioventricular junctions. A guide to electrophysiologic mapping. A Consensus Statement from the Cardiac Nomenclature Study Group, Working Group of Arrhythmias, European Society of Cardiology, and the Task Force on Cardiac Nomenclature from NASPE. *Circulation*. 1999;100(5):e31–e37.

Fitzpatrick AP, Gonzales RP, Lesh MD, et al. New algorithm for the localization of accessory atrioventricular connections using a baseline electrocardiogram. *J Am Coll Cardiol*. 1994;23(1):107–116.

Fitzsimmons PJ, McWhirter PD, Peterson DW, et al. The natural history of Wolff-Parkinson-White syndrome in 228 military aviators: A long-term follow-up of 22 years. *Am Heart J*. 2001;142(3):530–536.

Harper RW, Whitford E, Middlebrook K, et al. Effects of verapamil on the electrophysiologic properties of the accessory pathway in patients with the Wolff-Parkinson-White syndrome. *Am J Cardiol*. 1982;50(6):1323–1330.

Josephson ME. *Clinical cardiac electrophysiology*, 4th ed. Philadelphia: Lippincott Williams & Wilkins; 2008.

Klein GJ, Bashore TM, Sellers TD, et al. Ventricular fibrillation in the Wolff-Parkinson-White syndrome. *N Engl J Med*. 1979;301(20):1080–1085.

Milstein S, Sharma AD, Guiraudon GM, et al. An algorithm for the electrocardiographic localization of accessory pathways in the Wolff-Parkinson-White syndrome. *Pacing Clin Electrophysiol*. 1987;10(3 Pt 1):555–563.

Pappone C, Santinelli V. Should catheter ablation be performed in asymptomatic patients with Wolff-Parkinson-White syndrome? Catheter ablation should be performed in asymptomatic patients with Wolff-Parkinson-White syndrome. *Circulation*. 2005;112(14):2207–2215; discussion 2216.

Pappone C, Santinelli V, Manguso F, et al. A randomized study of prophylactic catheter ablation in asymptomatic patients with the Wolff-Parkinson-White syndrome. *N Engl J Med*. 2003;349(19):1803–1811.

Sellers TD Jr, Bashore TM, Gallagher JJ. Digitalis in the pre-excitation syndrome. Analysis during atrial fibrillation. *Circulation*. 1977;56(2):260–267.

Wellens HJ, Braat S, Brugada P, et al. Use of procainamide in patients with the Wolff-Parkinson-White syndrome to disclose a short refractory period of the accessory pathway. *Am J Cardiol*. 1982;50(5):1087–1089.

Wellens HJ, Brugada P, Roy D, et al. Effect of isoproterenol on the anterograde refractory period of the accessory pathway in patients with the Wolff-Parkinson-White syndrome. *Am J Cardiol*. 1982;50(1):180–184.

Wellens HJ, Durrer D. Wolff-Parkinson-White syndrome and atrial fibrillation. Relation between refractory period of accessory pathway and ventricular rate during atrial fibrillation. *Am J Cardiol*. 1974;34(7):777–782.

Ventricular Tachycardia

Ventricular tachycardias (VTs) include a spectrum of arrhythmias that range from nonsustained asymptomatic VT to a sustained arrhythmia that results in a cardiac arrest. VTs are defined by morphology and duration. They may be uniform in morphology (monomorphic) or polymorphic. They may be unsustained or sustained (defined arbitrarily as >15 to 30 seconds) unless cardioverted sooner because of hemodynamic intolerance). Sustained monomorphic VT most often occurs in the setting of prior myocardial infarction (MI). Sustained VTs (polymorphic or monomorphic) may also be seen in patients without structural heart disease or in a variety of disorders including cardiomyopathies, valvular disease, drug toxicity, metabolic disorders, and ion channelopathies (see Fig. 10-1).

Nonsustained VTs occur in many people without known heart disease. Although polymorphic VT can be seen in acute ischemia, this is rare except with associated marked ST segment changes (see Fig. 10-2). Most often these VTs occur in the setting of prior infarction or cardiomyopathy with small scars (i.e., insufficient slow conduction for production of monomorphic VT) or in normal ventricles due to functional reentry (e.g., Brugada syndrome, drug effect, long QT syndromes) which may be initiated by early afterdepolarizations (EADs) (see the following text) or catecholamine-induced triggered activity.

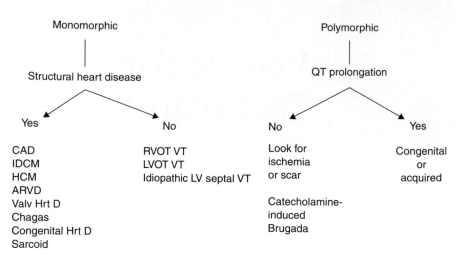

FIGURE 10-1. Differential diagnosis of ventricular tachycardia based on monomorphic and polymorphic ventricular morphology. CAD, coronary heart disease; IDCM, idiopathic dilated cardiomyopathy; HCM, hypertrophic cardiomyopathy; ARVD, arrhythmogenic right ventricular dysplasia; Valv Hrt D, valvular heart disease; RVOT, right ventricular outflow tract; LVOT, left ventricular outflow tract; LV, left ventricular; VT, ventricular tachycardia.

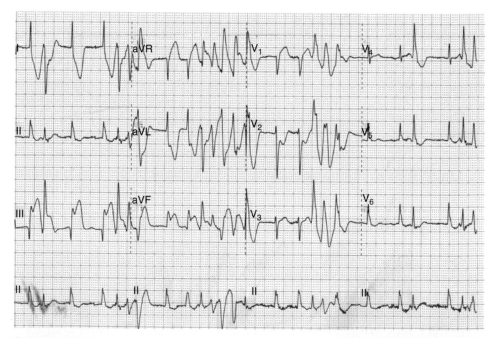

FIGURE 10-2. Acute ST elevation inferior myocardial infarction and polymorphic ventricular tachycardia. ST elevation in V_1 indicates associated right ventricular infarction.

IDENTIFYING THE MECHANISMS AND SUBSTRATE OF VENTRICULAR TACHYCARDIA

Mechanisms of Ventricular Tachycardia

Reentry: It is the most common mechanism of paroxysmal, sustained monomorphic VT in the setting of structural heart disease associated with scar, of which coronary artery disease (CAD) is most common. Reentry is characterized by:

- Initiation and termination by timed extrastimuli which are often site-specific (e.g., right ventricular apex [RVA], outflow tract, or left ventricle) (see Fig. 10-3)

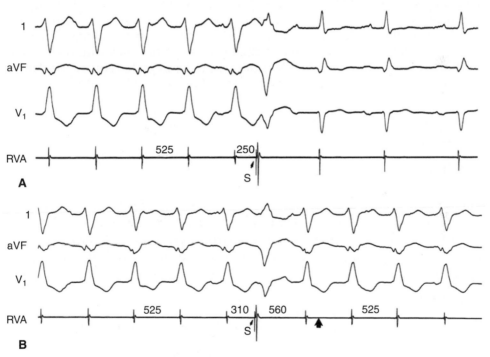

FIGURE 10-3. A: Demonstration of a timed ventricular extrastimulus at 250 msec resulting in termination of a reentrant VT. **B:** Demonstration of resetting of the same ventricular tachycardia. A ventricular extrastimulus is delivered at 310 msec after the preceding QRS complex. This extrastimulus enters the reentrant circuit and results in the next QRS complex occurring at 560 msec. This is 180 msec earlier than would have occurred had the ventricular premature depolarization (VPD) not affected the circuit (*black solid arrow*). RVA; right ventricular apex. (Adapted from Josephson ME. *Clinical Cardiac Electrophysiology*, 4th ed. 2008.)

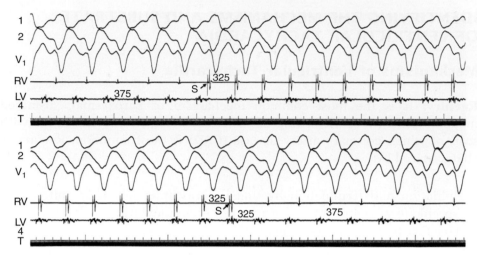

FIGURE 10-4. Entrainment of ventricular tachycardia. Ventricular tachycardia occurs at a cycle length of 375 msec. Pacing is initiated at a cycle length of 323 msec with a change in the surface electrocardiographic (ECG) morphology representing fusion of the paced and tachycardia morphology. Pacing is terminated in the bottom panel and the tachycardia resumes with the original morphology and cycle length. RV, right ventricle; LV, left ventricle. (Adapted from Josephson ME. *Clinical Cardiac Electrophysiology*, 4th ed. 2008.)

- Timed ventricular extrastimuli, which reset the tachycardia with fusion (Fig. 10-3)

- Entrainment of the tachycardia (see Fig. 10-4)

   Triggered rhythms due to delayed afterdepolarizations (DADs) are catecholamine sensitive and often occur during exercise. Such rhythms arise in otherwise normal tissue (Purkinje fibers, right ventricle [RV] and left ventricular outflow tract [LVOT], aorta in the right and left coronary cusp, and the mitral annulus), or in recently infarcted or reperfused and stunned myocardium.

Triggered VT

- Can be initiated by pacing more easily than by timed extrastimuli.

- Are more difficult to initiate on repeated attempts.

- Exhibit overdrive acceleration.

- Cannot be entrained or reset with fusion.

- Can be terminated by vagal maneuvers, adenosine, and by Na channel, β-adrenergic receptor or Ca channel blocking drugs.

   Digitalis-induced VT is also due to DADs, which are thought to be responsible for catecholamine-induced polymorphic tachycardias. Therefore, DADs can lead to monomorphic (e.g., RV/LVOT VTs) or polymorphic (e.g., ryanodine receptor defect) VTs.

Triggered rhythms initiated by EAD lead to polymorphic VTs associated with congenital and acquired long QT syndromes. These may also be seen in situations when there is calcium overload associated with short action potentials. This may explain polymorphic VTs following carotid sinus pressure or adenosine termination of supraventricular tachycardia (SVT).

Automatic VT: These are neither initiated nor terminated by programmed stimulation. They are seen in diseased tissue in which depolarized myocardial fibers develop phase 4 depolarization. Depending on the degree of depolarization overdrive suppression may or may not be seen. This mechanism may be seen after MI.

Substrate of Ventricular Tachycardia

The electrocardiogram (ECG) is useful in defining the underlying pathology. VT in patients with normal hearts (idiopathic VT) is characterized by tall, smoothly inscribed QRS complexes, whereas VTs in patients with diseased myocardium, particularly those with extensive scarring, have smaller, broader, and notched or splintered QRS' (see Fig. 10-5). Idiopathic VTs can have rapid initial forces whereas those VTs arising in scar have slower initial forces. A QS complex has no diagnostic value for underlying pathology. It can be seen in infarct-related VT, VT in cardiomyopathy, or even idiopathic VT arising on the epicardium (see the following text). A qR or QR complex in two anatomically adjacent leads is almost diagnostic of infarction. In many cases the infarct is more obvious during VT than in sinus rhythm.

The substrate of VT can be more accurately assessed by mapping the right and left ventricles during sinus rhythm. The normal heart has bipolar electrograms (EGMs) that are biphasic or triphasic, 1.5 mV (Carto) or 3 mV (standard Bard catheter) in amplitude, and which are <70 msec in duration. Abnormal EGMs can be classified as follows:

1. Low amplitude (<1.5 mV Carto)

2. Split (30 to 50 msec isoelectric interval)

3. Late (inscribed after the QRS)

4. Fractionated (low amplitude with multiple component)

Prior infarction scar is associated with low-amplitude signals ≤0.5 mV with a variable number of late, split, and fractionated signals. In patients with idiopathic cardiomyopathy the endocardium is less abnormal, with a smaller area of low-amplitude potentials, and a smaller percentage of split, late, and fractionated signals which are more frequent near the annuli. Such findings are more common on the epicardium in these patients. Arrhythmogenic RV

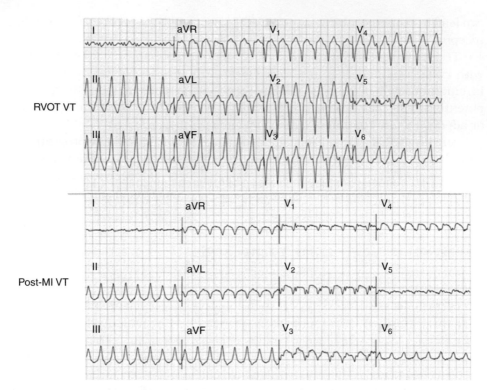

FIGURE 10-5. Idiopathic right ventricular outflow tract tachycardia (RVOT) compared with ventricular tachycardia (VT) due to underlying myocardial infarction (MI) and scar. RVOT VT is characterized by tall smoothly inscribed QRS complexes. The VT associated with prior myocardial infarction is characterized by lower amplitude and notched QRS complexes.

dysplasia is characterized by abnormal EGMs, primarily at the free wall of the RV. In approximately 15% to 20% of infarcts (primarily inferior) epicardial scar is more marked than endocardial scar.

Patients with sustained monomorphic VT have a greater number of abnormal EGMs than those with ventricular fibrillation (VF) or nonsustained VT, regardless of whether prior infarction or idiopathic cardiomyopathy is present. Because the abnormal EGMs are associated with slow conduction, these areas, not surprisingly, are the source of reentrant arrhythmias. Arrhythmias in apparently normal areas are more frequently due to triggered activity or automaticity. Such mechanisms can also be operative in diseased hearts.

DIFFERENTIATION OF VENTRICULAR TACHYCARDIA FROM SUPRAVENTRICULAR TACHYCARDIA WITH ABERRATION

Several ECG criteria have been proposed to diagnose VT (see Table 10-1). Although none are perfect, several generalizations can be made:

TABLE 10-1	**Electrocardiographic Criteria for Diagnosis of Ventricular Tachycardia**

Factors which favor Ventricular Iachycardia (VT) over Supraventricular tachycardia (SVT)

Atrioventricular (AV) Dissociation

QRS>0.14 with RBBB
QRS>0.16 with left bundle branch block (LBBB)

North west axis (−1, − aVF)
LBBB with axis +90 → +180

Concordance (+ or −)

QRS during tachycardia which is narrower than during sinus rhythm

Morphology as shown

Right bundle branch block (RBBB):
Monoplastic or biphasic complex in V_1
RS (only with left axis deviation)
or QS in V_6

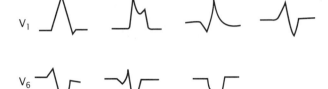

LBBB: Broad R wave in V_1 or V_2 ≥0.04 s
Onset of QRS to nadir of S wave in V_1 or V_2 of ≥0.07 s
Notched downslope of S wave in V_1 or V_2
Q wave in V_6

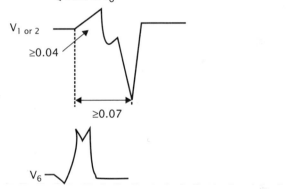

1. *A-V dissociation*, particularly when demonstrated by the presence of fusion and/or capture beats is virtually diagnostic of VT (see Figs. 10-6 and 10-7). Unfortunately capture beats are very uncommon and at very fast rates P waves may be difficult to see. Moreover one to one ventriculoatrial (VA) conduction may be seen in VT (usually at rates <200 bpm).

2. *QRS width* is useful in the absence of antiarrhythmic drugs or preexistent bundle branch block (BBB). Right bundle branch block (RBBB) aberration does not increase the QRS duration >0.14 seconds even with hypertrophy. Left bundle branch block (LBBB), which can produce a QRS of 0.14 seconds in a normal heart, can cause the QRS to reach 0.16 seconds in hypertrophy. Therefore, a RBBB-like complex >0.14 seconds and LBBB-like complex >0.16 seconds in the absence of drugs favors the diagnosis of VT. Of note somewhere between 2% and 5% of VTs have QRS' ≤120 msec.

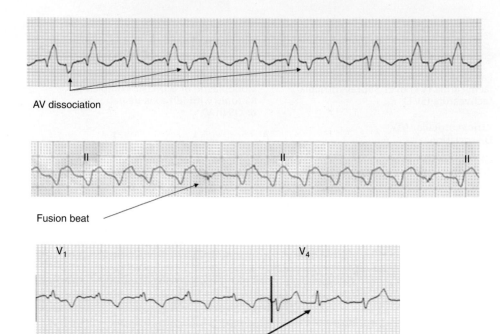

FIGURE 10-6. Characterization of atrioventricular (AV) dissociation with P waves clearly dissociated from the QRS complexes, fusion between normal QRS and QRS created by ventricular tachycardia (VT), and a capture beat demonstrated by a normal narrow QRS complex.

3. *Axis* may also be useful. An axis in the "northwest" quadrant is almost always VT in adults because no form of aberration has such a vector (see Fig. 10-8). In someone with a normal QRS in sinus rhythm, a LBBB-like wide complex tachycardia with a right axis (+90 to +180) is always VT because activation in LBBB aberration always goes from right to left.

4. **Concordance:** If *all* the precordial leads are positive (R) or negative (QS) the rhythm is very likely VT (see Fig. 10-9).

5. **V_1-V_2 morphology:** In RBBB-like tachycardias an RsR′ or rsR′ in V_1 favors SVT, whereas a monophasic R, Rr′ (Fig. 10-8), qR, or RS favors VT. In RBBB aberration the initial forces of the QRS are the same as in the narrow complex sinus rhythm. In LBBB-like tachycardias V_1 *and* V_2 require analysis because the initial forces in V_1 are often isoelectric. An R wave in V_1 *or* V_2 ≥40 msec favors VT. In addition, if the time from the onset of the QRS to the nadir of the S wave in V_1 *or* V_2 is ≥70 msec, VT is likely in the absence of Na channel blocking agents.

6. *V6* may be useful in diagnosis as well. A QS or rS favors VT in RBBB-like tachycardias, although this can be influenced by axis (it is almost always seen in VT with left axis deviation, but is seen in only approximately 50% of

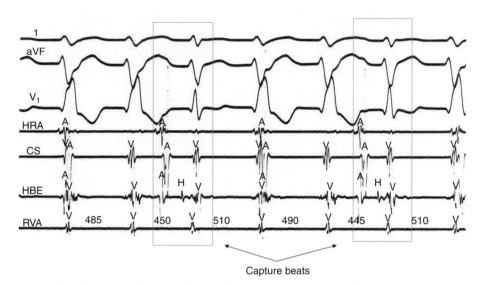

Capture beats

FIGURE 10-7. Ventricular tachycardia (VT) with a right bundle branch block morphology and northwest axis. The third and sixth beats demonstrate capture of the ventricle over the normal conduction system by sinus beats during VT. HRA, high right atrium; CS, coronary sinus; HBE, His bundle electrogram; RVA, right ventricular apex.

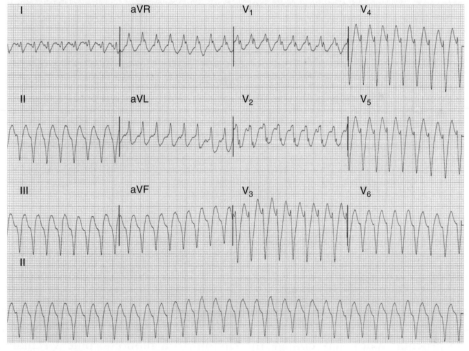

FIGURE 10-8. Ventricular tachycardia from the inferior wall of the left ventricle. The QRS complex has an Rsr' right bundle branch block morphology, a northwest axis, and a Q wave in V_6.

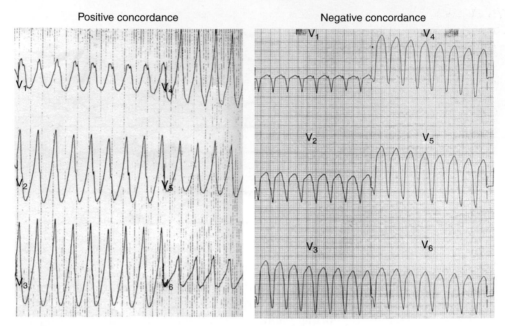

FIGURE 10-9. Positive (all R waves) and negative (all QS complexes) concordance.

VT with a normal axis, even in the same patient) (Fig. 10-8). In LBBB-like tachycardias, a qR or QS is highly predictive of VT.

7. If BBB or an intraventricular conduction disturbance (IVCD) is present in sinus rhythm, a wide QRS that is *narrower* must be VT because intraventricular conduction stays the same or gets slower at increasing rates.

ROLE OF THE ELECTROPHYSIOLOGY LABORATORY IN THE EVALUATION AND THERAPY OF VENTRICULAR TACHYCARDIA

The electrophysiology (EP) laboratory is useful for establishing the diagnosis and mechanism of VT, as well as localizing the site of origin (or exit) of the VT circuit and developing therapy. It is most useful for monomorphic VTs as polymorphic VTs do not pose a diagnostic challenge electrocardiographically, and are difficult to study by electrophysiology study (EPS). In these VTs the underlying substrate may be identified by mapping. In cases where a scar is present, but small, addition of an Na channel blocker (e.g., intravenous [IV] procainamide) may change the rhythm to a monomorphic VT that is inducible and able to be pace terminated, suggesting a reentrant arrhythmia. Catecholamine infusion may induce monomorphic as well as polymorphic VTs.

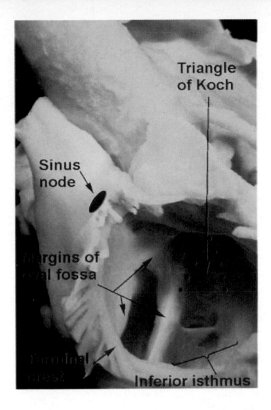

FIGURE 1-1. Right atrium opened, demonstrating the epicardial location of the sinus node in relation to the crista terminalis (terminal crest). The fossa ovalis and triangle of Koch are also demonstrated. (Courtesy Prof RH Anderson)

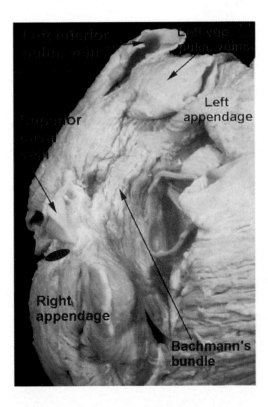

FIGURE 1-2. Right atrium demonstrating the location of the Bachmann bundle. The *blue oval* represents the sinus node. (Courtesy Prof RH Anderson)

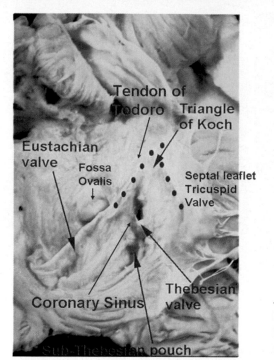

FIGURE 1-3. Demonstration of the boundaries of the triangle of Koch, right atrium, and fossa ovalis.

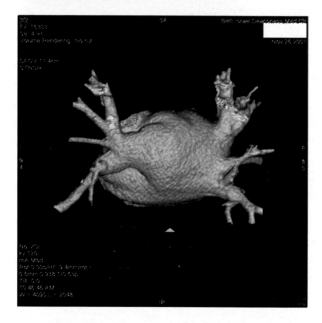

FIGURE 1-5. Computed tomographic angiogram of the posterior aspect of the left atrium.

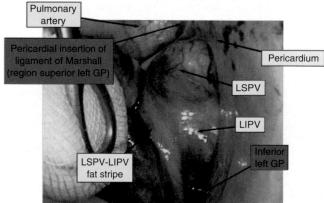

FIGURE 1-7. Epicardial exposure of the left atrium with the left superior pulmonary vein (LSPV), left inferior pulmonary vein (LIPV), ligament of Marshall, and ganglionic plexi (GP). (Courtesy Robert Hagberg, MD)

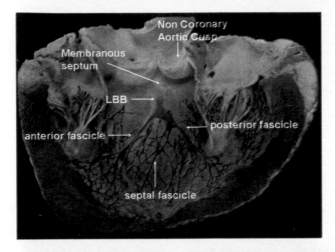

FIGURE 1-8.
A left ventricle with the membranous septum and the left bundle branch delineated. LBB, left bundle branch.

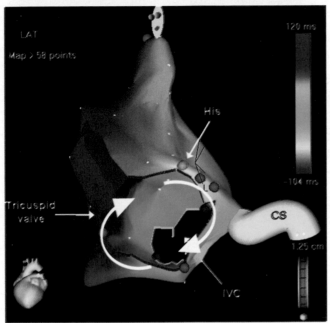

FIGURE 1-11.
Electroanatomic (CARTO) image of the activation sequence during clockwise atrial flutter. The "head" and "tail" of the reentrant circuit meet where red meets purple/blue. LAT, local activation time; CS, coronary sinus; IVC, inferior vena cava.

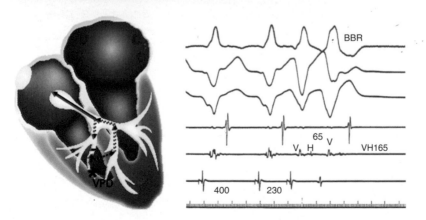

FIGURE 4-11. Demonstration of a bundle branch reentrant (BBR) beat. A ventricular extrastimulus blocks in the right bundle branch, conducts across the septum, and enters the left bundle branch. The impulse travels in a retrograde direction, activates the His bundle, and reenters the right bundle branch. The electrogram demonstrates the presence of a His bundle electrogram preceding activation of the right ventricle. VPD, ventricular premature depolarization.

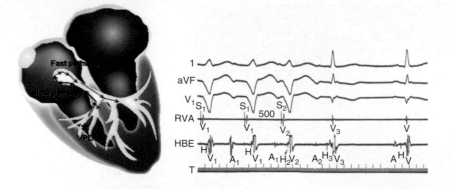

FIGURE 4-12. Ventricular pacing with ventricular extrastimulation resulting in an atypical atrioventricular (AV) nodal echo beat. VPD, ventricular premature depolarization; RVA, right ventricular apex; HBE, His bundle electrogram.

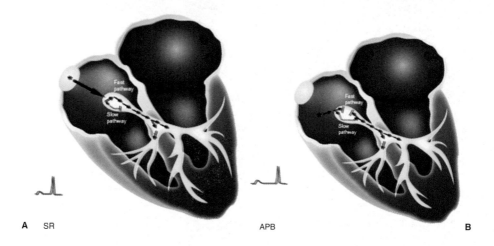

A SR

APB

B

FIGURE 5-2. Schema of dual atrioventricular (AV) nodal pathways.
A: Demonstrates conduction down both the fast and slow pathways with a normal PR interval of 160 msec. **B:** Demonstrates an atrial premature depolarization (APD) with block in the fast pathway and conduction down the slow pathway yielding a longer PR interval of 240 msec. SR, sinus rhythm.

Atrial remodeling = maintenance of AF
- Electrical (within hours) – rapid atrial activation → loss of nl shortening of atrial and PV myocyte refractory periods to rapid rates (decreases responsiveness to AADS)
- Mechanical (within weeks) – fibrosis and dilatation

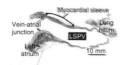

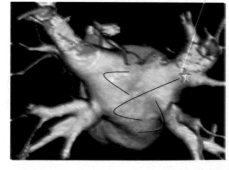

Inflammation
↑CRP
↑IL-6

FIGURE 6-1. Current understanding of the mechanisms of atrial fibrillation. AF, atrial fibrillation; nl, normal; PV, pulmonary vein; AAD, antiarrhythmic drugs; LSPV, left superior pulmonary vein; CRP, C-reactive protein; IL-6, interkeukin 6.

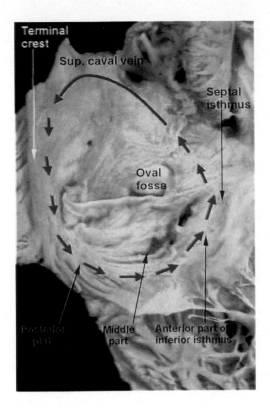

FIGURE 7-1. Anatomy of the right atrial flutter circuit.

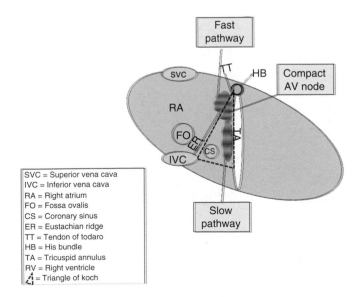

SVC = Superior vena cava
IVC = Inferior vena cava
RA = Right atrium
FO = Fossa ovalis
CS = Coronary sinus
ER = Eustachian ridge
TT = Tendon of todaro
HB = His bundle
TA = Tricuspid annulus
RV = Right ventricle
△ = Triangle of koch

FIGURE 8-1.
Schematic of the functional anatomy of the atrioventricular (AV) node in the right anterior oblique (RAO) view.

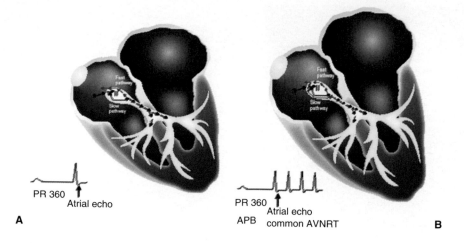

PR 360 ↑
Atrial echo

A

PR 360 ↑
Atrial echo
APB   common AVNRT

B

FIGURE 8-2. Diagrams of a typical atrioventricular (AV) nodal echo **(A)** and the initiation of atrioventricular nodal reentrant tachycardia (AVNRT) **(B)**. The *black arrow* represents initial conduction down the slow pathway. The *blue arrows* demonstrate retrograde conduction up the slow pathway (echo beat) with subsequent conduction back down the slow pathway with initiation of AVNRT.

Orthodromic AVRT
(concealed)

Antidromic AVRT
(pre-excited)

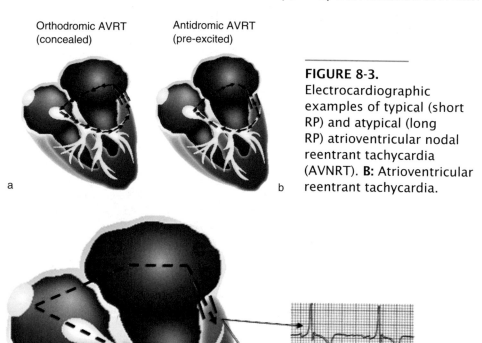

a

b

FIGURE 8-3.
Electrocardiographic examples of typical (short RP) and atypical (long RP) atrioventricular nodal reentrant tachycardia (AVNRT). **B:** Atrioventricular reentrant tachycardia.

FIGURE 9-1. Diagram of antegrade conduction over both the normal atrioventricular (AV) conducting system and a left-sided accessory pathway. The amount of conduction over the accessory pathway corresponds to the degree of ventricular preexcitation or delta wave.

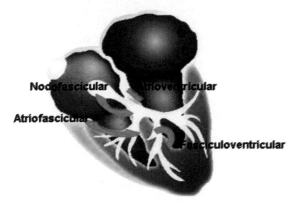

Nodofascicular

Atriofascicular

Atrioventricular

Fasciculoventricular

FIGURE 9-8.
Variants of preexcitation: atriofascicular, atrioventricular, nodofascicular, nodoventricular, and fasciculoventricular pathways connecting the respective structures are depicted.

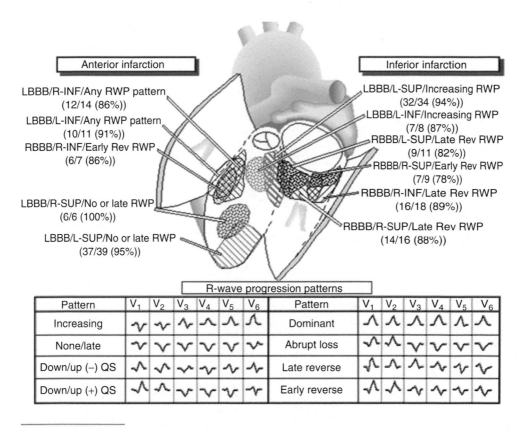

Anterior infarction
LBBB/R-INF/Any RWP pattern (12/14 (86%))
LBBB/L-INF/Any RWP pattern (10/11 (91%))
RBBB/R-INF/Early Rev RWP (6/7 (86%))
LBBB/R-SUP/No or late RWP (6/6 (100%))
LBBB/L-SUP/No or late RWP (37/39 (95%))

Inferior infarction
LBBB/L-SUP/Increasing RWP (32/34 (94%))
LBBB/L-INF/Increasing RWP (7/8 (87%))
RBBB/L-SUP/Late Rev RWP (9/11 (82%))
RBBB/R-SUP/Early Rev RWP (7/9 (78%))
RBBB/R-INF/Late Rev RWP (16/18 (89%))
RBBB/R-SUP/Late Rev RWP (14/16 (88%))

R-wave progression patterns

Pattern	V₁	V₂	V₃	V₄	V₅	V₆	Pattern	V₁	V₂	V₃	V₄	V₅	V₆
Increasing							Dominant						
None/late							Abrupt loss						
Down/up (−) QS							Late reverse						
Down/up (+) QS							Early reverse						

FIGURE 10-10. Patterns of surface QRS morphology associated with ventricular tachycardia related to prior inferior and anterior myocardial infarction. LBBB; left bundle branch block; R-INF, right inferior or positive axis; L-SUP, left superior or positive axis; RWP, R-wave progression; L-INF, left inferior or positive axis; RBBB; right bundle branch block; R-SUP, right superior axis; Rev, reverse. Courtesy of John Miller, MD.

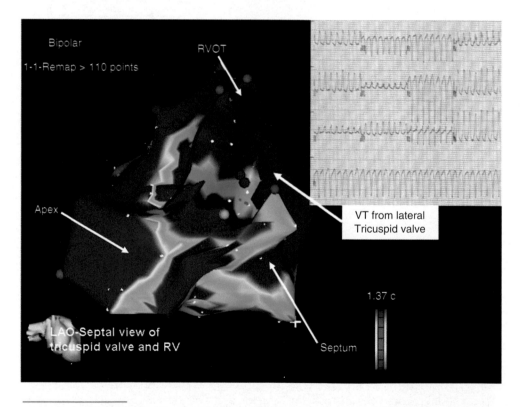

VT in Absence of structural heart disease

- ▨ RVOT- Septal
- ▨ RVOT- Free Wall
- ■ LVOT
- ▨ LV septal ("Purkinje")

Outflow tract-VT

Lead 1 more (−)

V_1–V_2

more (+)

R transition

V_3–V_4

Anterior

Basal — Septal

Lateral — Apical

Inferior

Outflow tract-VT

more (+) ← Lead 1 → more (−)

V_1–V_2

V_3–V_4 R transition

Anterior

Basal

Lateral — Septal

Apical

Inferior

FIGURE 10-11.
Schema of sites of idiopathic ventricular tachycardia (VT) [RVOT or right ventricular outflow tract VT, LVOT or left ventricular outflow tract VT, and left ventricular septal VT]. The image on the left represents the right anterior oblique view and on the right, the left anterior oblique view. The morphology in lead I and the point of transition at which the R wave becomes greater than the S wave in the right precordial leads is demonstrated. Courtesy of John Miller, MD.

Bipolar

1-1-Remap > 110 points

RVOT

Apex

VT from lateral Tricuspid valve

1.37 c

LAO-Septal view of tricuspid valve and RV

Septum

FIGURE 10-17. Electroanatomic map of a patient with arrhythmogenic right ventricular dysplasia (ARVD). The tricuspid valve is shown with areas of low voltage (red) representing characteristically affected regions with ARVD. This patient presented with the LBBB/inferior axis VT arising from an area lateral to the tricuspid annulus. LBBB, left bundle branch block; VT, ventricular tachycardia; LAO, left anterior oblique; RVOT, right ventricular outflow tract.

Diagnosis

VT is diagnosed by demonstrating that the atrium and atrioventricular (AV) junction (AV node and His bundle) are not required. This is best done by demonstrating AV dissociation with antegrade block below the His, intermittent or one to one relationship of ventricular and His potentials with shorter HVs than in sinus, or His potentials occurring after the QRS. Absence of visible His potentials and AV dissociation is also helpful, but obviously one must make sure that His potentials are recorded during sinus rhythm.

Mechanism

Monomorphic VTs are those most appropriately evaluated by EPS. A variety of responses characterize reentry (see Table 10-2). Reproducible initiation and termination by timed extrastimuli are the easiest to establish. In the setting of prior infarction, initiation of monomorphic VT can be accomplished in approximately 90% to 95% of patients. Both may be site dependant (RVA vs. right ventricular outflow tract [RVOT] vs. LV) for ability and/or ease of initiation and termination. The standard protocol for induction of

TABLE 10-2 Techniques Used for Mapping Ventricular Tachycardia Based on Arrhythmia Mechanism

Mapping of Ventricular Tachycardia

Mapping Technique	Mechanisms		
	Reentry	TA	AUTO
Activation mapping ("earliest site")	++	+++	+++
Stimulus response (SR) mapping (abnl EGMs)	++	–	–
Pace mapping			
12-lead ECG	–	++	++
+ activation pattern	–	+++	+++
Entrainment mapping (Pacing during VT)	+++	–	–
Target	Vulnerable Component	Focus of origin	

TA, triggered activity; AUTO, automatic; EGM, electrogram; ++, moderately useful; +++, very useful.

VT involves stimulating at two basic drive cycle lengths for 8 beats followed by the introduction of premature stimuli (i.e., 600/380, 600/360 etc. and 400/360, 400/340 etc.). This protocol is carried out until the refractory period is reached at both drive cycles and at two distinct sites in the RV (i.e., RVA and RVOT).

If no arrhythmias are induced, a second premature stimuli is introduced at two cycle lengths at two sites. If no arrhythmias are induced, the protocol is repeated using three extrastimuli. The protocol is done this way because of the site specificity noted earlier. In this way the least aggressive stimulation is used for initiation. Using up to three extrastimuli from one site may induce an untolerated, nonclinical VT or VF when a single extrastimulus from another site would have induced the clinical VT. The physicians use 180 msec as the tightest premature stimulus introduced. Occasionally LV stimulation or rapid ventricular pacing is required to induce VT. The introduction of a premature impulse followed by a relative pause and then another premature impulse (short-long-short) sequence is particularly useful for inducing bundle branch reentry (BBR) tachycardia (see the following text).

As noted earlier, polymorphic VT, particularly in the setting of a prior scar, can occasionally be transformed into monomorphic VT that is able to be reproducibly initiated and terminated by an Na channel blocker (e.g., IV procainamide). Termination is accomplished by the introduction of synchronized timed extrastimuli or bursts of rapid pacing beginning at approximately 90% of the VT cycle length and gradually reducing the paced cycle length to avoid acceleration of VT or degeneration to VF. The ability to reset (single beat) or entrain (overdrive pacing producing continuous resetting) with fusion is diagnostic of reentry (see Chapter 3). The requirement of conduction delay for initiation suggests reentry. Mapping reentrnt excitation is also possible but not easily achievable.

VT caused by triggered activity due to DADs may be initiated and terminated by overdrive pacing (more readily than timed extrastimuli), but less reliably than reentry. Pacing can be from the ventricles or atrium. It is often more difficult to induce repeatedly due to activation of the Na/K exchanger which suppresses DADs. Catecholamines, atropine, aminophylline, and Ca may be needed to induce these VTs. There is often a direct relationship between the drive cycle or premature stimulus that initiates the VT and the coupling interval to the onset of the VT and the initial cycles of the VT, but this is not universal. The VTs tend to exhibit overdrive acceleration in response to pacing, but *cannot* be reset with fusion or entrained. Vagal maneuvers, adenosine, β-blockers, calcium blockers, or nonspecific Na channel blockers can terminate these VTs because the DADs responsible for the VTs are caused by adenyl cyclase–mediated calcium overload leading to a Na/Ca exchange.

LOCALIZING THE SITE OF ORIGIN (OR EXIT)—ELECTROCARDIOGRAM AND MAPPING

The 12-lead ECG is a useful tool to help identify the site of origin of VT. Despite the limitations of scarring and fibrosis, aneurysm, chest wall deformities, metabolic and drug effects, and so on, analysis of the QRS patterns and vectors can regionalize the site of activation of viable myocardium. Obviously it is easier in normal hearts than in scarred hearts (see Figs. 10-10 and 10-11).

General Principles of Electrocardiogram Localization

The ECG pattern is a manifestation of the way in which the heart is activated by the VT. Most reentrant VTs arise from reentrant circuits associated with

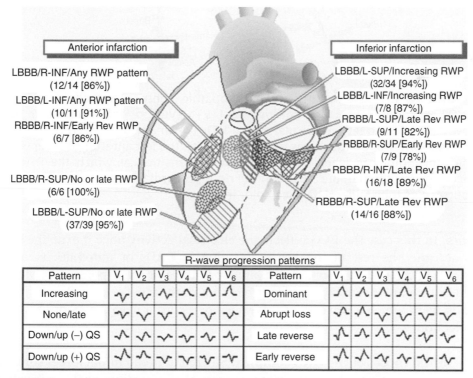

FIGURE 10-10. Patterns of surface QRS morphology associated with ventricular tachycardia related to prior inferior and anterior myocardial infarction. LBBB; left bundle branch block; R-INF, right inferior or positive axis; L-SUP, left superior or positive axis; RWP, R-wave progression; L-INF, left inferior or positive axis; RBBB; right bundle branch block; R-SUP, right superior axis; Rev, reverse. Courtesy of John Miller, MD. (See color insert.)

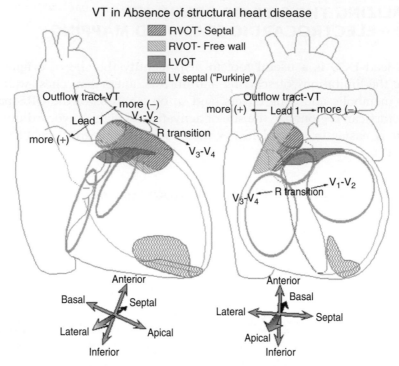

FIGURE 10-11. Schema of sites of idiopathic ventricular tachycardia (VT) [RVOT or right ventricular outflow tract VT, LVOT or left ventricular outflow tract VT, and left ventricular septal VT]. The image on the left represents the right anterior oblique view and on the right, the left anterior oblique view. The morphology in lead I and the point of transition at which the R wave becomes greater than the S wave in the right precordial leads is demonstrated. Courtesy of John Miller, MD. (See color insert.)

scars. In this case the ECG reflects the electrical activity once it exits the scar to activate the rest of the heart. VTs due to DADs or automaticity arise from a focal site and spread radially from the initiating point. ECG leads which face an oncoming wavefront record a positive deflection (R wave) and leads from which a wave front travels away record a negative (S or Q wave) deflection.

1. **Initial forces of the QRS complex:** Slurred or broad initial forces suggest that the tachycardia is arising from scarred myocardium or the epicardial surface, whereas rapid (normal) initial forces suggest a normal myocardial substrate (Fig. 10-5).

2. **QS waves in VT complexes:** qR or qr complexes suggest underlying MI and can help localize the site of origin of the VT to the area of the infarct. QS complexes are less specific for substrate and do not necessary localize the site of origin of VT because they can just represent a cavity potential

overlying a transmural scar. They always suggest that the wavefront is moving away from the recording electrodes, which in the setting of a normal heart helps localize the origin, particularly epicardial.

3. **QRS morphology:** VTs arising from the RV have a LBBB-like morphology because the RV is activated before the LV. Similarly most VTs arising from the LV will have a RBBB-like morphology; however, VTs arising on or adjacent to the LV septum can have a LBBB morphology if VT exits from the septum to the RV. In CAD, >95% of those with LBBB-like patterns arise from the LV (Fig. 10-10).

4. **The width of the QRS complex:** The QRS is generally wider in VTs which arise on the free wall (particularly epicardial) compared with those that arise closer to the septum. This is because free wall VTs activate the ventricles sequentially while those arising in or near the septum activate them more simultaneously. A caveat is that the presence of markedly slowed conduction in septal infarcts can lead to wide QRSs in VTs arising in the septum.

5. **QRS axis:** The axis is related to the superior/inferior and right/left direction the VT travels away from its site of origin or exit to activate the remainder of the heart. VT arising from the superior aspects of the heart (i.e., RVOT, superior aspects of the LV septum, and lateral wall) will have an inferior axis. VTs arising from the inferior wall will have a superior axis. VTs arising from the inferobasal septal LV and inferior RV will have a left superior axis (Fig. 10-10). VTs arising from the inferoapical LV will often have a QS in leads I, II, and III leading to a right superior axis ($-90 \rightarrow -180$). Lateral LV sites have a right inferior or superior axis.

6. **Anterior (apical) versus basal sites:** VTs arising at the base will have vectors pointing anteriorly so that R waves dominate the precordium, even during LBBB-like patterns (Fig. 10-9). VTs arising near the apex will have posteriorly directed forces leading to negative complexes in the precordial leads. Positive concordance (R waves in V_1-V_6) indicates that the wave front is traveling from back to front. It is associated with VTs from the base of the heart near the aortic-mitral continuity as well as the basal aspect of the LV septum. Negative concordance (QS complexes in V_1-V_6) indicates VT from the apical septum and typically anterior infarction (Fig. 10-9).

Mapping Ventricular Tachycardia

The mapping techniques used to localize VT depend on the mechanism of VT. The available techniques include activation mapping, pace mapping, and entrainment mapping. These techniques are used alone or in combination to guide ablative procedures. When no target is available (noninducible VT or induction of hemodynamically untolerated VT or multiple VTs) substrate mapping can be used to guide ablation of scar-related VTs. The utility of each mapping technique is shown in Table 10-2.

Activation mapping is an attempt to find the earliest recorded electrical activity during VT. In the case of VT due to enhanced automaticity or triggered activity, both focal mechanisms, the earliest site should be the site of origin of the arrhythmia and therefore the target for ablation. Such sites are rarely earlier than 60 msec before the surface QRS. The physicians also suggest simultaneous unipolar recordings to make sure that the ablating electrode (the tip) is the one recording earliest activity. In reentrant VT there is continuous activation of a reentrant pathway; therefore, the concept of an "earliest site" does not apply. Nevertheless appropriate target sites for reentrant VT are usually 100 to 200 msec before the QRS. The prematurity of a site does not guarantee that it will be a good site to ablate because many such regions represent pathways connected to but not critical to the tachycardia circuit ("dead-end pathways"). Other means are necessary to identify critical sites in a reentrant circuit (see the following text).

Pace mapping similarly is only useful for identifying the origin of focal tachycardias. It is based on the hypothesis that if one can find a site in the ventricles at which pacing reproduces the identical QRS configuration of the VT, it must be the site of spontaneous impulse formation. Unfortunately pacing from over an area of 1 to 2 cm^2 can yield similar morphologies because the virtual pacing electrode (unipolar or bipolar) exceeds the size of the focus. Using additional intracardiac recordings (e.g., RVOT, RVA, V in His bundle electrogram [HBE]) as reference EGMs improves the accuracy somewhat, making ablation delivered at a site with a good pace-map and similar activation to other ventricular sites likely to be successful.

Reentrant VT requires identification of a critical isthmus of conduction that is vulnerable to ablation. In the vast majority of cases the target will precede the QRS by at least 80 msec; typically by between 25% and 75% of the VT cycle length. On the basis of models of resetting and entrainment (see Fig. 10-12) pacing from a critical isthmus (central common pathway) is called *entrainment mapping* and is characterized by:

1. An *identical* QRS as the VT (see Fig. 10-13)

2. A postpacing interval (PPI) equal to the VT cycle length (within 10 to 30 msec) (see Fig. 10-14)

3. A stimulus-QRS equal to the spontaneous target EGM to QRS (Fig. 10-14)

If all three criteria are met there is a high likelihood that ablation at that site (±1 cm will terminate the VT and prevent its initiation. There are limitations to this and other mapping techniques. They include stimulating and recording far field, poor contact, inability to define the local EGM, production of conduction delays due to too rapid pacing thereby exceeding PPI

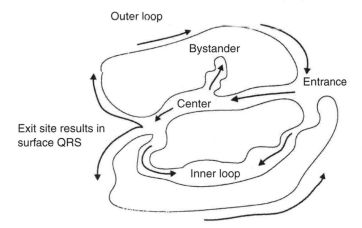

FIGURE 10-12. Schema of an area of scar, which generates a circuit for ventricular tachycardia (VT). The center is a protected region, which represents an isthmus for the VT circuit. Pacing from this area with entrainment of the tachycardia, which produces an exact 12-lead morphology as the clinical VT is called *concealed entrainment* and identifies an excellent site for ablation. The exit site results in the surface QRS morphology. (Modified with permission from William Stevenson, MD.)

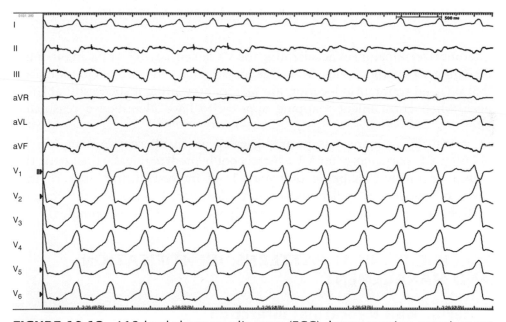

FIGURE 10-13. A 12-lead electrocardiogram (ECG) demonstrating entrainment (first 6 beats) with a complete match of the clinical ventricular tachycardia (VT) morphology.

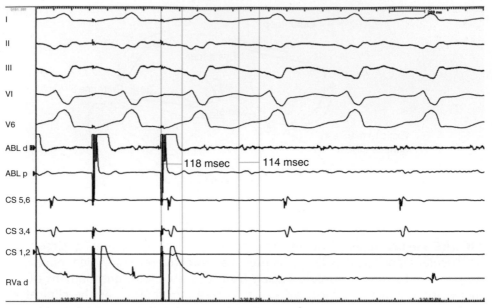

Paced QRS morphology is identical to VT QRS morphology
Postpacing interval = VT cycle length (440 msec)
Stimulus to QRS = spontaneous electrogram to QRS (118 msec)

FIGURE 10-14. Demonstration of all three criteria for an excellent ablation site in the same ventricular tachycardia (VT) shown in Figure 10-13.

tolerance, terminating or accelerating the VT during pacing, or pacing-induced changing VT morphologies. Too large an isthmus, endocardial clot or epicardial fat, and intramural location are factors preventing a successful ablation even when entrainment mapping appears to have identified a reasonable site.

Substrate mapping has been suggested as an alternative approach for ablating VT, particularly for VT which is not hemodynamically tolerated. This technique involves mapping the ventricle of interest during sinus rhythm. Areas of low voltage indicating scar are identified. Lesions are then created between areas of scar and anatomic barriers (e.g., mitral valve annulus).

SPECIFIC CLINICAL PATTERNS: IDENTIFICATION AND MANAGEMENT

Anterior Wall Myocardial Infarction

Anterior wall MIs cover a large potential mass of myocardium and the ECG patterns associated with these infarcts can be quite varied (Fig. 10-10). LBBB-like patterns arising from the septum can have a superior or inferior axis. Apical septal VTs with superior axis can show negative concordance. In this case there are Q waves in lead I and aVL. LBBB-like patterns and inferior axis have a right and inferior axis and Qs in I and aVL.

Concordance is rarer in this variety. Anterior MIs with RBBB morphology always have a qR morphology in the midprecordium. QS complexes can be seen in I, II, and III whenever VTs arise at the inferoapical region. It is difficult to distinguish septum from free wall when there is an R in aVR and aVL. When there is a diminution of R in aVL versus aVR the exit is on the free wall. Inferior axis is usually directed rightward.

Inferior Myocardial Infarction

Compared with anterior infarctions, inferior MIs are associated with more focal myocardial damage and related VTs are easier to locate from the ECG. In general these VTs activate the heart from back to front and result in large R waves in the precordial leads (V_2-V_4 or V_5) regardless of the BBB pattern. There are no Q waves in I or aVL. The R waves may decrease in size toward the lateral leads (V_4-V_6) if the infarct is in the posterolateral left ventricle.

VT due to CAD can be treated with ablation during the tachycardia if the rhythm is hemodynamically tolerated or substrate-based ablation if the rhythm is not tolerated. Antiarrhythmic drugs that are effective and commonly employed in CAD-based VT include amiodarone, sotalol, and dofetilide.

Right Ventricular Outflow Tract Ventricular Tachycardia

These are triggered VTs due to DADs that are characterized by a LBBB morphology with an inferior axis. These VTs often occur in settings of catecholamine excess (e.g., during stress testing).

The RVOT is described as anterior or posterior and septal or free wall (Figs. 10-5 and 10-11). Septal sites are associated with a more narrow QRS (<140 msec) whereas free wall sites tend to have a wider QRS in V_1. Similarly, the R wave in the inferior leads is often of lower amplitude and notched in free wall tachycardias presumably because the RV and LV are activated in sequence. Conversely, the R wave associated with septal tachycardias is often monophasic due to simultaneous activation of both ventricles.

The anterior (septal) aspect of the RVOT is both anterior and leftward and VTs arising there have a right inferior axis (negative in lead I and aVL, 90 to 180 degrees), whereas posterior sites in the RVOT are both posterior and rightward and more likely to cause a VT with a left inferior axis (positive in lead, 0 to 90 degrees). The precordial lead in which the R wave becomes greater than the S wave is described as the site of R wave *transition*. In RVOT VT the transition occurs at V_3 or V_4. This transition may occur earlier with sites close to the RV inflow tract posteriorly and later with anterior and free wall sites (Figs. 10-5 and 10-11).

Left Ventricular Outflow Tract Ventricular Tachycardia

These VTs most often originate from the posterior aspect of the left ventricular septal outflow tract below the aortic valve, the region of the aortomitral continuity on the epicardium, or in the left or right coronary cusp (Fig. 10-11). LVOTs from the basal septum or from the right coronary cusp have an rS, RS, or R in I with a vertical or slightly left inferior axis because the LVOT is inferior, posterior, and rightward from the RVOT (especially the superior aspect of the RVOT). Those arising from the left coronary cusp have a right inferior axis and an rS in I. They frequently have a w-shaped QRS in V_1. All LVOTs with a LBBB configuration have a transition that occurs earlier than that seen with RVOT VT (by V_2-V_3). The R in V_1-V_2 is larger and broader than seen in RVOT VTs. LVOT VTs which arise from the aortomitral continuity on the epicardium usually have a RBBB with a qR or RS in V_1 with a regression of the R in V_2 and a relatively narrow QRS. In these LVOT VTs there is no S in V_6.

Fascicular and Mitral Annular Ventricular Tachycardia

Triggered VT due to DADs can occur from other sites in the ventricle in addition to the RVOT and LVOT. Two common sites are the fascicles of the left bundle branch (LBB) and the mitral annulus. They behave like other VTs described earlier in that they are catecholamine sensitive. They may be seen early after MI, following reperfusion (either produced by coronary artery bypass graft [CABG] or angioplasty/stenting), and in particular, due to digitalis intoxication.

Fascicular VTs are relatively narrow, and typically have a classic RBBB/left anterior hemiblock (LAH) or RBBB/left posterior hemiblock (LPH) configuration (see Fig. 10-15). The initial forces are rapidly inscribed. On some occasions they have an intermediate axis because of retrograde conduction in the fascicle of origin and antegrade conduction down the other fascicle and even the right bundle branch (RBB). In the setting of infarction the fascicular rhythm originates closer to the infarcted myocardium and, consequently, the QRS complexes are a little wider and almost always exhibit a classical fascicular block pattern. Digitalis-induced fascicular rhythms can progress to a bidirectional tachycardia, with alternating inferior and superior axes. The physicians have also seen bidirectional tachycardias in the absence of digitalis. More recently, catecholamine-induced polymorphic VTs have been described due to ryanodine receptor or calsequestran receptor defects that are often initiated by a bidirectional VT.

VTs arising from the mitral annulus all have RBBB patterns with the axis dependent on whether the origin is superior, lateral (posterior), or inferior. In all cases R waves persist through V_6. In those VTs arising superiorly near the aortic valve there is concordance of the QRS' with no S wave in V_6. These may be endocardial or epicardial.

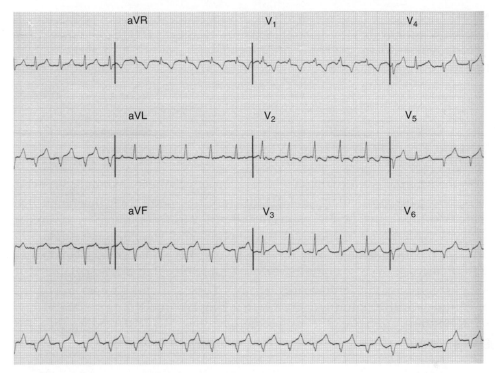

FIGURE 10-15. A 12-lead electrocardiogram of a fascicular ventricular tachy-cardia (VT) coming from the top of the left posterior fascicle. The third complex from the end of the tracing demonstrates a capture beat.

Idiopathic Verapamil-Sensitive Ventricular Tachycardia

This form of tachycardia is characterized by a RBBB with left axis deviation most often and less frequently, RBBB with right superior axis deviation. It occurs most often in young men and is not exercise or catecholamine dependent. There is some evidence that a similar VT can also occur in patients with organic heart disease. This tachycardia is frequently called *fascicular tachycardia*, but this is believed to be inappropriate because this VT is due to reentry and it is not clear whether the Purkinje system is actually a necessary component of the reentrant circuit. In most one can demonstrate an inverse relationship of the coupling interval of the ventricular premature complex (VPC) initiating the VT or the drive-paced cycle length and the interval to the onset of the VT. Most importantly these VTs can be entrained with fusion from either the ventricle or atrium, a diagnostic feature of reentry.

In many cases a late potential can be observed on the LV septum which can be traced to an exit site on the inferior septum. Purkinje spikes are often seen near the onset of the QRS, but the earliest Purkinje fiber and terminal late potential do not always correlate. Furthermore, these VTs can be entrained from the atrium with normalization of the QRS and HV interval.

Na channel blockers, but not vagal maneuvers or adenosine, can also terminate this VT. Chronic therapy includes calcium channel blockers or other forms of antiarrhythmic drugs. Alternatively, ablation is an excellent option but the best mapping technique is debatable. Pace mapping, entrainment mapping, earliest Purkinje fiber, and earliest ventricular activation have all been used with success. Multiple techniques are most often used.

Bundle Branch Reentrant Ventricular Tachycardia

BBR tachycardia is a form of VT which incorporates the main bundle branches or occasionally, particularly in CAD, the fascicles (intrafascicular reentry) as critical components of the reentrant circuit. Most commonly it occurs in patients with severe myocardial dysfunction and His-Purkinje conduction disease, but occasionally may be seen in patients with primary conduction system disease. It is a common type of monomorphic VT associated with idiopathic dilated cardiomyopathy (IDCM). These patients have an incomplete or complete LBBB pattern in sinus with a long HV interval.

Reentrant excitation goes anterogradely down the RBB and up the LBB, giving rise to a LBBB pattern with a left superior axis (see Fig. 10-16). In

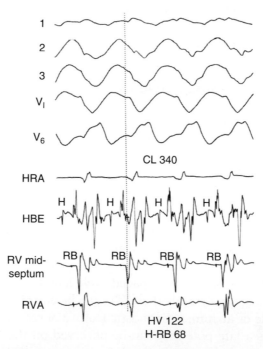

FIGURE 10-16. Bundle branch reentry ventricular tachycardia (VT). The His bundle electrogram (HBE) is shown preceding the RB (right bundle) electrogram. The morphology of the VT is left bundle branch with left axis deviation. HRA, high right atrium; RV, right ventricle, RVA, right ventricular apex.

this instance, the HV interval approximates the HV in sinus rhythm, but may be slightly longer if there is delay in the RBB. The H precedes the RBB and follows the LBB. More rarely the circuit is reversed in which case incomplete RBBB is seen in sinus rhythm. Ablation is easy and is highly successful in macroreentrant bundle branch reentry by targeting the RBB just distal to the location of the His potential.

Intrafascicular Reentry

This is the rule in patients with anterior MI complicated by RBBB and fascicular block. RBBB is fixed; therefore, reentry occurs down the apparently unblocked fascicle and up the "blocked" fascicle. Activation retrogradely goes to the LBB and His while simultaneously going down a fascicle. This gives rise to an "HV" interval much shorter than in sinus, usually 60 msec, with a reversal of sequence of His and LBB. Ablation is much more difficult in intrafascicular reentry. In either case, those patients with diseased hearts often have multiple additional intramyocardial reentrant VTs and require concomitant implantable cardioverter defibrillator (ICD) placement.

ARRHYTHMOGENIC RIGHT VENTRICULAR DYSPLASIA

Arrhythmogenic right ventricular dysplasia (ARVD) or RV cardiomyopathy is characterized by fibrofatty infiltration of the RV. RV tachycardia associated with ARVD must be distinguished from idiopathic RVOT VT. VTs associated with ARVD may arise in the RVOT (see Fig. 10-17) and can be difficult to differentiate from RVOT VT. Clues to the presence of ARVD include multiple morphologies of VT or VPCs from different sites within the RV, T wave inversions in the right precordial leads, a delay in the upstroke of the S in V_1 >60 msec, an epsilon wave, a positive signal average ECG and evidence of fatty infiltration, and RV dysfunction by magnetic resonance imaging (MRI).

In the physicians' experience VTs most commonly occur at the RV inflow tract, using the tricuspid annulus as a fixed boundary of the reentrant circuit. ICDs are used in high-risk patients. The role of ablation ranges from adjunctive to ICDs to primary therapy in patients with extensive scar and tolerated monomorphic VT. Sotalol is frequently used as a first-line antiarrhythmic drug in ARVD. (See Chapter 13 for more detail.)

Tetralogy of Fallot

VT occurs in 12% of patients and sudden death in 8% of patients by the age of 35 with corrected tetralogy of Fallot. Common VT circuits in this population involve the ventricular septal defect (VSD) patch as well as the RVOT (infundibular) scar. Ablation can be successful but is difficult. If VT is

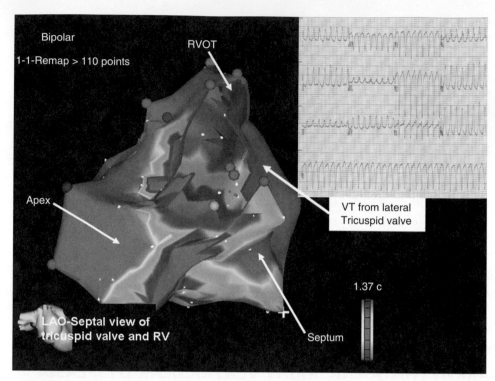

FIGURE 10-17. Electroanatomic map of a patient with arrhythmogenic right ventricular dysplasia (ARVD). The tricuspid valve is shown with areas of low voltage (red) representing characteristically affected regions with ARVD. This patient presented with the LBBB/inferior axis VT arising from an area lateral to the tricuspid annulus. LBBB, left bundle branch block; VT, ventricular tachycardia; LAO, left anterior oblique; RVOT, right ventricular outflow tract. (See color insert.)

not successfully ablated ICD placement is warranted in patients who present with sustained ventricular arrhythmias, sudden death, or unexplained syncope. Some data suggests that a QRS duration >180 msec portends an increased risk of ventricular arrhythmias.

DIFFERENTIAL DIAGNOSIS

Common entities in the differential diagnosis of left and RBBB morphology wide complex rhythms include:

LBBB morphologies

- RV VT
- CAD-related VT from the septum

- BBR VT (most commonly LBBB with left superior axis)

- SVT with aberration

- Atriofascicular tachycardia (LBBB with normal axis)

RBBB morphologies

- CAD-related VT

- LVOT VT

- Intrafascicular tachycardia (RBBB with either left or right axis deviation)

- SVT with aberration

SELECTED BIBLIOGRAPHY

Delacrataz E, Stevenson W. Catheter ablation of ventricular tachycardia in patients with coronary heart disease, part 1 and 2. *Pacing Clin Electrophysiol*. 2001;24:1261–1277.

Gatzoulis M, Balaji S, Webber S, et al. Risk factors for arrhythmia and sudden cardiac death late after repair of tetrology of Fallot: A multicenter study. *Lancet*. 2000;356:975–981.

Josephson ME. *Clinical cardiac electrophysiology*, 4th ed. Philadelphia: Lippincott Williams & Wilkins; 2008.

Miller JM, Das MK, Yadav AV, et al. Value of the 12-lead ECG in wide QRS tachycardia. *Cardiol Clin*. 2006;24:439–451.

Stevenson W, Friedman PL, Sager PT, et al. Exploring postinfarction reentrant ventricular tachycardia with entrainment mapping. *J Am Coll Cardiol*. 1997;29:1180–1189.

Bradycardias

CLINICAL SYNDROME

Sinus node dysfunction is characterized by disorders of impulse formation in and conduction out of the sinus node (see Table 11-1). Electrocardiographically these abnormalities in sinus node function are characterized by sinus bradycardia or pauses. The most common cause of apparent sinus node dysfunction is sinus arrhythmia. Sinus arrhythmia is defined by a maximum of 160 msec difference between the shortest and longest PP intervals. Respiratory sinus arrhythmia is common in the young but dissipates with aging. It is manifested as a gradual increase in heart rate with inspiration and decrease with expiration. Sinus arrhythmia may be present in older age but in this instance is not a respiratory phenomenon. Ventriculophasic sinus arrhythmia is a unique arrhythmia associated with complete heart block. In this case the PP interval surrounding the QRS complex is shorter than the PP interval following the QRS complex (see Fig. 11-1). Heightened vagal tone (VT) from any cause can result in sinus bradycardia or pauses. Common clinical circumstances associated with vagal surges include sleep (particularly during the apneic phase of obstructive sleep apnea), nausea, vomiting, hiccups, coughing, or gagging. In the hospitalized patient on a ventilator, suctioning of the airway is a frequent cause of sinus bradycardia and pauses.

Common causes of nonvagally induced sinus node dysfunction include aging (fibrosis) and suppression by medications (e.g., β-blockers,

163

TABLE 11-1 Sinus Node Dysfunction

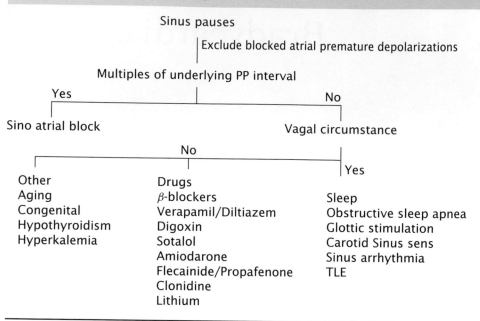

Sinus pauses

Exclude blocked atrial premature depolarizations

Multiples of underlying PP interval

Yes | No

Sino atrial block | Vagal circumstance

No | Yes

Other	Drugs	Sleep
Aging	β-blockers	Obstructive sleep apnea
Congenital	Verapamil/Diltiazem	Glottic stimulation
Hypothyroidism	Digoxin	Carotid Sinus sens
Hyperkalemia	Sotalol	Sinus arrhythmia
	Amiodarone	TLE
	Flecainide/Propafenone	
	Clonidine	
	Lithium	

TLE, temporal lobe epilepsy.

nondihydropyridine calcium channel blockers, digoxin, antiarrhythmic drugs, and the chronic use of lithium). Sick sinus syndrome refers to sinus node dysfunction often in association with atrial fibrillation. This commonly manifests as sinus bradycardia after conversion of atrial fibrillation. Tachybrady syndrome is similar to sick sinus syndrome (SSS) but includes other forms of supraventricular tachycardia such as atrial tachycardia. These syndromes may be associated with conduction abnormalities in the atrioventricular (AV) node as well as the sinus node.

Hypothyroidism, hyperkalemia, and hypothermia are less common causes of sinus bradycardia. Trauma to the sinus node associated with cardiac

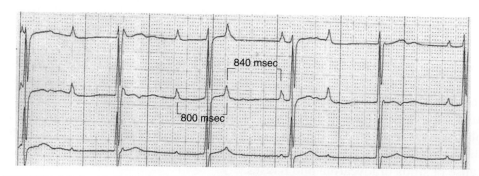

840 msec

800 msec

FIGURE 11-1. Ventriculophasic conduction during complete atrioventricular (AV) block with a shorter PP interval surrounding the QRS than between the QRS complexes.

surgery can cause sinus node dysfunction (if the right atrium is entered). This can occur in adults, particularly with redo valve surgery or in children following correction of congenital heart disease (e.g., Fontan procedure). Familial sinus node dysfunction is an autosomal dominant disorder. It is characterized by a familial pattern of sinus node dysfunction at young age (e.g., early 20s) with an associated mutation in a gene, HCN 4, which codes for a pacemaker ion channel.

ATRIOVENTRICULAR CONDUCTION DISEASE

AV conduction disease can occur in the AV node or below the AV node (infranodal) within the His bundle or Purkinje system. Occasionally extrasystoles arising from the His bundle can result in AV block. These may be difficult to identify on the surface electrocardiogram (ECG) as they can conduct retrogradely to the atrium but not antegradely to the ventricle (i.e., concealed) (see Fig. 11-2). The most common causes of complete heart block are fibrocalcific degeneration (Lev disease) and idiopathic degeneration (LeNegre disease) of the conduction system, which is genetically based. A common clinical example of fibrocalcific destruction of the conduction system is heart block related to calcification of the mitral annulus. Other causes of heart block are discussed in the following text.

Infection

Endocarditis with abscess formation in the region of the AV node and His-Purkinje system (HPS) can result in conduction abnormalities including heart

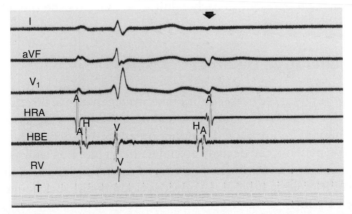

FIGURE 11-2. Demonstration of a concealed His extrasystole. A His potential precedes the atrial electrogram. The surface leads show a negative P wave in lead 2 due to retrograde conduction through the AV node. Antegrade conduction to the ventricle does not occur resulting in the absence of an associated QRS complex. AV, atrioventricular; HRA, high right atrium; HBE, His bundle electrogram; RV, right ventricular.

block. Abscesses involving the right and noncoronary cusp regions of the aortic valve are most often responsible for conduction abnormalities due to invasion of the AV node (noncoronary cusp) or proximal HPS (right coronary cusp). Lyme disease is an important cause of AV nodal block, which presents as a secondary manifestation of infection. It rarely if ever involves the infranodal conduction system and is generally reversible with antibiotic treatment.

Acute myocarditis can present with complete heart block in any region of the conduction system. When this occurs it is usually accompanied by a fulminant myocarditis which may or may not recover.

Infiltrative diseases such as sarcoidosis and benign tumors such as rhabdomyomas or malignancy can cause conduction disease.

Congenital Atrioventricular Block

Congenital AV block may be associated with maternal systemic lupus erythematosus (with anti-Rho and anti-La antibodies) or may occur as an independent entity. It causes AV nodal conduction disease ranging from a prolonged PR interval to complete heart block. It is increasingly recognized in infancy with improved prenatal diagnostic testing. It is not unusual for prolonged AV nodal Wenckebach periodicity or 2:1 block to persist for years and then deteriorate into complete heart block. Patients will often present with diminished exercise tolerance. Predictors of mortality in these patients include ventricular ectopy particularly in association with a prolonged QT interval, mitral regurgitation, and progressive left ventricular dysfunction.

Corrected (L type) transposition of the great vessels is associated with complete heart block. Some forms of familial dilated cardiomyopathy are also associated with progressive conduction disease. In this latter disorder the conduction disease may present in early adulthood and precede the development of ventricular dysfunction.

Neurodegenerative Disorders

Myotonic dystrophy is the most common neurodegenerative disease associated with conduction disease. It is an autosomal dominant disorder associated with the development of an infranodal conduction abnormality (without cardiomyopathy). These patients can develop complete heart block as well as ventricular tachycardia due to bundle branch reentry. Conduction disease may present with modest PR prolongation or the new development of a fascicular or bundle branch block (BBB).

Emery Dreifuss syndrome is a severe form of X-linked muscular dystrophy associated with complete heart block, atrial fibrillation, and dilated cardiomyopathy. Duchenne and Beckers muscular dystrophy are also associated dilated cardiomyopathy and varying degrees of AV conduction abnormality and atrial dysrhythmias. Limb Girdle muscular dystrophy is also associated with

AV conduction disease. Other forms of neuromuscular disease associated with conduction abnormalities include Erb dystrophy and Kearns-Sayre syndrome.

Heart Block Associated with Trauma

The AV node or His bundle can be damaged during aortic valve surgery. Mitral valve surgery may result in damage to the His bundle. This damage may be permanent or reversible if due to edema. The physicians typically wait 4 to 7 days for recovery of conduction before placing a permanent pacemaker in these patients. Closure of ventricular septal defects (VSDs), whether surgical (particularly with AV canal repairs) or catheter-based can also result in HPS damage.

Paroxysmal Atrio Ventricular Block

This disorder is characterized by the abrupt development of AV block associated with the slowing of impulses reaching the HPS. This can be due to slowing of the sinus rate following premature atrial, His, or ventricular beats, or during posttachycardia pauses (see Fig. 11-3). It is an important cause of unrecognized syncope and is a manifestation of infranodal conduction disease that caused phase 4 depolarization in abnormal tissue.

Conduction Disease Associated with Myocardial Infarction

The conduction disease associated with inferior myocardial infarction (IMI) occurs in two main stages. High-degree AV block, even associated with sinus tachycardia, may be seen in the first 24 hours following infarction (see Figs. 11-4 and 11-5). This is likely due to the Bezold Jarsch reflex and is

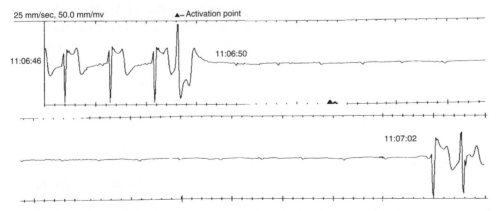

FIGURE 11-3. Ventricular premature depolarization results in paroxysmal atrioventricular (AV) block.

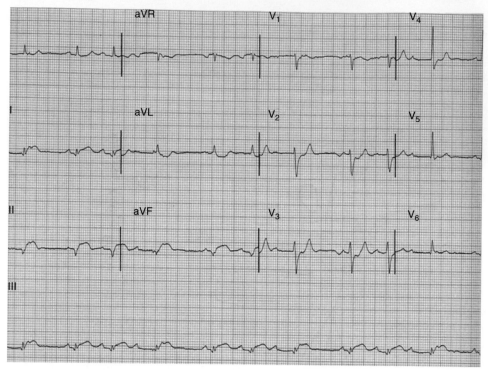

FIGURE 11-4. Inferior myocardial infarction with ST elevation in leads II and III and aVF with atrioventricular (AV) Wenckebach with a sinus rate of 100 beats per minute (bpm).

atropine sensitive. A second, later stage begins day 2 or 3 after myocardial infarction (MI) and occurs in a predictable sequence (PR prolongation, followed by type 1 second degree AV block followed by complete heart block). These abnormalities occur predominantly with occlusion of the proximal right coronary artery (RCA) and may have concomitant right ventricular (RV) infarction. Occlusion of the sinus node branches of the RCA can rarely result in sinus bradycardia or atrial fibrillation. More often sinus bradycardia results from heightened Vagal tone. The RCA supplies the AV node, which may produce PR prolongation, Mobitz 1, and complete heart block with a narrow complex escape rhythm. Conduction abnormalities present within the first few hours of infarction and are due to ischemia and heightened Vagal tone. Abnormalities that persist beyond 24 to 48 hours are due to edema and almost always normalize after 7 to 10 days. In this setting, the loss of AV synchrony can result in significant hemodynamic compromise. Temporary pacing may be helpful but the risk of RV perforation must be considered.

Conduction disease with anterior MI affects the conduction system below the AV node. Conduction abnormalities with anterior MI occur abruptly, are irreversible, and only develop with large infarctions. These abnormalities most commonly include left anterior fascicular block (LAFB), bifascicular

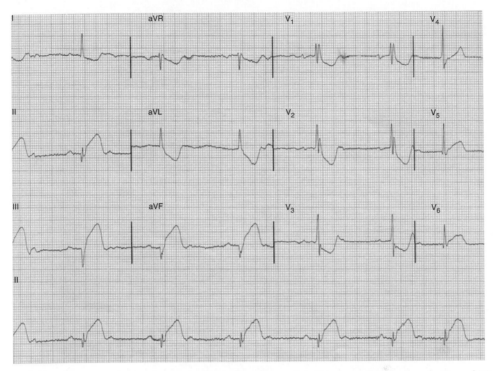

FIGURE 11-5. Inferior myocardial infarction with ST elevation in leads II and III and aVF with 2:1 block. The sixth QRS complex is brought in with a long PR interval.

block (most commonly LAFB and right bundle branch block [RBBB]) (see Fig. 11-6A), and complete heart block with a wide complex escape. Conduction abnormalities with acute myocardial infarction (AMI) are related to the size of the infarction as opposed to autonomic reflexes. They typically occur 24 to 48 hours into an infarction, in an unpredictable manner, and are associated with large infarctions and severe hemodynamic compromise. Left BBB may occur with anterior MI but is often a transient occurrence. If it persists it is indicative of extensive tissue necrosis.

DIAGNOSIS

Symptoms/Signs

The diagnosis and appropriate management of bradyarrhythmias rely primarily on the electrocardiographic demonstration of the arrhythmia and correlation with symptoms.

Sinus pauses and bradycardia are often asymptomatic and do not necessarily warrant intervention unless symptoms correlate with electrocardiographic

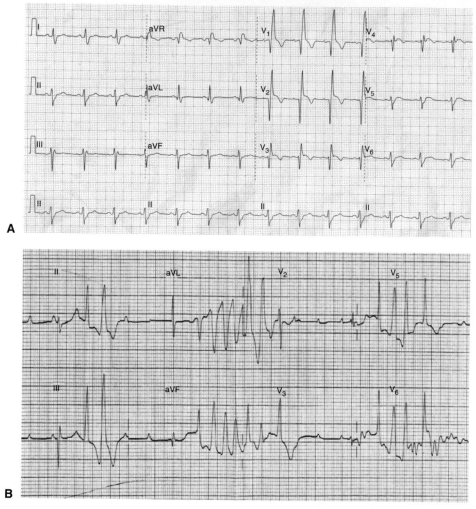

FIGURE 11-6. A: Electrocardiogram displaying right bundle branch block (RBBB) and left anterior fascicular block (LAFB) with q waves in the precordial leads indicative of prior anterior wall myocardial infarction (MI). **B:** Complete heart block with QT prolongation and polymorphic ventricular tachycardia.

demonstration of conduction disease. Symptoms, when they occur, vary from fatigue to syncope. The optimal way to demonstrate a symptom-rhythm correlation is with an ambulatory event recorder. Patients with exercise-related symptoms such as fatigue should have a stress test. This is the optimal way to identify chronotropic incompetence due to sinus node dysfunction. Chronotropic incompetence refers to the inability to augment the sinus rate in response to demand. There is no absolute definition of this abnormality but in general it can be inferred by the inability to reach a heart rate of 100 bpm in response to maximal exertion. Intra-His disease can also be identified with exercise by the development of conduction block at increasing heart rate. The most common complaints associated with complete heart block are fatigue and decreased exercise tolerance. A particularly common scenario is the elderly patient with complete AV block who presents with lethargy, preserved or elevated systolic blood pressure, and renal insufficiency due to a low output state. Heart block can also result in hypotension and syncope (Stokes Adams attack) or polymorphic Vagal tone associated with bradycardia-related QT prolongation (see Fig. 11-6B).

Electrocardiogram Clues to Diagnosis

Sinoatrial (SA) exit block can occur in two forms, first and second degree. First degree is impossible to discern on the surface ECG. Second degree has two types, type 1 and 2. Type 1 demonstrates Wenckebach periodicity with progressively shorter PP intervals before a longer PP interval (pause) including the blocked sinus beat. Type 2 is characterized by a pause that is an exact multiple of the underlying PP intervals. There may be an up to 10 msec variation in the intervals and still qualify as SA exit block (see Fig. 11-7). Sinus pauses are generally not considered significant if <3 seconds.

Conduction disease in the AV node typically manifests as a prolonged PR interval (e.g., "first-degree AV block") or Mobitz 1 AV block. Markedly prolonged PR intervals (e.g., >300 msec) are almost always due to AV nodal disease. This is illustrated by the example that if a PR interval of 200 msec represents an AH interval of 150 msec with an HV of 50 msec, an increase in the PR interval to 300 msec would be more likely to have resulted from an increase in the AH interval to 250 msec compared with a threefold prolongation in the HV interval to 150 msec.

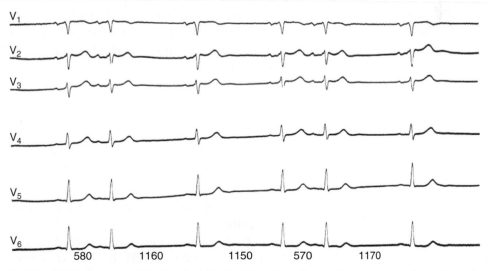

FIGURE 11-7. Sinoatrial exit block. The duration of the pause is twice the sinus rate of identified P waves.

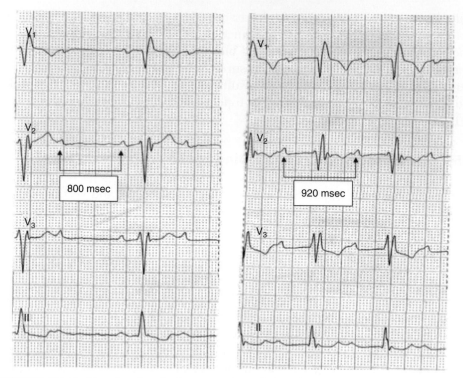

FIGURE 11-8. Conduction is improved at slower heart rates (920 msec) compared with 2:1 conduction at more rapid rates (800 msec).

Block below the AV node is often associated with a normal or minimally prolonged PR interval (i.e., Mobitz 2).

Block in the AV node and sometimes in the His bundle is generally associated with a narrow complex escape rhythm. Infranodal block below the His bundle has a wide complex escape rhythm. Block at faster sinus heart rates, which improves at slower sinus heart rates suggests block below the AV node (see Fig. 11-8).

The presence of retrograde conduction with pacing or ventricular premature depolarizations (VPDs) in the setting of antegrade heart block is consistent with antegrade block below the AV node, whereas AV nodal antegrade block is never associated with intact retrograde conduction. An understanding of these clinical findings can help identify the location of block in patients with 2:1 AV block (see Table 11-2).

Bifascicular block refers to RBBB with either left anterior or posterior fascicular block. This is not an indication for pacing unless it develops in the setting of AMI (see subsequent text). Trifascicular block is a misnomer in that it represents bifascicular block with prolonged conduction rather than true block in the AV node or His bundle (prolonged PR interval). Trifascicular block is not an indication for pacing unless it is a consequence of AMI or it is associated with unexplained syncope.

TABLE 11-2	**Determining the Site of Block from the Electrocardiogram (ECG)**

The ECG can be helpful in determining the site of AV block. Factors which favor a site of AV block in the AV node include the following:

1. Narrow QRS duration (suggesting an absence of baseline infranodal conduction disease)
2. Long PR interval (>0.30 sec) on the conducted beats. PR durations of >0.30 suggest predominant delay in the AV node because prolongation of the HV interval to that degree is very unlikely
3. Improvement in conduction with maneuvers which reduce vagal tone, e.g., atropine, exercise

Factors which favor an infranodal site of AV conduction delay include the following:

1. Wide QRS duration (suggest underlying His-Purkinje disease)
2. Normal or mildly increased duration PR interval
3. Worsened conduction with maneuvers which reduce vagal tone or increase heart rate (e.g., atropine, exercise) and improvement in conduction with slowing of the heart rate

AV, atrioventricular.

Electrophysiology Laboratory Evaluation

Sinus node dysfunction: The electrophysiologic (EP) laboratory evaluation of sinus node dysfunction is limited.

The standard evaluation of the sinus node in the electrophysiology study begins with carotid sinus massage. The corrected sinus node recovery time (CSNRT) is assessed at multiple pacing cycle lengths and is considered abnormal if >500 msec. Further evidence of sinus node dysfunction is a lack of response to atropine.

AV nodal conduction: An AV nodal Wenckebach cycle length of >600 msec (heart rates of slower than 100 bpm) are abnormal but are often influenced by Vagal tone.

Prolongation of the HV interval to >100 msec following the infusion of intravenous procainamide as is block in or below the His bundle at pace cycle lengths <400 msec (heart rates of <150 bpm) (see Figs. 11-9 and 11-10).

TREATMENT

The context in which bradycardia occurs influences the aggressiveness of therapy. If sinus pauses, sinus bradycardia or higher-degree conduction abnormalities in the AV node occur only during sleep; particularly if associated with periods of apnea, pacemaker implantation is rarely required.

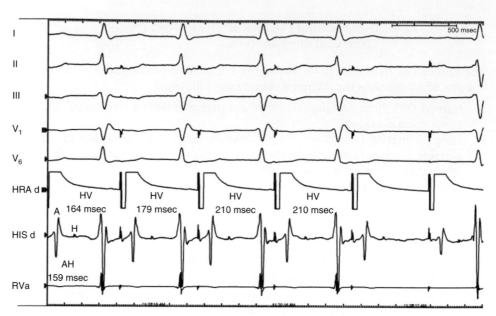

FIGURE 11-9. High right atrial pacing at 500 msec results in progressive HV prolongation and block below the His bundle.

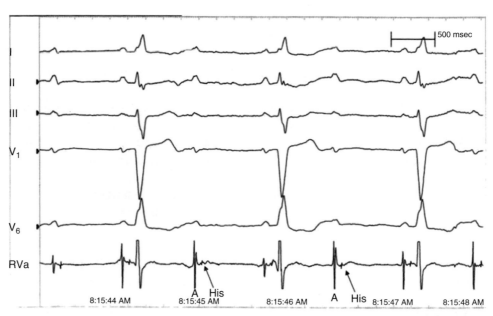

FIGURE 11-10. A 2:1 conduction with block demonstrated after the His potential.

T A B L E 11-3 Potentially Reversible Causes of Complete Heart Block

Causes	Management
Medications	Withdraw and wait
Lyme disease	Antibiotics, temporary pacing
↑ Vagal tone	None unless repetitive and disabling
Ischemia (IMI)	Observation, temporary pacing
Trauma (e.g., PA catheter, CT surgery, ablation)	Observation for up to 5 d, temporary pacing

↑, increasing; IMI, inducible myocardial ischemia; PA, pulmonary artery; CT, computed tomography.

T A B L E 11-4 Indications for Pacemaker Implantation

Class 1
Sinus node
  Symptomatic sinus bradycardia (usually <40)
  Sinus pauses (usually >3 s) unassociated with sleep
  Symptomatic chronoscopic incompetence (usually <100 bpm at peak exertion)
  In patients with syncope felt due to carotid hypersensitivity—pause of >3 s with carotid sinus massage.
AV block
  Third-degree AV block
  High-grade AV block
  Symptomatic Mobitz 1 or 2 AV block
  Mobitz 2 with wide QRS or bifascicular block irrespective of symptoms
  In patients with congenital AV block: symptoms due to bradycardia, wide QRS escape rhythm, complex ventricular ectopy, LV dysfunction.
  In patients with neuromuscular disease: second- or third-degree AV block

Class 2 (weaker evidence than class 1 but reasonable if felt clinically indicated)
Chronic sinus rates <30 bpm during daytime with minimal symptoms
Prolonged PR intervals (>300 msec) with associated hemodynamic compromise
Bifascicular or trifascicular block with syncope not attributed to other causes (e.g., vasovagal mechanism or ventricular tachycardia)
In patients with neuromuscular disease: prolonged PR interval
Drug-induced bradycardia without alternative to discontinue offending medication
aParoxysmal AV block—generally identified during the evaluation of syncope

Class 3
SA exit block/sinus arrest without symptoms
Asymptomatic bradycardia during sleep
Carotid sinus hypersensitivity in the absence of symptoms
Bifascicular block without symptoms

aNot listed in formal American College of Cardiology (ACC)/American Heart Association (AHA) guidelines.
AV, atrioventricular; LV, left ventricular; SA, sinoatrial.

TABLE 11-5 Indications for Pacing Associated with Myocardial Infarction (MI)

Class	Temporary Pacing	Permanent Pacing
IMI class 1	Symptomatic bradycardia (including sinus bradycardia Mobitz 1 block or third AV block with hypotension or ventricular arrhythmias	Persistent symptomatic bradycardia beyond 7 to 10 d
AMI class 1	Bilateral BBB (alternating BBB or right BBB alternating with LAFB or LPFB)	Persistent second-degree AV block in the His-Purkinje system, with bilateral BBB or third-degree AV block within or below the His-Purkinje system post MI
	Bifascicular block that is new or of indeterminate age	
	(right BBB with LAFB or LPFB or LBBB) with a prolonged PR interval	
	Mobitz 2 block	
IMI class 2a	Recurring sinus pauses not responsive to atropine	None
AMI class 2a	RBBB and LAFB or LPFB that is new or age indeterminate	None
	RBBB with a prolonged PR interval	
	LBBB that is new or age indeterminate	
IMI 2b	None	None
AMI 2b	Bifascicular block of indeterminate age	None
	Isolated RBBB that is new or of indeterminate age	

IMI, inducible myocardial ischemia; AV, atrioventricular; AMI, acute myocardial infarction; BBB, bundle branch block; LAFB, left anterior fascicular block; LPFB, left posterior fascicular block; LBBB, left bundle branch block; RBBB, right bundle branch block.

(Modified from American College of Cardiology and the American Heart Association for Temporary and Permanent Implantation of Pacemakers in Patients with Acute Myocardial Infarction.)

Bradycardia due to medications should be managed with dose reduction or discontinuation if possible. Attempts at substituting β-blockers with sympathomimetic activity (pindolol, bisoprolol) for standard β-blockers can be attempted but is rarely clinically helpful. Reversible causes of conduction disease such as medications, infections such as Lyme disease or ischemia (inferior infarction) should always be excluded before permanent pacemaker implantation (see Table 11-3). Society-sponsored guidelines should be followed for pacemaker implantation (see Tables 11-4 and 11-5).

SELECTED BIBLIOGRAPHY

Josephson ME. *Clinical cardiac electrophysiology*, 3rd ed. Philadelphia: Lippincott Williams & Wilkins; 2003.

Josephson ME. *Clinical cardiac electrophysiology*, 4th ed. Philadelphia: Lippincott Williams & Wilkins; 2008.

Michaelsson M, Jonzon A, Riesenfeld T. Isolated congenital complete atrioventricular block in adult life. A prospective study. *Circulation*. 1995;92:442–449.

Syncope

Syncope will occur in up to 50% of the population and is defined by the abrupt loss of consciousness due to cerebral hypoperfusion. Syncope must be distinguished from seizures, in which case loss of consciousness occurs without cerebral hypoperfusion, falls, drop attacks without loss of consciousness, falling asleep, and psychogenic episodes. In the vast majority of instances there is insufficient monitoring (blood pressure, pulse) at the time of the clinical event to clearly identify the cause. It is therefore necessary to rely heavily on the description of the event from the patient and witnesses as well as the medical history of the patient and first-degree family members. Close attention to these factors will help guide a focused clinical evaluation.

DIFFERENTIAL DIAGNOSIS

Reflex Syncope

Neurally mediated or reflex syncope accounts for >50% of syncope diagnoses (see Table 12-1). This category of diseases includes neurocardiogenic syncope (a term which encompasses vasovagal and vasodepressor syncope); carotid sinus hypersensitivity; and situational causes such as syncope associated with prolonged standing, micturition, defecation, or coughing. Vasovagal syncope can occur at any age. It may or may not be associated with a prodrome of

TABLE 12-1 General Categories of Syncope

Reflex Syncope	Obstructive Causes	Arrhythmias	Orthostasis	Seizures
Neurocardiogenic	Aortic stenosis	Bradycardia	Blood loss	Grand mal
Carotid sinus hypersensitivity	HCM	Tachycardia	Autonomic insufficiency	—
	Pulmonary embolus	—	—	—
Situational	Pulmonary HTN	—	Drug-induced	—
	Atrial myxoma	—	Adrenal insufficiency	—

HCM, hypertrophic cardiomyopathy; HTN, hypertension.

nausea and/or vomiting. The mechanism is believed to be related to autonomic activation. In most instances, a decrease in venous filling such as occurs with peripheral venous pooling results in a compensatory sympathetic activation to maintain blood pressure. This activates peripheral baroreceptors, most notably those in the aorta and occasionally C fibers in the inferoposterior aspect of the left ventricle (LV) (also activated with inferior myocardial ischemia as part of the Bezold-Jarisch reflex). There is a resultant central and eventual peripheral withdrawal of sympathetic tone and increase in parasympathetic tone. This may manifest in a number of ways including the following:

1. Bradycardia with sinus arrest and/or varying degrees of atrioventricular (AV) nodal block resulting in hypotension (cardioinhibitory response)

2. Marked vasodilation with a normal or slightly increased sinus rate (vasodepressor response)

3. Mixture of vasodilation and bradycardia

When bradycardia is noted, there is often gradual slowing of the sinus rate with or without AV block or a ventricular escape rhythm (see Fig. 12-1).

This disorder can develop at any age and may be associated with multiple affected family members. It is not unusual for recurrent episodes of neurally mediated syncope to occur over decades of life. Patients may experience these episodes in clusters. Attempts at preventing neurocardiogenic syncope are generally unsuccessful. Fortunately, this form of syncope rarely occurs in circumstances which could pose a high risk for damage such as driving a car. One exception is syncope in the bathroom where hard surfaces can inflict significant injury.

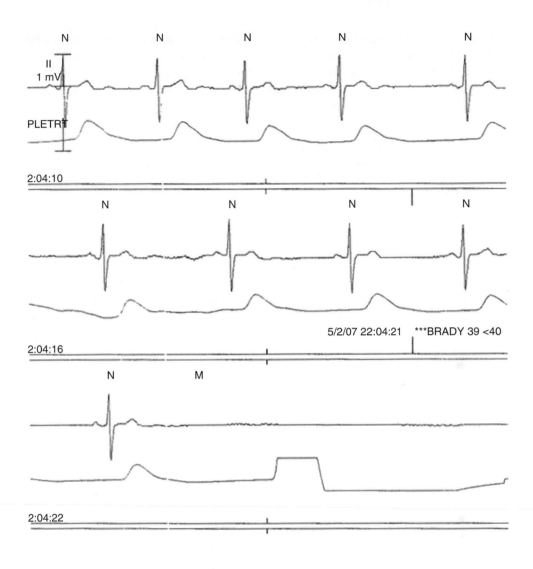

FIGURE 12-1. Sinus slowing and pause related to heightened vagal tone.

Carotid sinus hypersensitivity occurs through activation of an overly sensitive carotid body and is associated with prolonged periods of asystole and secondary hypotension. This disorder is rarely seen before the age of 40 and occurs most often in those older than 60 years of age.

Obstructive: Cardiopulmonary

Syncope can occur due to a drop in cardiac output in the setting of fixed or dynamic cardiovascular or pulmonary obstruction. Syncope can occur with critical aortic stenosis when vasodilation occurs and cardiac output cannot be sufficiently augmented. Hypertrophic obstructive cardiomyopathy can cause syncope particularly when associated with an acute drop in preload such as standing up quickly, often in the setting of dehydration. Rarely, intermittent obstruction of the mitral valve with a mobile mass such as a myxoma can result in syncope. Severe fixed pulmonary hypertension or pulmonary obstruction associated with a large pulmonary embolus can also result in syncope due to reduced LV filling and cardiac output.

Arrhythmic

Ventricular and less commonly supraventricular tachycardia (SVT) can cause syncope. Syncope in association with ventricular tachycardia (VT) is generally related to diminished output in a poorly functioning ventricle. Syncope due to VT can be the initial manifestation of acute myocardial infarction. Non-sustained polymorphic VT associated with acquired or congenital long QT syndrome is also an important cause of syncope. Children with unrecognized long QT syndrome may carry a history of syncope or seizure disorder until the QT interval is recognized to be abnormal. Non sustained polymorphic VT or VF can also be seen in patients without structural heart disease and can present with syncope or sudden death (see Fig. 12-2). Syncope in association with SVT (e.g., atrioventricular nodal reentrant tachycardia [AVNRT]) is very unusual but when it occurs it is felt likely due to a baroreceptor response and generally occurs immediately after the onset of SVT. Syncope in association with atrial fibrillation (AF) is a special circumstance. AF with preexcitation can result in syncope or sudden death due to the induction of ventricular arrhythmia. More commonly, AF is associated with syncope due to a pause at the time of conversion of AF to sinus rhythm (see Fig. 6-3). Atrial flutter associated with

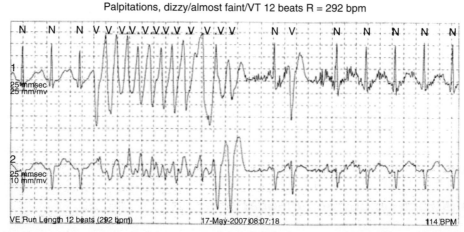

FIGURE 12-2. Polymorphic VT or VF associated with presyncope (see symptom log above the tracing). VT, ventricular tachycardia; BPM, beats per minute.

sodium channel blocking drugs such as flecainide or propafenone can produce a wide QRS complex and impaired myocardial contraction which can result in syncope.

Bradyarrhythmias can cause syncope due to sinus pauses or AV block. In general sinus pauses are >3 to 5 seconds when associated with syncope. AV block can occur in the AV node or below and if an escape rhythm is absent can result in syncope. A cause of high-grade AV block in the absence of apparent preexisting conduction disease is paroxysmal AV block. This disorder is characterized by the abrupt development of AV block with slight changes in the sinus rate or following a premature atrial or ventricular beat (see Chapter 11). It is a sporadic and unpredictable event.

Bradyarrhythmias, particularly complete heart block, can also result in QT prolongation and *torsade de pointes*.

Neuropsychiatric

The major neurologic causes of syncope include seizure disorder and autonomic insufficiency (discussed in subsequent text). Seizure disorder is an important cause of loss of consciousness, which must be distinguished from myoclonus which can occur with all forms of true syncope. It is important to stress that strokes and transient ischemic attacks (TIAs) *do not* cause syncope unless there is global cerebral hypoperfusion or a seizure as a consequence of a prior stroke. Vertebrobasilar insufficiency causes "drop attacks" which are manifested as a fall due to unsteadiness or feeling as though ones "legs gave out" *without* a loss of consciousness.

Psychogenic or pseudosyncope are witnessed or reported episodes of feigned syncope. Patients with this disorder frequently have a psychiatric history.

Orthostasis

Any cause of orthostasis can result in syncope. This is particularly common if the supine blood pressure already starts low (e.g., 100 mm Hg). Volume depletion, often caused by diuretic use, gastrointestinal bleeding, or viruses (with vomiting and/or diarrhea), or vasodepression due to medication use (antihypertensive drugs) are common reversible causes. More unusual causes of volume depletion and vasodepression include Addison disease and pheochromocytoma.

Autonomic insufficiency represents a neurologic cause of vasoregulatory syncope. This disorder can be divided into pure autonomic failure and multiple system atrophy. Pure autonomic failure occurs with Shy-Drager and Bradbury-Eggleston syndromes. The most common example of multiple system atrophy is Parkinson disease. Within the spectrum of these disorders is a recently described but relatively uncommon entity called the *postural orthostatic tachycardia syndrome (POTS)*. This disorder is characterized by an increase in heart rate associated with a gradual and modest reduction in blood pressure. It is distinguished from pure orthostasis with reflex tachycardia by the more modest drop in blood pressure and more protracted increase in heart rate (see Chapter 17). It is most common in young women and appears to be associated with lower extremity sympathetic denervation.

THE CLINICAL HISTORY

Symptoms and Circumstances

A detailed history of the event, including a description by onlookers, is extremely helpful in determining the mechanism of syncope (see Table 12-2). The description of vagal symptoms such as nausea and diaphoresis before, during, or after a syncopal episode is highly associated with a vasovagal etiology. The authors find that a description of fatigue or a feeling of being "washed out" after the event is highly correlated with a vagal etiology. In contrast to other causes of syncope, the vagal discharge with vasovagal syncope may result in a more prolonged period of hypotension. This often leads to recurrent syncope if a patient tries to stand up soon after a vasovagal episode. Vasovagal syncope can occur in clusters over the course of days.

Common circumstances associated with the development of reflex or "situational" syncope include prolonged standing in a hot crowded space (e.g., church, train), the sight of blood, micturition or defection, coughing, gagging,

---

TABLE 12-2   Useful Clinical Points

Syncope from any cause can result in significant injury; benign causes of syncope (reflex syncope) can occur abruptly and result in trauma

Stroke and TIAs do not cause syncope

Repetitive extremity movements do not necessarily mean seizure disorder; they can represent hypoxia driven myotonic movements from syncope due to any cause

Urinary incontinence can occur with any form of syncope not only seizure disorder

Syncope while driving is virtually never vasovagal in origin

Syncope associated with atrial fibrillation is usually from a conversion pause not tachycardia

Gray complexion favors arrhythmia

Green or pale complexion favors vasovagal mechanism

TIA, transient ischemic attack.

or drinking a cold beverage, following the termination of vigorous exercise or during extreme exercise. Witnesses will often describe the patient as appearing green or very pale in complexion.

Carotid sinus hypersensitivity resulting in prolonged bradycardia often occurs in association with neck turning. This disorder should be suspected in the setting of syncope while driving (e.g., looking over the shoulder to merge) or other circumstances in which pressure is applied to the neck.

If palpitations are described with syncope it is critical to have the patient define if they were very rapid (i.e., tap out different rates). Rapid palpitations suggest SVT or VT. In the rare circumstance in which syncope is due to AF with preexcitation it is usually associated with exertion or another high catecholamine state. This is because catecholamines reduce the refractory period of the accessory pathway (AP) and promote antegrade conduction over the AP. Atrial flutter with 1:1 conduction due to a class 1C antiarrhythmic drug can also result in hemodynamic collapse and syncope. In the physicians' experience this often occurs during abrupt exertion such as walking up a steep incline on a golf course. Bradyarrhythmias due to conduction disease rather than vagal triggers are difficult to identify by symptoms or circumstance. Witnesses of patients with tachyarrhythmia- or bradyarrhythmia-mediated syncope will often describe an ashen or gray complexion.

Syncope associated with driving is particularly concerning and should not be ascribed to a vasovagal mechanism. As noted earlier, carotid sinus hypersensitivity should be strongly considered. Other forms of arrhythmic syncope are also very possible. Falling asleep at the wheel is amongst the most common reasons for motor vehicle accidents felt to be due to syncope and can be suggested by a description of the accident site. Patients with arrhythmic syncope rarely recover in time to depress the brakes while a patient who has fallen asleep at the wheel will likely awaken in time to depress the brakes (and produce skid marks). Profound somnolence, particularly in the late afternoon, is characteristic of obstructive sleep apnea and should always be considered in patients who have met with unexplained motor vehicle accidents.

Psychogenic syncope should be considered in patients with repeated episodes of syncope and a complete absence of trauma, particularly if there is a history of a psychiatric disorder.

Syncope During Pregnancy

Syncope can be associated with pregnancy for all of the reasons described earlier. Many arrhythmias appear to occur in increased frequency during pregnancy (e.g., AVNRT, idiopathic VT) and may be less well tolerated due to a baseline reduced blood pressure as part of the normal physiology of pregnancy. Reflex syncope is common during pregnancy and may be related to decreased preload from uterine obstruction of the inferior vena cava. This is often associated with position such as lying supine or less commonly on the right side and may be relieved by avoiding these positions.

Syncope in the Athlete

Syncope on exertion in the conditioned athlete is uncommon but may represent the presenting sign for a lethal condition. In a series of athletes with sudden death, a history of prior syncope was obtained in approximately 20% of cases. Athletes are subject to all the causes of syncope mentioned earlier but the excess adrenergic activity favors the generation of arrhythmias in certain conditions including Wolff-Parkinson-White (WPW) syndrome, catecholaminergic polymorphic VT, hypertrophic obstructive cardiomyopathy, arrhythmogenic right ventricular cardiomyopathy, cardiac ischemia resulting from an anomalous coronary, premature coronary artery disease, or Kawasaki disease. The assessment of the electrocardiogram (ECG) and echocardiogram can be difficult in this population. Precordial ST elevation may be a normal finding. Deep horizontal ST depression with T-wave inversion should suggest an underlying cardiovascular abnormality. Bradyarrhythmias including sinus bradycardia and AV block are common at rest and are due to heightened vagal tone. They should resolve with activity. The echocardiogram in this population commonly shows findings consistent with an "athlete's heart." This condition is associated with an increase in LV mass manifested by increased LV cavity size (LV diastolic dimension) and thickness. In general, the hypertrophy is ≤12 to 13 mm but can be thicker and is often greater in the septum than the other walls making it difficult to distinguish from hypertrophic cardiomyopathy (HOCM). Most importantly, diastolic function by echocardiography is normal in the athlete's heart in contradistinction to the abnormal diastolic function generally associated with HOCM. Postexercise postural hypotension is common, particularly in highly conditioned runners and may result in syncope.

Distinguishing Syncope with Motor Movements from Epilepsy

As noted, it is not unusual for syncope from any cause to be associated with repetitive motor movements (i.e., myoclonus) or for the syncope to be unwitnessed and the diagnosis of seizure disorder empirically assigned. The erroneous diagnosis of seizure disorder is made often, particularly in children. Clinical characteristics that favor seizure disorder rather than syncope include lateral tongue biting and post–event profound somnolence of a greater degree than seen with reflex syncope (Todd paralysis). Urinary incontinence may occur in both situations and is not a useful discriminating feature. Witnesses will not generally note a change in complexion with seizures in contradistinction to vasovagal or arrhythmic causes of syncope.

DIAGNOSTIC EVALUATION

After a detailed history, the physical examination is important to identify murmurs associated with aortic stenosis or HOCM (see Table 12-3A). Orthostatic blood pressure measurements should be performed as should carotid sinus massage (CSM). Before CSM, the presence of carotid bruits must be excluded and a continuous ECG should be running. Family members should also be asked to leave the room. The carotid sinus is massaged at the level of the cricoid cartilage for 5 to 10 seconds. A positive result is defined by a >3 second pause and/or a drop in blood pressure of ≥50 mm Hg.

A 12-lead ECG is mandatory in all patients in whom reflex syncope is not the clear diagnosis (Table 12-3B). In young individuals, the evaluation should exclude WPW, Brugada syndrome, long QT syndrome, and abnormal voltage and ST changes suggestive of hypertrophic obstructive cardiomyopathy. Q waves should suggest VT as an etiology. Epsilon waves can identify arrhythmogenic right ventricle (RV) dysplasia. The presence of conduction disease (e.g., right bundle branch block [RBBB] and left anterior fascicular block [LAFB]) indicates infranodal conduction disease but by itself is not conclusive evidence of a bradyarrhythmic cause of syncope.

Ambulatory Monitoring

The goal of all syncope evaluation is to obtain a symptom-rhythm correlation. Unfortunately, the yield from standard ambulatory monitors (24- to 48-hour Holter, 14- to 30-day continuous or post–event recorders) is low because of the remote likelihood that the patient will have a recurrent syncopal event during that period of monitoring. Newer mobile cardiac outpatient telemetry (MCOT) devices allow long-term (e.g., event recorders) and continuous (e.g., Holters) monitoring with wireless download to a monitoring station. These devices provide the most comprehensive external monitoring available; however, the yield for identifying a cause of syncope is still likely to be low given the relatively short duration of monitoring (up to 1 month).

When an arrhythmic cause of syncope is suspected but the frequency of events is low, a long-term insertable loop recorder (ILR) is recommended. These devices have a total memory of 40 minutes with capacity for patient-triggered events as well as programmable automatic triggers for bradycardia and tachyarrhythmias including AF.

Exercise Testing

This is useful if the syncopal episode occurred during or immediately after exertion. The presence of heart block can be elucidated if there is His-Purkinje system (HPS) disease and polymorphic VT may be identified. Neurocardiogenic syncope may be identified post exercise.

TABLE 12-3 Evaluation Algorithm

A

Syncope

- Vital signs stable blood pressure (BP), pulse, and oxygen saturation
- No complaints of chest pain or shortness of breath
- Absence of significant trauma

Yes   No

Current syncopal episode associated with

1. Micturition/defecation
2. Eating
3. Pre-or postevent nausea or vomiting
4. Stationary position/crowded space
5. History of syncopal episode(s) >1 yr before current episode
6. Standing up (orthostatic change in BP)
7. Postevent fatigue–feeling "washed out"

Consider cardiology or Electctrophysiologic consult

Yes   No

No further evaluation required   Proceed with algorithm

B

Presence of:

1. Rapid palpitations

2. Multiple recent syncopal episodes (within 6 mo)

3. History of Coronary artery disease, hypertrophic, or dilated cardiomyopathy

4. History of congestive heart failure or left ventricular dysfunction

5. Family history (first-degree relative) with sudden death HOCM, Brugada's syndrome, or long QT syndrome

6. High grade or complete heart block

7. Sinus rate <50

8. QT interval >500 msec

9. Antiarrhythmic medications

10. History of or current ventricular tachycardia

11. Implantable cardioverter-defibrillation

12. Pacemaker

Electrophysiology or cardiology consultation

Yes

No

Likely low-risk syncope and no further evaluation required

HOCM, hypertropohic obstructive cardiomyopathy.

Tilt Table Testing

It is of limited value given a low sensitivity (30% to 70%) and specificity (60% to 80%). A positive test may be seen in up to 45% of those with no history of syncope. Furthermore, the pattern of positive response in patients with clear neurocardiogenic syncope often does not correlate with the clinical pattern. The reproducibility of the test is also limited (70%) and it is therefore unhelpful in assessing the success of therapy. It is found most helpful in patients who are unable to provide a specific history of symptoms but in whom a neurocardiogenic cause is suspected. A positive tilt response that completely reproduces the clinical symptoms can be helpful in confirming a suspected diagnosis.

Electroencephalograms are of low yield between seizures and should not be routinely performed. Similarly, brain imaging is not recommended in the evaluation of syncope unless a source for a possible seizure is being investigated.

ELECTROPHYSIOLOGY STUDY

Electrophysiology (EP) studies are of limited utility in the evaluation of syncope. They should be considered in patients with electrocardiographic evidence of conduction disease, a history consistent with rapid palpitations, or underlying structural heart disease with a probable history of tachycardia. The standard EP protocol should begin with CSM followed by a determination of sinus node function, atrioventricular node (AVN) function, and His-Purkinje function. Once this is completed, a full atrial stimulation protocol is performed to identify the presence of SVT. The laboratory staff must be prepared to assess the blood pressure immediately (or an arterial catheter should be placed) given that hypotension with SVT generally occurs at the onset of the arrhythmia. A standard ventricular stimulation protocol is also performed. The specificity for ventricular stimulation in patients with unexplained syncope is highest when restricted to single and double extra stimulation from two sites.

MANAGEMENT

The management of reflex syncope is generally frustrating. Avoidance of common triggers is the best advice. Patients should be instructed to sit or optimally lie down as soon as symptoms reminiscent of those associated with prior syncopal episodes develop. Friends and family should be cautioned against trying to stand the patient up immediately following the syncopal episode. Isometric activities such as handgrip or clenching the leg muscles may be of some preventative value.

Multiple medical therapies including β-blockers, fludrocortisone, serotonin reuptake inhibitors, disopyramide have all been tried with variable and

TABLE 12-4 Management Options for Neurocardiogenic Syncope

Treatment	Instructions	Precautions/Adverse Reactions
Hydration	At least 2 L/d	—
Elastic stockings	Apply in the morning	Difficult to put on
Salt loading	120 mmol/d	—
Fludrocortisone	0.1–0.2 mg b.i.d.	Hypokalemia, headaches, volume overload, hypertension
Midodrine	5–10 mg t.i.d.	Supine hypertension (do not use after 7 pm), scalp tingling, nausea
β-blockers	Depends on the drug	Fatigue, bronchospasm, depression, bradycardia
Disopyramide	200 mg b.i.d.	Anticholinergic side effects, QT prolongation, TDP
Fluoxetine	20 mg q.d.	Insomnia, nausea, diarrhea
Pacemakers	Must have algorithms designed to pace rapidly in response to abrupt drop in heart rate	—

TDP, *torsade de pointes.*

disappointing results (see Table 12-4). Midodrine, an α-agonist, is sometimes helpful in predominantly vasodepressor syncope. Pacemakers are generally of no value unless a clear and repetitive mechanism of asystole (cardioinhibitory response) is confirmed. In this instance, a pacemaker with the ability to detect a rapid drop in heart rate and pace rapidly for a prolonged period of time (rate drop function) should be implanted.

Situations in which implantable cardioverter defibrillator (ICD) implantation should be considered with or without further evaluation include unexplained syncope with HOCM (i.e., not felt to be due to obstruction), noncoronary dilated cardiomyopathy, long QT syndrome, Brugada syndrome, arrhythmogenic right ventricular dysplasia (ARVD), or convincing evidence of idiopathic ventricular fibrillation (VF) or catecholaminergic polymorphic VT.

Driving Restrictions

Driving regulations vary by region. In general, it is recommended that patients avoid driving for 6 months following an unexplained syncopal episode. If a reversible cause of syncope is identified and managed definitively, driving can be resumed more quickly at the discretion of the treating physician. As noted, neurocardiogenic syncope rarely occurs with driving, therefore, the physicians make no restrictions on this activity.

SELECTED BIBLIOGRAPHY

Alboni P, Brignole M, Menozzi C, et al. Diagnostic value of history in patients with syncope or without heart disease. *J Am Coll Cardiol*. 2001;37:1921.

Farine D, Seaward PG. When it comes to pregnant women sleeping, is left right? *J Obstet Gynaecol Can*. 2007;29:841–842.

Josephson ME. *Clinical cardiac electrophysiology*, 4th ed. Philadelphia: Lippincott Williams & Wilkins; 2008.

Olshansky B. A pepsi challenge. *N Engl J Med*. 1999;340(25):2006.

Pelliccia A, Di Paolo F, Quattrini F, et al. Outcomes in athletes with marked ECG repolarization abnormalities. *N Engl J Med*. 2008;358:152–161.

Sutton R, Brignole M, Menozzi C, et al. Dual-chamber pacing in the treatment of neurally mediated tilt- positive cardioinhibitory syncope : Pacemaker versus no therapy: a multicenter randomized study. The Vasovagal Syncope International Study (VASIS) Investigators. *Circulation*. 2000:102:294–299.

Sudden Death Syndromes

The most common etiology of sudden cardiac death (SCD) is acute ischemia or ventricular tachycardia (VT) resulting from prior myocardial infarction. Dilated cardiomyopathy from a nonischemic cause is another important substrate for ventricular arrhythmias and sudden death. These two entities are discussed in separate chapters. The sudden death syndromes due to inherited arrhythmias or acquired electrical abnormalities are discussed in this chapter. The inherited arrhythmia syndromes are physiologically diverse disorders. They are, however, often considered as a group because of important shared clinical features:

- An increased risk of malignant ventricular arrhythmias and sudden cardiac arrest (SCA)

- Presentation in children, adolescents, and young adults

- In most syndromes, an absence of overt structural heart disease

In practice, the cardiologist or electrophysiologist is often asked to consider all of these diagnoses in young, otherwise healthy, individuals who present with palpitations, presyncope, syncope, nonsustained ventricular arrhythmias, or cardiac arrest.

Because of the serious implications of the diagnoses and the nonspecific nature of the common presenting complaints, a disciplined, systematic

193

approach to the consideration of these disorders is necessary. The corner-stones of such an evaluation remain the clinical history and close evaluation of the electrocardiogram (ECG) although advanced testing including cardiac magnetic resonance imaging (MRI), genetic testing, electrophysiology (EP) testing, and microvolt T wave alternans (TWA) also have a role in selected cases.

The list of disorders included in the inherited arrhythmia syndromes varies and it has evolved over the last 20 to 30 years, reflecting the ongoing recognition, definition, and characterization of these diseases. In this discussion, we will include six disorders in two general groups; ion channelopathies and diseases of the myocardium:

Ion channelopathies

Congenital long QT syndrome (LQTS)

Short QT syndrome

Brugada syndrome (BSM)

Catecholaminergic polymorphic VT

Myocardial diseases

Arrhythmogenic right ventricular dysplasia (ARVD)

Hypertrophic cardiomyopathy (HCM)

Less common diseases, including Rett syndrome, and Timothy syndrome, are also associated with an increased risk of SCA. Owing to their rarity and/or their association with other, more prominent, noncardiac abnormalities, these disorders are not discussed in detail here.

LONG QT SYNDROME

The congenital LQTS is a disorder of myocardial repolarization. It is characterized by prolongation of the QT interval, morphologic abnormalities of the T wave, and an increased risk of *torsade de pointes* (TDP). Traditionally, the congenital LQTS has been characterized as an autosomal dominant disorder called the *Romano-Ward syndrome* or an autosomal recessive disorder called the *Jervell and Lange-Nielsen (JLN) syndrome*. The latter syndrome has associated congenital sensorineural deafness. It is now recognized that most forms of congenital LQTS result from mutations in the genes responsible for the cardiac potassium and sodium channels. The acquired form of long QTS is often related to electrolyte depletion or drug exposure, particularly with antiarrhythmic agents that block potassium channels (see Table 13-1). It is currently

TABLE 13-1 Common Causes of Acquired Long QT Syndrome (LQTS)

Antiarrhythmic drugs: quinidine, procainamide, disopyramide, sotalol, dofetilide, amiodarone, ibutilide

Antihistamines (particularly in association with erythromycin): terfenadine, astemizole

Psychotropic drugs: thioridazine, haloperidol (Haldol), tricyclic antidepressants, methadone, risperidone, SSRIs, phenothiazines

Antibiotics: erythromycin, clarithromycin, azithromycin,

Metabolic causes: hypokalemia, hypomagnesemia (particularly, in association with diuretics), anorexia nervosa, liquid protein diets

Bradyarrhythmias: AV block

HIV protease inhibitors

SSRI, selective serotonin reuptake inhibitor; AV, atrioventricular; HIV, human immunodeficiency virus.

believed that many patients with acquired LQTS have a partial abnormality in the HERG potassium channel, which is clinically inapparent until exposure to a potassium channel blocking drug or severe electrolyte depletion results in marked QT prolongation.

The accuracy of data on the epidemiology of the congenital LQTS is limited by both variable penetrance of the clinical phenotype and incomplete genetic characterization of the disease. Estimates of the incidence of LQTS range between 1 in 2,500 and 1 in 10,000.

Seven genes have been linked to congenital LQTS (see Table 13-2). Five encode proteins that are components of cardiac potassium channels, one the cardiac sodium channel, and one the plasma membrane protein ankyrin B. Mutations in at least one of these loci have been detected in up to 70% of patients with congenital LQTS.

In addition to LQT 1 to 7, QT prolongation and malignant ventricular arrhythmias have been identified in patients with other genetic disorders, including Rett syndrome, a neurodevelopmental disorder affecting approximately 1/20,000 females; and Timothy syndrome, a rare multisystem disorder with a total of 17 described cases.

Long QT Clinical Syndrome

The clinical presentation of congenital LQTS is most often syncope, seizures, or sudden death due to TDP. The average age of clinical presentation is 7 with one third of patients having a family history of LQTS. LQT-associated TDP can be misdiagnosed as a seizure disorder particularly in children. The circumstances

| | | | Action | | Percentage |
Syndrome	Gene	Current	Potential Effect	LQTS Syndrome	of LQTS (%)
LQT 1	KvLQ1	IKs	Delayed phase 3	RW/JLN	42–55
LQT 2	HERG	IKr	Delayed phase 3	RW	35–45
LQT 3	SCN5A	Ina	Prolonged phase 2	RW	8–10
LQT 4	Ankyrin B	—	—	RW	—
LQT 5	KCNE1	IKs	Delayed phase 3	RW/JLN	—
LQT 6	KCNE2	IKr	Delayed phase 3	RW	—
LQT 7	KCNJ2	KIr2.1	Delayed phase 3	HPP	—

TABLE 13-2   Genes Linked to Congenital Long QT Syndrome (LQTS)

RW, Romano Ward; JLN, Jervell and Lange-Nielsen; HPP, Hereditary periodic paralysis.

associated with the cardiac event (i.e., syncope, sudden death) are also helpful. Patients with LQT 1 often have exercise-related events. TDP associated with swimming is typical with LQT 1 and may be a cause of unexplained drowning. LQTS 2 is unique in that startling auditory stimuli can precipitate arrhythmic events (e.g., "alarm clock syncope"). LQT 3 is characterized by arrhythmias occurring at rest or during sleep.

Long QT Syndrome Diagnosis

A variety of tests and algorithms have been proposed for diagnosing LQTS including the Schwartz score. This score comprises the most clinically important factors associated with risk of clinical events with LQTS and assigns points for the degree of QT prolongation (e.g., $\geq$480 msec, family history, personal history of syncope, and T-wave morphology).

In genotypically confirmed LQTS, longer QT intervals, particularly those >500 msec, are associated with a higher frequency of cardiac events. Importantly, 6% of patients with LQTS will have cardiac events with a normal QT interval. The T-wave morphology can help predict the specific type of LQT. Specifically, a broad T wave suggests LQT 1, a notched T wave suggests LQT 2, and a long isoelectric ST segment and T wave, LQT 3 (see Fig. 13-1).

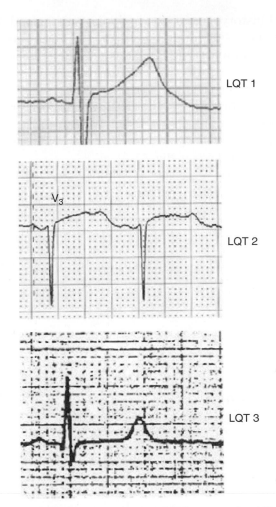

FIGURE 13-1. A broad T wave suggests LQT 1, a notched T wave LQT 2, and a long isoelectric ST segment and T wave, LQT 3.

Our strategy for the diagnosis of the congenital LQTS is based on a careful personal and family history and close inspection of the resting ECG:

- In patients with a history of presyncope, syncope, or SCA, the clinical details of the event are carefully examined to discern the likelihood of a ventricular arrhythmia.

- A careful family history is obtained, asking specifically about SCD at an early age in first-degree relatives.

- The ECG is examined for the duration of the QTc interval and the morphology of the T wave. ECGs from first-degree family members should also be obtained when possible.

If the clinical history suggests arrhythmic syncope and the QTc is significantly prolonged (i.e., >480 msec), no further testing is necessary to give the diagnosis of LQTS. Similarly, if the QTc is normal and the history is benign, no further testing is necessary to exclude the diagnosis.

In many cases, the diagnosis will remain uncertain, owing to an equivocal personal or family history and/or a borderline QTc. In such cases, an exercise test with assessment of microvolt TWA should be performed. If the QT interval fails to shorten appropriately during exercise or if TWA is present, the patient is considered to have LQTS (see Fig. 13-2).

Additional tests including electrophysiology study (EPS), pharmacologic provocation (e.g., epinephrine challenge), and facial immersion do not have established diagnostic accuracy and are not routinely included in the diagnostic evaluation for LQTS.

Genetic testing is currently commercially available to identify the most common genes involved in LQTS. When feasible, the patient of interest and first-degree family members with suspicious phenotypes (ECGs) should be genotyped.

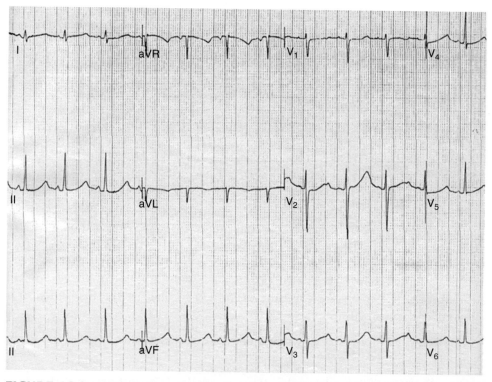

FIGURE 13-2. ECG demonstrating characteristic T wave alternans associated with the long QT syndrome (LQTS).

Management of Congenital Long QT Syndrome

The common components in the management of patients with LQTS include:

Activity restriction: All patients with a diagnosis of LQTS should refrain from competitive athletics and from vigorous recreational sporting activities.

β-Blockers: The authors recommend β-blocker therapy in all patients with a diagnosis of LQTS regardless of whether or not symptoms are present. They have shown significant decrease in the rate of recurrent syncope and sudden death but are not effective enough in symptomatic patients to obviate the use of an implantable cardioverter defibrillator (ICD). β-Blockers should be titrated to blunt the maximal heart rate during exertion. It would be expected that these agents would be particularly useful in LQT 1 and less beneficial in LQT 3.

Potassium supplementation, particularly in LQT 2, has demonstrated a reduction in QTc duration but data pertaining to clinical events is not yet available. It is prudent to keep the potassium replete in patients with LQTS.

Mexiletine has been proposed for patients with LQT 3. Once again, clinical validation for this approach does not yet exist.

Sympathetic denervation: Left cardiac sympathetic denervation involves removal of the left stellate ganglion. This approach has been shown to reduce but not eliminate the risk of recurrent cardiac events and is associated with the development of Horner syndrome. It is rarely performed in the current era.

ICD implantation: Comprehensive indications for ICD implantation in patients with LQTS have not been defined. ICD therapy is appropriate for the secondary prevention of SCD in all LQTS patients with a history of SCA. In addition, the authors recommend ICD implantation in patients with recurrent syncope or TDP despite β-blocker therapy. Finally, ICD implantation is reasonable in selected high-risk patients, such as those with a strong family history of SCD or those with JLN.

Acute Management of Acquired Long QT Syndrome

Discontinuation of causative agent
Magnesium sulfate: 2 g bolus of 50% magnesium sulfate over 2 minutes
Consider isoproterenol to accelerate sinus rate and shorten the QT interval
Sodium bicarbonate if quinidine-related TDP
Consider placement of temporary pacing system with pacing at >80 bpm

SHORT QT SYNDROME

The short QT syndrome is a recently described disorder of SCD in association with a QTc of <300 msec. The frequency of this disorder is unknown. At present, genetic abnormalities involving an increase in function of KVLQT1, HERG, and a decrease in function of Ik1 have all been described in association with a shortened action potential duration and surface QT interval. In addition to a short QT interval, there is relative absence of the ST segment and symmetric tall T waves in the precordial leads.

There is no role for EP testing in this disorder and the current management is an ICD in symptomatic individuals. The role for an ICD in first-degree relatives of symptomatic individuals who have the phenotype but no symptoms is uncertain.

BRUGADA SYNDROME

The BS is a primary electrical disorder characterized by an ECG pattern of a pseudo-right bundle branch block with ST elevation in the right precordial leads (V_1 to V_3) and a history of documented or suspected ventricular arrhythmias and/or a family history of the disorder. Both clinical and ECG features are necessary to make a diagnosis of BS.

BS displays an autosomal dominant inheritance pattern. A single gene, encoding the cardiac sodium channel SCN5A, has been linked to BS. However, mutations of the *SCN5A* gene have been found in only 18% to 30% of BS families, and the genetic defect is unknown in most cases.

Most of the available epidemiologic data describe only the prevalence of Brugada ECG abnormalities. As the ECG findings are insufficient for the diagnosis of BS, and the penetrance of disease is incomplete, these data do not reflect the prevalence of either the clinical syndrome or the underlying genetic defect. The prevalence of a typical (type 1 see—subsequent text) Brugada-type ECG varies in different ethnic populations, ranging from up to 0.16% in Asian populations to <1 in 3,000 in a European cohort.

- BS occurs in men more frequently than women.

- The average age at diagnosis is late 30s or early 40s.

- Events are not typically exercise induced and may occur during sleep.

- The ECG manifestations may represent an early form of ARVD.

The pathophysiologic model of BS is based on reduced function of the cardiac sodium channel. Reduction of the inward sodium current during phase 0 of the myocardial action potential reduces the depolarization voltage peak. This defect in turn affects the impact of the repolarizing transient potassium current I(to) in phase 1. Because the phase 0 peak is lower than normal, I(to) can drive phase 1 voltage lower below the level necessary to activate the calcium channels that maintain depolarization during phase 2. Without the influence of these calcium currents, the phase 2 "dome" of the action potential is lost, resulting in a dramatic shortening of action potential duration. Because I(to) is more prominent in the epicardium and M cells than it is in the endocardium (particularly, in the right ventricle), the impact of the sodium channel defect varies between myocardial layers. Therefore, a transmural voltage gradient develops during phase 2, producing the characteristic ST elevation in the right precordial leads. This heterogeneous loss of the phase 2 action potential "dome" can also produce the electrophysiologic substrate for arrhythmias through a process called *phase 2 reentry*. A full description of phase 2 reentry is detailed elsewhere, but is beyond the scope of this text.

Brugada Diagnosis and Management

A Brugada-type ECG is not sufficient to make a diagnosis of BS; clinical features are required. Three types of ST-T wave abnormalities have been described in patients with BS. These findings must be present in at least two of the right precordial leads to qualify for the diagnosis of a Brugada-type ECG. The classic pattern, or type 1 ECG, has downsloping ST elevation of at least 2 mm with inverted T waves. This pattern is referred to as the *coved-type* Brugada ECG. In type 2 and type 3 Brugada ECGs, the elevated ST segment, after initially sloping downward, reflects upward into an upright T wave, referred to as a *saddleback* configuration (see Fig. 13-3). The distinction between type 2 and 3 ECGs is based on the magnitude of this ST elevation; ≥1 mm for type 2 and <1 mm

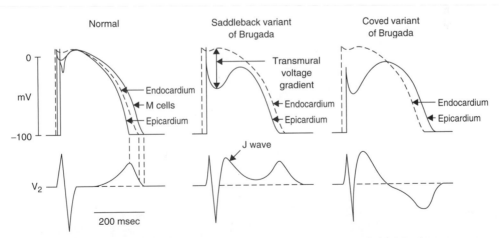

FIGURE 13-3. Proposed electrophysiology of the Brugada ECG demonstrating the mechanism of the saddleback and coved variants. (Adapted with permission from Scheinman MM and Keung E. *J Am Coll Cardiol*. 2007;49: 2061–2069.)

for type 3. Attention must be placed to the positioning of the precordial leads (particularly, V_1 and V_2) because placement of these leads in inappropriately high interspaces can cause a pseudo-Brugada pattern. In a consensus report from the Study Group on the Molecular Basis of Arrhythmias of the European Society of Cardiology, it was proposed that the diagnosis of BS should be strongly considered in patients who meet the following criteria:

A type 1 ST Brugada ECG plus at least one of the following clinical features:

a) Documented ventricular fibrillation (VF)

b) Self-terminating polymorphic ventricular tachycardia (PMVT)

c) Family history of SCD in those younger than 45 years

d) Type 1 ST segment elevation in family members

e) Electrophysiologic inducibility of VT

f) Unexplained syncope suggestive of a tachyarrhythmia

g) Nocturnal agonal respiration

Among patients with a type 2 or 3 ECG, drug challenge with a sodium channel blocker (e.g., flecainide 400 mg PO, or procainamide 10 mg per kg IV over 10 minutes) can convert the ECG to a type 1 pattern (see Fig. 13-4). According to many experts, and the ESC consensus statement, patients with

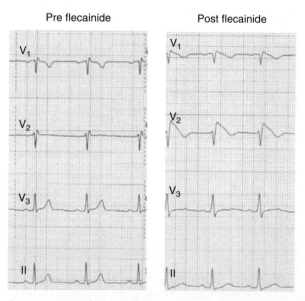

FIGURE 13-4. Conversion of Brugada type 2 ECG to a type 1 pattern following the administration of 300 mg of flecainide.

a type 2 or 3 ECG should only be diagnosed with BS if the ECG converts to type 1 following drug challenge. However, drug challenge is probably unnecessary in patients with a type 2 or 3 ECG who have documented VF, self-terminating polymorphic VT, unexplained syncope suggestive of a tachyarrhythmia, or nocturnal agonal respiration (clinical features a, b, f, and g). Most such patients will receive an ICD regardless of the results of drug testing.

Therefore, the main indication for drug challenge is the presence of a type 2 or 3 ECG with clinical features (c) and (d) or (f). If the drug challenge is positive, EP testing can be performed to further risk stratify individuals. In this group, the authors favor ICD implantation if there is a history of syncope very consistent with an arrhythmic cause or a first-degree family member with sudden death.

Currently, there is no pharmacologic therapy, which has established efficacy for reducing SCD risk in patients with BS.

ARRHYTHMOGENIC RIGHT VENTRICULAR DYSPLASIA

ARVD, also referred to as *arrhythmogenic right ventricular cardiomyopathy (ARVC)*, is characterized pathologically by fibrofatty replacement of myocardium, primarily in the right ventricle (RV) and less commonly in the left ventricle (see Chapter 10). The true prevalence of ARVD is unknown, but estimates range from 1 in 5,000 to 1 in 1,000. The disorder has been diagnosed more frequently in athletes experiencing SCD in northern Italy (22%), than in similar series from other parts of the world. However, Italy has had a uniquely comprehensive athletic screening program for several decades. Therefore, it is not clear if these data reflect a true increased prevalence of this disorder in Italy, or if they are due to varying degrees of awareness and recognition in different regions. The authors do not, at this point, base their diagnostic suspicion of ARVD on a patient's ethnicity.

A growing number of gene mutations have been linked to ARVD (see Table 13-3). Both autosomal dominant and autosomal recessive forms of the disease have been described. The dominant forms, which are more common, exhibit variable penetrance. In the less common recessive forms (Naxos disease and Carvajal syndrome), ARVD is accompanied by noncardiac manifestations including hyperkeratosis of the palms and soles and woolly hair.

The five genes that are most strongly linked to ARVD all encode desmosomal proteins. This observation is the basis for the evolving model for the pathogenesis of ARVD: impaired desmosome function, when subjected to mechanical stress, results in myocyte detachment and cell death, which is followed by inflammation and ultimately the fibrofatty replacement of damaged myocytes.

A number of the clinical features of ARVD are consistent with this pathogenic hypothesis. The characteristic pathology, fibrofatty replacement

TABLE 13-3 **Genes Linked to Arrhythmogenic Right Ventricular Dysplasia (ARVD)**

Gene Product	Inheritance Pattern
Plakoglobin	Autosomal recessive
Plakophilin-2	Autosomal dominant
Desmoplakin	Autosomal dominant and recessive
Desmoglien-2	Autosomal dominant
Desmocolin-2	Autosomal dominant
Ryanodine receptor-2	Autosomal dominant[a]
TGF-β-3	Autosomal dominant[b]

[a]Ryanodine receptor-2 mutation identified in a single family with clinical features consistent with catecholaminergic polymorphic ventricular tachycardia (PMVT).
[b]Identified in single family.
TGF, transforming growth factor.

of myocardium, is most prominent in the region of the RV that is the thinnest, and therefore subject to the greatest degree of mechanical stress. This area is referred to as the *triangle of dysplasia* (defined by the RV apex, inflow tract, and outflow tract). In addition, trained athletes often have severe pathologic manifestations of the disease and also appear to be more susceptible to malignant arrhythmias compared to other patients with ARVD. These observations could be explained by the intensity of the mechanical stress associated with physical training. Finally, the variable penetrance of ARVD may be the result of variations in the stress placed on the diseased myocardium among different family members with the same mutation. Patients present with ventricular ectopy, sustained VT, and SCD. The presence of multifocal right ventricular premature depolarizations (VPDs) (e.g., left bundle branch block [LBBB]/left axis deviation and LBBB/right axis deviation) and sustained left bundle branch VT (not thought to be idiopathic right ventricular outflow tract VT) should prompt an evaluation for ARVC. Eventually, patients with ARVC can also develop severe right-sided heart failure.

Arrhythmogenic Right Ventricular Dysplasia Diagnosis

Important factors in the diagnosis of ARVD include the clinical and family history, the ECG and imaging evidence of an RV cardiomyopathy by echocardiography or cardiac MRI. The typical ECG finding is T-wave inversions in the right precordial leads. Marked fractionation of the terminal component of the QRS complex is called an *epsilon wave* and is consistent with ARVD (see Fig. 13-5).

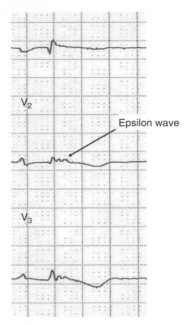

FIGURE 13-5. Classical ECG associated with arrhythmogenic right ventricular dysplasia. Marked fractionation of the terminal component of the QRS complex is called an *epsilon wave*.

In 1994, a task force from the European Society of Cardiology and the International Society and Federation of Cardiology proposed criteria for the diagnosis of ARVD (see Table 13-4).

The diagnosis of ARVD is based on the presence of two major criteria, one major plus two minor criteria, or four minor criteria. Owing to concerns that these criteria underdiagnosed ARVD in family members of confirmed probands, modified criteria specific to potentially affected family members were proposed in 2002 (see Table 13-5).

Both the original and modified criteria can be helpful guidelines, but should not be considered gold standards for the diagnosis of ARVD.

In addition to the echocardiogram, MRI is emerging as a useful tool to identify fatty infiltration of the right ventricle consistent with ARVD.

EPS: Voltage mapping of the right ventricle can be useful to confirm the diagnosis of ARVC. In particular, areas of markedly reduced voltage in regions consistent with the triangle of dysplasia support a diagnosis of ARVD.

Management of Arrhythmogenic Right Ventricular Dysplasia

The management of patients with ARVD includes the following:

- Restriction from all competitive athletics and most vigorous recreational sporting activities (Table 13-9).

206

TABLE 13-4 Criteria for the Diagnosis of Arrhythmogenic Right Ventricular Dysplasia (ARVD)

	Major	*Minor*
Family history	• Familial disease confirmed at autopsy	• Family history of SCD, in those younger than 35 yrs, caused by suspected ARVD • Family history of ARVD based on clinical criteria
Depolarization/conduction abnormalities	• Epsilon waves V_1 to V_3 • Localized QRS prolongation (>110 msec) V_1 to V_3	• Late potentials on SAECG
Repolarization abnormalities		• Inverted T waves in V_2 or V_3 in people older than 12 yr without RBBB
Tissue characterization	• Fibrofatty replacement detected on myocardial biopsy	
Myocardial structure and functional abnormalities on imaging	• Severe RV dilation and reduction in ejection fraction with no or mild LV involvement • Localized RV aneurysms • Severe segmental dilation of the RV	• Mild global RV dilation and/or ejection fraction reduction with normal LV • Mild segmental dilation of the RV • Regional RV hypokinesis
Arrhythmias		• Sustained or nonsustained VT of LBBB morphology, either spontaneously or with exercise. • >1,000 VPC/24 h on Holter monitoring

SCD, sudden cardiac death; ARVD, arrhythmogenic right ventricular dysplasia; SAECG, signal averaged electrocardiogram; RBBB, right bundle branch block; RV, right ventricle; LV, left ventricle; VT, ventricular tachycardia; VPC, ventricular premature complex.

(Data from McKenna WJ, Thiene G, Nava A, et al. Diagnosis of arrhythmogenic right ventricular dysplasia/cardiomyopathy. Task Force of the Working Group Myocardial and Pericardial Disease of the European Society of Cardiology and of the Scientific Council on Cardiomyopathies of the International Society and Federation of Cardiology. *Br Heart J.* 1994;71:215.)

TABLE 13-5 **Proposed Modification of Task Force Criteria for the Diagnosis of Familial Arrhythmogenic Right Ventricular Cardiomyopathy (ARVC)**

ARVD in a first-degree relative *and*

One of the following:

- T-wave inversion in right precordial leads (V_2 and V_3)
- Late potentials seen on signal-averaged ECG
- LBBB-type VT on ECG, Holter monitoring or during exercise testing
- >200 VPCs over a 24-h period
- Mild global RV dilatation and/or EF reduction with normal LV
- Mild segmental dilatation of the RV
- Regional RV hypokinesia

ARVD, arrhythmogenic right ventricular dysplasia; ECG, electrocardiogram; LBBB, left bundle branch block; VT, ventricular tachycardia; VPC, ventricular premature complex; RV, right ventricle; EF, ejection fraction; LV, left ventricle.

(Modified from Hamid MS, Norman M, Quraishi A, et al. Prospective evaluation of relatives for familial arrhythmogenic right ventricular cardiomyopathy/dysplasia reveals a need to broaden diagnostic criteria. *J Am Coll Cardiol.* 2002;40(8):1445–1450.)

- ICD implantation for the secondary prevention of SCD in patients with a history of SCA or sustained VT.

- ICD implantation for the primary prevention of SCD for individuals with high-risk clinical features (extensive RV disease, LV involvement, one or more affected family members with SCD, or unexplained syncope consistent with a tachyarrhythmia).

- Antiarrhythmic therapy, usually with amiodarone or sotalol, has a limited role, either as primary therapy for patients who have an indication for ICD implantation but refuse or are not candidates for a device, or as adjunctive therapy for patients with an ICD who experience frequent shocks.

- Catheter ablation is an important tool for the elimination of symptomatic ventricular arrhythmias associated with ARVD. These procedures can be challenging and the progressive nature of this disorder, with risk for recurrent arrhythmias, should prompt consideration of ICD implantation even in patients who the authors believe have had a successful VT ablation.

HYPERTROPHIC CARDIOMYOPATHY

HCM is an inherited disease of the cardiac sarcomere. Clinically, it is characterized by left ventricular hypertrophy (LVH), most notably in the intraventricular

TABLE 13-6 Genes Linked to Hypertrophic Cardiomyopathy (HCM)

Genetic Mutation	Frequency among HCM Patients
Cardiac myosin-binding protein C	14%–26%
β-Cardiac myosin heavy chain	13%–25%
Troponin I	5%–10%
Troponin T	5%–10%
α-Tropomyosin	5%–10%
Myosin regulatory (essential light chain)	Rare
α-Cardiac myosin heavy chain	Rare
α-Cardiac actin	Rare
Titin	Rare
Titin-cap	Rare
Muscle LIM protein (MLP)	Rare
Ventricular essential myosin light chain	Rare

Genetic disorders with similar phenotype: PRKAG2 and LAMP2; α-galactosidase A.

A more complete listing can be obtained at: genetics.med.harvard.edu/~seidman/cg3/.

septum, left ventricular outflow tract obstruction, and ventricular arrhythmias. The prevalence of HCM has been reported to be as high as 1 in 350 adults, although clinically significant disease is much less common.

HCM is inherited in an autosomal dominant pattern with variable penetrance. A growing number of genes have been linked to HCM (see Table 13-6). With rare exceptions, these genes encode components of the myocardial contractile apparatus. In cohorts of patients with a clinical diagnosis of HCM, genetic abnormalities have been identified in 30% to 61% of cases.

Hypertrophic Cardiomyopathy Diagnosis

Although specific diagnostic criteria have not been established, the diagnosis of HCM can usually be made through a careful personal and family history, inspection of the ECG, and an echocardiogram.

ECG abnormalities are common in patients with HCM, with LVH and repolarization abnormalities being the most common findings. Left axis deviation, prominent Q waves in the inferior and lateral leads, and left atrial or biatrial enlargement can also be seen. In patients with the apical variant of HCM, deeply inverted T waves (so-called giant negative T waves) may be seen in the anterolateral leads. However, both the sensitivity and specificity of ECG findings are low in a general population of patients with palpitations or syncope, and imaging studies are required to establish the diagnosis.

Echocardiography is the recommended imaging modality for the evaluation of the patient with suspected HCM. The usual diagnostic criterion for HCM is LV wall thickness ≥15 mm in the absence of alternative explanations of LVH (e.g., hypertension, aortic stenosis). HCM may present with lesser degrees of LVH or even normal wall thickness. Therefore, repeat imaging tests are appropriate in patients with other clinical features suggestive of HCM. Cardiac MRI is also emerging as a useful tool for the diagnosis of HCM.

Moderate degrees of LVH can develop in trained athletes, the so-called athlete's heart. This can be an important clinical distinction in a young athlete with palpitations or syncope (see Table 13-7).

TABLE 13-7 Distinguishing Hypertrophic Cardiomyopathy (HCM) from "Athlete's Heart"

Parameter	Findings in HCM	Findings in Athlete's Heart
LV wall thickness/morphology	Can be >16 mm; can be heterogeneous or asymmetric across segments	Typically <16 mm, especially in women; symmetric
Diastolic LV cavity	<45 mm (except in late, dilated phase)	>55 mm
LA size	Enlarged	Normal
LV diastolic filling pattern	Impaired relaxation (E:A ratio <1, prolonged diastolic deceleration time)	Normal
Response to deconditioning	None	LV wall thickness decreases
ECG findings	• Very high QRS voltages • Q waves • Deep negative T waves	Criteria for LVH but without unusual features
Family history of HCM	Present (except *de novo* mutations)	Absent

LV, left ventricle; LA, left atrium; ECG, electrocardiogram; LVH, left ventricular hypertrophy.

(Adapted from Maron BJ, Pellicia A, Spirito P. Cardiac disease in young trained athletes. Insights into methods for distinguishing athlete's heart from structural disease, with particular emphasis on hypertrophic cardiomyopathy. *Circulation.* 1995;91:1596.)

Hypertrophic Cardiomyopathy Risk Stratification

SCA is the most feared complication of HCM. Across the spectrum of patients with HCM, the average annual incidence of SCA is approximately 1%. However, this risk is heterogeneous, and there are high-risk subgroups that have identifiable clinical characteristics including:

- Prior cardiac arrest

- Spontaneous sustained VT

- Family history of sudden death

- Syncope consistent with a ventricular arrhythmia, particularly if it is repetitive, occurs with exertion and is not felt consistent with left ventricular outflow tract obstruction

- Massive LVH defined as wall thickness ≥30 mm

It is important to realize that although severe LVH (≥30 mm) is an independent risk factor for sudden death, there are highly lethal variants of HCM which are associated with minimal LVH. It is possible that genetic analysis will eventually be able to help stratify which variants are at the highest risk for sudden death.

Other findings that are sometimes considered major risk factors for arrhythmia but are less well defined include the following:

- Abnormal blood pressure (BP) response to exercise, variably defined (e.g., a fall below baseline BP during or immediately following exercise or a drop of >20 mm Hg from peak BP during exercise)

- Nonsustained VT

Hypertrophic Cardiomyopathy Management

Medical therapy for HCM is primarily focused on the management of symptoms associated with outflow tract obstruction. For patients with HCM who are considered to be at an increased risk of SCD, implantation of an ICD is indicated.

ICD therapy is indicated in the following patients with HCM:

- For the secondary prevention of SCD in patients with a prior SCA or sustained ventricular arrhythmias

- For the primary prevention of SCD in patients with two or more major risk factors

- For the primary prevention of SCD in selected patients with a single major risk factor (e.g., a history of multiple affected family members with SCA)

- For the primary prevention of SCD in patients with HCM who develop the end-stage phenotype, which is characterized by left ventricular dilation, wall thinning, and systolic dysfunction

CATECHOLAMINERGIC POLYMORPHIC VENTRICULAR TACHYCARDIA

Familial catecholaminergic polymorphic ventricular tachycardia (CPVT) is an inherited disorder characterized by adrenergically mediated polymorphic ventricular tachyarrhythmias. Malignant arrhythmias can occur during periods of either emotional or physical stress. Patients with CPVT generally have no evidence of structural heart disease and usually have no resting ECG abnormalities.

The disease is relatively rare and comprehensive epidemiologic data do not exist. The authors' clinical understanding of this disorder comes from individual case reports and several cohorts of up to approximately 30 affected families.

Genetic studies have led to an evolving appreciation of CPVT as a disorder of calcium handling by the cardiac myocytes. The more common form of the disease is autosomal dominant. In this dominant form of the disease, mutations in the cardiac ryanodine receptor have been identified in up to 47% of probands. A less common homozygous form of the disease has been linked to mutations in the calsequestrin gene.

Catecholaminergic Polymorphic Ventricular Tachycardia Diagnosis

Diagnostic criteria have not been established. In contrast to the other disorders discussed earlier, resting ECG abnormalities are not a typical component of this disorder although sinus bradycardia has been reported. The diagnosis is based on the clinical history of a personal and/or family history of syncope or SCD related to exertion or emotional stress. Exercise stress testing is an important diagnostic tool in suspected cases of CPVT, and up to 80% of patients will have characteristic onset of PMVT with exertion and resolution with rest. Bidirectional VT is often seen in patients with CPVT. In this arrhythmia there is a beat-to-beat 180-degree alteration of the QRS axis (see Fig. 13-6).

Catecholaminergic Polymorphic Ventricular Tachycardia Clinical Course and Management

Data are limited, but CPVT appears to have a particularly malignant natural history. Patients often present in childhood (as opposed to adolescence or adulthood in LQT and ARVD). Mortality in untreated patients is as high as 50% by age 40.

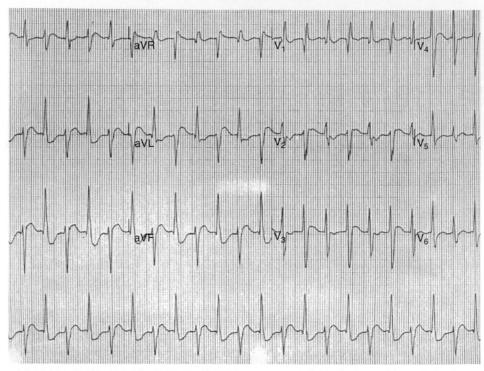

FIGURE 13-6. Bidirectional ventricular tachycardia (VT): With bidirectional VT there is a beat-to-beat 180-degree alteration of the QRS axis.

β-Blockers are the cornerstone of treatment and observational data suggest that they are effective in suppressing recurrent syncope in symptomatic patients. Patients who continue to have symptoms or exercise-induced arrhythmias on β-blocker therapy are candidates for ICD therapy. It is important to note that patients with ICDs still require β-blockers to prevent arrhythmic storm.

GENERAL DIAGNOSTIC APPROACH

Exclusion of these inherited syndromes is an important concern in the patient, particularly a young healthy patient, with nonspecific complaints such as palpitations, low-grade ventricular ectopy, or syncope. Even in a referral center, most patients referred for evaluation of such symptoms will not have a malignant diagnosis. However, a careful, disciplined approach is necessary, and with appropriate attention to the clinical history and ECG, extensive testing is usually unnecessary.

The details of the presenting complaint should be clearly defined. Syncope warrants particular attention, as the suspicion of a malignant arrhythmia derived from the history will often guide the extent of the diagnostic evaluation. For example, in a patient with antecedent and postevent symptoms consistent with a vasovagal mechanism, the family history and ECG, if similarly benign, are often adequate to complete the evaluation. In contrast, in a patient with a syncopal event strongly suggestive of a ventricular arrhythmia (e.g., abrupt loss of consciousness and recovery, without antecedent or postevent symptoms, particularly if in the midst of vigorous physical activity), will often warrant more extensive testing (e.g., echocardiography, cardiac magnetic resonance [MR], and/or exercise testing).

The family history is the second important component of the general evaluation. It is important to recognize that many lay people refer to any sudden death as a "heart attack." In many cases this distinction is not critical, but if a patient with a suspicious personal history or ECG reports that a first-degree or second-degree relative died at a young age of a "heart attack," it may be helpful to try to clarify that history (i.e., did the patient have an established diagnosis of coronary artery disease [CAD], did he or she undergo cardiac catheterization, was an autopsy performed?).

The ECG is the third element of this general evaluation. Exclusion of the inherited arrhythmia syndromes requires specific inspection for the hallmark findings of each disorder, and it is appropriate to comment specifically on the QT interval and the absence of epsilon waves and Brugada-type ECG abnormalities (see Table 13-8).

SPECIAL CONSIDERATIONS IN ATHLETES

The inherited arrhythmia syndromes, with the possible exception of BS, carry an increased risk of malignant arrhythmic events during vigorous exercise. This risk poses two challenges: defining the appropriate approach to preparticipation screening of athletes for these disorders and restriction of competitive and recreational athletic activity in patients with these diagnoses.

American Heart Association guidelines for preparticipation screening of competitive athletes includes a personal and family history and a physical examination performed preferably by licensed physicians, before training and competition begin (see Table 13-9). A 12-lead ECG is not routinely recommended due to a low specificity and sensitivity but should be considered in the presence of a concerning personal or family history.

With regard to activity restriction, patients with any of these diagnoses should be restricted from competitive athletics, which are defined as any organized team or individual sport in which there is regular competition, placing a premium on achievement.

The approach to recreational sports and activities is more complicated. In general sports associated with burst or intensive activity such as sprinting (e.g., singles tennis, squash, basketball, etc.) are not recommended.

TABLE 13-8 Hallmarks of Various Sudden Death Syndromes

	QRS Complex	ST Interval	QT Interval, T Wave	Arrhythmias and Circumstances in Which They Occur
HCM	• Increased voltages in midleft precordial leads • Abnormal Q waves in inferior and/or lateral leads • LAD, LBBB • Delta wave	• Downsloping • Upsloping	• Inverted in midleft precordial lead • Giant and negative in the apical variant	• Atrial fibrillation • VT • VPCs Circumstances: Exercise and rest
ARVD	• Prolonged: >110 msec in right precordial leads • Epsilon wave in right precordial leads • Reduced voltages ≤0.5 mV in frontal leads • RBBB	• Upsloping in right precordial leads	• Inverted right in precordial leads	• VPCs with an LBBB pattern • VT with an LBBB pattern Circumstances: Often with exercise

LQTS	Normal	Normal	• Bifid or biphasic in all leads	• VPCs • *Torsade de pointes* Circumstances: Exercise (e.g., swimming), emotionally startling event, rest/sleep
Brugada syndrome	• S1S2S3 pattern • RBBB/LAD	• Upsloping in coved-type right precordial leads	• Inverted in right precordial leads	• Polymorphic VT • Atrial fibrillation • Sinus bradycardia Circumstances: Rest/sleep

HCM, hypertrophic cardiomyopathy; VT, ventricular tachycardia; VPC, ventricular premature complex; LAD, left axis deviation; LBBB, left bundle branch block; ARVD, arrhythmogenic right ventricular dysplasia; RBBB, right bundle branch block; LQTS, long QT syndrome.

(Modified with permission from: Corrado D, Pelliccia A, Bjornstad HH, et al. Cardiovascular pre-participation screening of young competitive athletes for prevention of sudden death: Proposal for a common European protocol. Consensus statement of the Study Group of Sport Cardiology of the Working Group of Cardiac Rehabilitation and Exercise Physiology and the Working Group of Myocardial and Pericardial Diseases of the European Society of Cardiology. *Eur Heart J.* 2005;26:516. Copyright © 2005 Oxford University Press.)

TABLE 13-9 The 12-Element American Heart Association (AHA) Recommendations for Preparticipation Cardiovascular Screening of Competitive Athletes

Medical history[a]

Personal history

1. Exertional chest pain/discomfort
2. Unexplained syncope/near syncope[b]
3. Excessive exertional and unexplained dyspnea/fatigue, associated with exercise
4. Prior recognition of a heart murmur
5. Elevated systemic blood pressure

Family history

6. Premature death (sudden and unexpected, or otherwise) before age 50 yr due to heart disease, in one relative
7. Disability from heart disease in a close relative younger than 50 yr of age
8. Specific knowledge of certain cardiac conditions in family members: hypertrophic or dilated cardiomyopathy, long QT syndrome or other ion channelopathies, Marfan syndrome, or clinically important arrhythmias

Physical examination

9. Heart murmur[c]
10. Femoral pulses to exclude aortic coarctation
11. Physical stigmata of Marfan syndrome
12. Brachial artery blood pressure (sitting position)[d]

---

[a]Parental verification is recommended for high school and middle school athletes.

[b]Judged not to be neurocardiogenic (vasovagal); of particular concern when related to exertion.

[c]Auscultation should be performed in both supine and standing positions (or with Valsalva maneuver), specifically to identify murmurs of dynamic left ventricular outflow tract obstruction.

[d]Preferably taken in both arms.

(Reproduced with permission from: Maron BJ, Thompson PD, Ackerman MJ, et al. Recommendations and considerations related to preparticipation screening for cardiovascular abnormalities in competitive athletes: 2007 update: A scientific statement from the American Heart Association Council on Nutrition, Physical Activity, and Metabolism: endorsed by the American College of Cardiology Foundation. *Circulation.* 2007;115:1643. Copyright ©2007 Lippincott Williams & Wilkins.)

SELECTED BIBLIOGRAPHY

Antzelevitch C, Brugada P, Borggrefe M, et al. Brugada syndrome: Report of the second consensus conference: Endorsed by the Heart Rhythm Society and the European Heart Rhythm Association. *Circulation*. 2005;111:659.

Chen Q, Kirsch GE, Zhang D, et al. Genetic basis and molecular mechanism for idiopathic ventricular fibrillation. *Nature*. 1998;392:293.

Corrado D, Pelliccia A, Bjornstad HH, et al. Cardiovascular pre-participation screening of young competitive athletes for prevention of sudden death: Proposal for a common European protocol. Consensus Statement of the Study Group of Sport Cardiology of the Working Group of Cardiac Rehabilitation and Exercise Physiology and the Working Group of Myocardial and Pericardial Diseases of the European Society of Cardiology. *Eur Heart J*. 2005;26:516.

Gussak I, Brugada P, Brugada J. Idiopathic Short QT interval: A new clinical syndrome? *Cardiology*. 2000;94:99–102.

Hamid MS, Norman M, Quraishi A, et al. Prospective evaluation of relatives for familial arrhythmogenic right ventricular cardiomyopathy/dysplasia reveals a need to broaden diagnostic criteria. *J Am Coll Cardiol*. 2002;40:1445.

Josephson ME. *Clinical cardiac electrophysiology*, 4th ed. Philadelphia: Lippincott Williams & Wilkins; 2008.

Laitinen PJ, Brown KM, Piippo K, et al. Mutations of the cardiac ryanodine receptor (RyR2) gene in familial polymorphic ventricular tachycardia. *Circulation*. 2001;103:485.

Maron B, Chaitman BR, Ackerman MJ, et al. Recommendations for physical activity and recreational sports participation for young patients with genetic cardiovascular diseases. *Circulation*. 2004;109:2807.

Maron BJ, Mathenge R, Casey SA, et al. Clinical profile of hypertrophic cardiomyopathy identified de novo in rural communities. *J Am Coll Cardiol*. 1999;33:1590.

Maron BJ, McKenna WJ, Danielson GK, et al. American College of Cardiology/European Society of Cardiology clinical expert consensus document on hypertrophic cardiomyopathy. A report of the American College of Cardiology Foundation Task Force on Clinical Expert Consensus Documents and the European Society of Cardiology Committee for Practice Guidelines. *J Am Coll Cardiol*. 2003;42:1687.

Maron BJ, Thompson PD, Ackerman MJ, et al. Recommendations and considerations related to preparticipation screening for cardiovascular abnormalities in competitive athletes: 2007 update: A scientific statement from the American Heart Association Council on Nutrition, Physical Activity, and Metabolism: Endorsed by the American College of Cardiology Foundation. *Circulation*. 2007;115:1643.

McKenna WJ, Thiene G, Nava A, et al. Diagnosis of arrhythmogenic right ventricular dysplasia/cardiomyopathy. Task Force of the Working Group Myocardial and Pericardial Disease of the European Society of Cardiology and of the Scientific Council on Cardiomyopathies of the International Society and Federation of Cardiology. *Br Heart J*. 1994;71:215.

Modell SM, Lehmann MH. The long QT syndrome family of cardiac ion channelopathies: A Huge review. *Genet Med*. 2006;8:143.

Priori SG, Napolitano C, Memmi M, et al. Clinical and molecular characterization of patients with catecholaminergic polymorphic ventricular tachycardia. *Circulation*. 2002;106:69.

Richard P, Charron RP, Carrier L, et al. Hypertrophic cardiomyopathy: Distribution of disease genes, spectrum of mutations, and implications for a molecular diagnosis strategy. *Circulation*. 2003;107:2227.

Schwartz PJ, Moss AJ, Vincent GM, et al. Diagnostic criteria for the long QT syndrome. An update. *Circulation*. 1993;88:782.

Sen-Chowdhry S, Syrris P, McKenna WJ. Genetics of right ventricular cardiomyopathy. *J Cardiovasc Electrophysiol*. 2005;16:927.

Splawski I, Shen J, Timothy KW, et al. Spectrum of mutations in long-QT syndrome genes: KVLQT1, HERG, SCN5A, KCNE1, and KCNE2. *Circulation*. 2000;102:1178.

Wilde AA, Antzelevitch C, Borggrefe M, et al. Proposed diagnostic criteria for the Brugada syndrome. *Eur Heart J*. 2002;23:1648.

Zipes DP, Camm AJ, Borggrefe M, et al. ACC/AHA/ESC 2006 Guidelines for management of patients with ventricular arrhythmias and the prevention of sudden cardiac death-executive summary a report of the American College of Cardiology/American Heart Association Task Force and the European Soc iety of Cardiology Committee for practice guidelines (writing committee to develop guidelines for management of patients with ventricular arrhythmias and the prevention of sudden cardiac death). *J Am Coll Cardiol*. 2006;48:1064.

Implantable Cardioverter Defibrillator Indications

GENERAL PRINCIPLES

Current indications for implantable cardioverter defibrillator (ICD) therapy are derived from the inclusion criteria of several pivotal clinical trials. Each of these studies demonstrated mortality benefit with ICD therapy in a specific patient cohort (see Table 14-1). Applying these results to individual patients, however, requires not only a knowledge of these data, but also an appreciation for the unique clinical features of ICD therapy (see Table 14-2).

Recommendations regarding patient selection for ICD therapy were included in the 2006 American College of Cardiology/American Heart Association/European Society of Cardiology (ACC/AHA/ESC) guidelines for the management of ventricular arrhythmias and the prevention of sudden cardiac death (SCD). Although these recommendations provide the framework for a standardized approach to ICD utilization, decisions regarding ICD implantation are unique to each patient.

Clinical Trials

Clinical trials have definitively established that ICD therapy dramatically reduces the risk of arrhythmic death, and that in specific patient cohorts this reduced rate of arrhythmic death results in improved overall survival. Since the publications of Multicenter Automatic Defibrillator Implantation

TABLE 14-1 **Studies Demonstrating Mortality Benefit with Implantable Cardioverter Defibrillator (ICD) Therapy in a Specific Patient Cohort**

Trial	Patient Population	Inclusion Criteria	Results[a]
AVID (1997)	Secondary	Resuscitated VF; symptomatic VT requiring cardioversion with an LVEF <40%	31% RRR, 11% ARR in overall mortality at 36 mo compared to class III antiarrhythmics (most commonly amiodarone)
CASH (2000)	Secondary	Resuscitated SCA	23% RRR, 8% ARR (nonsignificant) in overall mortality at 57 mo compared to amiodarone or metoprolol
CIDS (2000)	Secondary	VF; out-of-hospital SCA requiring defibrillation or cardioversion; sustained VT causing syncope; VT (>150 bpm) causing presyncope or angina, with an LVEF <35%; syncope with subsequent spontaneous or induced monomorphic VT	20% annual RRR; 2% annual ARR (nonsignificant) in overall mortality compared to amiodarone
MUSTT (1999)	Primary	LVEF ≤40, prior MI, NSVT, (+) EPS (inducible VT)	[a]50% RRR, 24% ARR in overall mortality at 5 yr for ICD compared to conventional medical therapy
MADIT (1996)	Primary	LVEF ≤35, prior MI, NSVT, (+) EPS (inducible monomorphic VT that was not suppressible with procainamide)	54% RRR and 23% ARR for overall mortality at 27 mo compared to antiarrhythmic therapy
MADIT II (2002)	Primary	Prior MI, LVEF ≤30	35% RRR, 5.6% ARR in overall mortality at 20 mo compared to conventional medical therapy

SCD-HeFT (2005)	Primary	LVEF ≤35, NYHA class II or III HF (cardiomyopathy was ischemic or nonischemic in 52% and 48% of patients, respectively)	23% RRR, 7% ARR in overall mortality at 5 yr compared to conventional medical therapy
COMPANION (2004)	Primary	LVEF ≤35, NYHA class III or IV HF, and QRS >120 msec (Patients were randomly assigned to standard medical therapy, CRT alone, or CRT with an ICD)	36% RRR, 7% ARR in overall mortality at 12 mo for CRT plus an ICD compared to conventional medical therapy

[a]Risk reduction for ICD versus control, except for MUSTT (see note[b]). Results are statistically significant unless noted.

[b]MUSTT was not a randomized comparison of ICD therapy to AADs or conventional medical therapy. Rather it compared EPS-guided therapy (AAD or ICD) to conventional medical therapy. There was a nonsignificant improvement in survival among patients assigned to EPS guided therapy (6% ARR) that was entirely due to substantially reduced mortality in patients treated with an ICD. Patients in the EPS-guided arm who were treated with AADs had outcomes similar to the control arm (conventional medical therapy without EPS).

AVID, antiarrhythmics versus implantable defibrillators; CASH, Cardiac Arrest Study Hamburg; CIDS, Canadian Implantable Defibrillator Study; MUSTT, Multicenter Unsustained Tachycardia Trial; MADIT, Multicenter Automatic Defibrillator Implantation Trial; SCD–HeFT, Sudden Cardiac Death in Heart Failure Trial; COMPANION, Comparison of Medical Therapy, Pacing,and Defibrillation in Heart Failure; VF, ventricular fibrillation; VT, ventricular tachycardia; LVEF, left ventricular ejection fraction; bpm, beats per minute; MI, myocardial infarction; NSVT, nonsustained ventricular tachycardia; EPS, electrophysiologic study; HF, heart failure; NYHA, New York Heart Association; CRT, cardiac resynchronization therapy; AAD, antiarrhythmic drug; ARR, absolute risk reduction; RRR, relative risk reduction.

T A B L E 14-2 Complications Associated with Implantable Cardioverter Defibrillator (ICD) Therapy	
Device-related issues	
Implantation risk (standard transvenous approach in a typical patient)	The reported incidence of serious complications (e.g., serious infection, cardiac perforation, pneumothorax, or bleeding/hematoma) varies from ~1%–7%. Patient-specific issues (e.g., complicated access or increased infectious risk) can increase these risks
Long-term device-related risks	Infection/erosion requiring explantation Inappropriate shocks Device or lead failure
Patient-specific concerns	
Competing mortality Goals of care and quality of life	Many ICD candidates have substantial comborbidities in addition to advanced cardiac disease; therefore, the benefit of a reduced risk of arrhythmic death may be mitigated by an increased incidence of nonarrhythmic death (e.g., heart failure)
Infectious risks	Conditions associated with an increased incidence of infection and bacteremia (e.g., hemodialysis, chronic immunosuppression), may increase the long-term risk of device infection.

VT, ventricular tachycardia.

Trial (MADIT) (primary prevention) and antiarrhythmics versus implantable defibrillators (AVID) (secondary prevention) in 1996 and 1997 respectively, ICD indications have evolved rapidly.

General Concerns Related to Implantable Cardioverter Defibrillator Therapy

Once it is recognized that a patient's clinical profile justifies consideration of an ICD, a number of additional issues also need to be considered (Table 14-2). Because the benefit of ICD therapy is straightforward (improved survival), these additional issues are largely factors that could mitigate the expected benefit from and/or the patient's desire for a device. All cardiologists who refer patients for consideration of ICD implantation should have at least a general knowledge of these issues. Physicians directly responsible for recommending

ICD implantation should have a firm understanding of each of these concerns and be comfortable discussing them with prospective patients with ICD and their families.

For most ICD candidates, the potential mortality benefit of the device outweighs these concerns. It is not possible to define specific circumstances in which competing mortality or reduced quality of life make ICD therapy inappropriate. However, the ACC/AHA/ESC guidelines addressed this issue by including in all statements recommending ICD implantation the stipulation that the patient should "have reasonable expectation of survival with good functional status for more than one year." Ultimately, it is the responsibility of the physician recommending ICD therapy to individualize this assessment and decision process, ensuring that each patient makes a well-informed decision.

SECONDARY PREVENTION

Patients who survive sudden cardiac arrest (SCA) or symptomatic ventricular tachycardia (VT) are at an increased risk for recurrent malignant arrhythmias and SCD. Most such patients should be treated with an ICD, regardless of the nature of underlying heart disease (see Table 14-3).

The rationale for this approach is based on the results of three randomized trials (AVID, Cardiac Arrest Study Hamburg [CASH], and Canadian Implantable Defibrillator Study [CIDS]) that compared the efficacy of the ICD to that of antiarrhythmic drugs (AADs), most commonly amiodarone (Table 14-1). A meta-analysis that included these three trials and a fourth

---

TABLE 14-3   Treatment with an Implantable Convertible Defibrillator (ICD)

Events for which an ICD is indicated for secondary prevention of SCD

Resuscitated SCA due to ventricular fibrillation or ventricular tachycardia (VT)

Symptomatic ventricular tachycardia (e.g., syncope, presyncope, chest pain, SOB), particularly in patients with reduced systolic function

Exceptions

Reversible triggers, most commonly acute ischemia (documented NSTEMI, or STEMI within 48–72 h of the arrhythmic event)

Limited life expectancy (e.g., <1-2 yr) or poor quality of life

Asymptomatic/hemodynamically tolerated VT in patients with structurally normal hearts (e.g., RV outflow tract VT)

SCA, superior cerebellar artery; SOB, shortness of breath; NSTEMI, non-ST segment elevation; STEMI, ST-segment elevation; RV, right ventricular.

smaller trial showed that ICD therapy resulted in relative and absolute mortality reductions of 25% and 7%, respectively.

Reversible Causes

In some cases, SCA is attributed to a transient or reversible cause. Ischemic events (both non–ST-segment elevation myocardial infarction [NSTEMI] and ST-segment myocardial infarction [STEMI]), are the most commonly cited reversible triggers of malignant arrhythmias. Additional reversible causes include drugs, particularly antiarrhythmics and other drugs that prolong the QT interval, and metabolic or electrolyte disorders. The physicians approach such patients in the following manner:

- Polymorphic VT or ventricular fibrillation (VF) that occurs in the setting (i.e., within 48 to 72 hours) of myocardial ischemia can be attributed to the ischemic event. Management should focus on ischemia and such patients are not considered candidates for secondary prevention therapy. If such a patient suffers a large myocardial infarction (MI) with resulting left ventricular (LV) dysfunction and heart failure (HF), the usual approach to risk stratification for primary prevention should be pursued.

- Monomorphic VT usually reflects stable arrhythmic substrate (e.g., myocardial scar from a prior MI), and not acute ischemia. If monomorphic VT is documented in the setting of an ischemic event, the patient should be evaluated for the presence of preexisting substrate and if found, secondary prevention should be considered.

- Polymorphic VT that occurs in the setting of QT prolongation due to known QT prolonging medications should be treated with avoidance of such medications. An ICD for secondary prevention is not indicated.

- Electrolyte abnormalities, in isolation, are an unusual cause of malignant arrhythmias. In addition, transient electrolyte abnormalities (e.g., hyperkalemia) can develop during cardiac arrest and resuscitation. Therefore, unless there is compelling evidence, SCA events should not be attributed to mild or moderate electrolyte abnormalities.

PRIMARY PREVENTION

Because initial SCA events are usually fatal, it is preferable to identify patients at risk for malignant arrhythmias before the first event occurs. Therefore, extensive work has been done to define the clinical profiles of patients who would benefit from ICD implantation for the primary prevention of SCD. The clinical characteristics that have proved to be the most powerful predictors of SCD risk include a prior MI, moderate-to-severe systolic dysfunction, and clinical HF. Additional predictors include nonsustained VT, single-averaged electrocardiogram (SAECG) abnormalities, T wave alternans (TWA), and inducible monomorphic VT at electrophysiologic study (EPS).

The Multicenter Unsustained Tachycardia Trial (MUSTT), MADIT, MADIT-II, and SCD-HeFT trials each demonstrated improved survival with ICD therapy in specific cohorts of primary prevention patients. In broad terms, these categories include patients with moderate-to-severe LV dysfunction due to a prior MI (MUSTT, MADIT, and MADIT-II) and patients with HF due to moderate-to-severe systolic dysfunction of any etiology (SCD-HeFT). In addition, selected patients with inherited arrhythmia syndromes are also candidates for ICD implantation for primary prevention. Specific criteria are presented in Table 14-4.

The authors' approach to primary prevention is somewhat more conservative than that outlined in the 2006 ACC/AHA/ESC guidelines, which suggest consideration of ICD therapy in patients with less severe systolic dysfunction (e.g., left ventricular ejection fraction [LVEF] up to 40%) or HF (e.g., some New York Heart Association [NYHA] class I patients). These discrepancies reflect the challenges and controversies involved in identifying appropriate candidates for primary prevention ICD implantation. Many patients outside of the profiles defined by clinical trials criteria will experience SCD. Therefore, there is interest in expanding ICD indications to include patients with less severe LV dysfunction and/or fewer risk factors. However, because such patients have a lower arrhythmic risk, liberalization of ICD indications will greatly increase the number of patients needed to treat in order to save one life. This dilution of ICD efficacy will expose substantially more patients to the risks of an implanted device and will also greatly increase the societal costs of ICD therapy. For these reasons, the physicians favor a closer adherence to the patient profiles defined in the clinical trials while further research is done to guide a rational expansion of ICD indications.

Prior Myocardial Infarction and Left Ventricular Systolic Dysfunction

Myocardial scar from a prior MI provides the electrophysiologic substrate for ventricular arrhythmias, usually monomorphic VT. Both the likelihood of such arrhythmias and the risk of associated hemodynamic collapse increase with progressive degrees of systolic dysfunction. Therefore, patients with a prior MI and significant reductions in systolic function are at a high risk of fatal arrhythmias.

MUSTT and MADIT evaluated the role of ICD implantation for primary prevention of SCD in patients with a prior MI, at least moderate LV systolic dysfunction (LVEF ≤35% to 40%), and inducible monomorphic VT at electrophysiology (EP) study. Although the designs of these two trials differed, each demonstrated significant mortality benefit with ICD implantation in these

TABLE 14-4 Specific Criteria for ICD Implantation

Indications for ICD implantation for primary prevention of SCD

Prior MI and LV systolic dysfunction (MI >4 wk prior)

LVEF ≤30% due to prior infarction(s)

LVEF 30%–40% due to prior infarction(s) and

Inducible monomorphic VT at EPS *or*

(+) TWA and abnormal SAECG *or*

Widened QRS *or*

LVH *or*

Unrevascularized 3VD

LV systolic dysfunction and heart failure (HF) (cardiomyopathy present for >9 mo)

LVEF ≤35% and NYHA class II or III HF[a]

Indications for an ICD combined with biventricular pacing

LVEF ≤35% and evidence of intraventricular dyssynchrony[b] and NYHA class III or IV HF[a]

Special cases/inherited arrhythmia syndromes

HCM: If two of five are present—family history of SCD, NSVT, syncope, abnormal BP response, LVH >30 mm; there are differing opinions regarding the utility of an ICD in patients with a single prominent risk factor (e.g., multiple affected family members with SCD)

Brugada syndrome: Spontaneous type 1 ECG and a history of syncope; there are differing opinions regarding the utility of an ICD in patients with a type 1 ECG and other risk factors (e.g., strong family history of SCD and/or inducible VT)

LQTS: Syncope of unclear etiology; there are differing opinions regarding the utility of an ICD in patients with other risk factors (e.g., strong family history of SCD and/or Jervell and Lange-Neilson)

ARVC: Syncope of unclear etiology; there are differing opinions regarding the utility of an ICD in patients with other risk factors (e.g., strong family history of SCD, extensive RV involvement and/or LV involvement)

---

[a]Persistent HF symptoms of this class after optimization of medical therapy.

[b]Widened QRS, and/or echocardiographic evidence of dyssynchrony (no standard defined at present).

ICD, implantable convertible defibrillator; SCD, sudden cardiac death; MI, myocardial infarction; LV, left ventricular; LVEF, left ventricular ejection fraction; VT, ventricular tachycardia; EPS, electrophysiologic study; TWA, T wave alternans; SAECG, signal-averaged electrocardiography; LVH, left ventricular hypertrophy; VD, vessel disease; NYHA, New York Heart Association; HCM, hypertrophic cardiomyopathy; SCD, sudden cardiac death; NSVT, nonsustained ventricular tachycardia; BP, blood pressure; ECG, electrocardiogram; LQTS, long QT syndrome; ARVC, arrhythmogenic right ventricular cardiomyopathy; RV, right ventricular.

populations. These results were advanced by the MADIT II and SCD-HeFT, which demonstrated mortality benefit with ICD therapy in patients with either severe LV dysfunction due to a prior MI (LVEF ≤30%) or moderate LV dysfunction of any etiology (LVEF ≤35%) and symptomatic HF (Table 14-1). These results form the basis for current ICD indications in patients with a prior MI (Table 14-4).

Heart Failure and Left Ventricular Systolic Dysfunction

Like those with severe LV dysfunction due to a prior MI, patients with nonischemic cardiomyopathy are also at an increased risk for malignant ventricular arrhythmias and SCD. This risk increases with more severe LV dysfunction and more advanced HF. However, important differences between ischemic and nonischemic cardiomyopathy have direct implications on the utility of ICD therapy. First, the arrhythmic substrate differs significantly in these conditions. For this reason, some of the variables that predict arrhythmic risk in patients with a prior MI (e.g., nonsustained ventricular tachycardia [NSVT], inducible VT) are not predictive in patients with nonischemic cardiomyopathy. Second, patients with severe cardiomyopathy and advanced HF have substantial mortality rates due to HF. Therefore, a reduction in arrhythmic death rates with the ICD is less likely to result in substantial improvement in overall mortality.

Despite these challenges, SCD-HeFT demonstrated improved survival with ICD therapy in patients with either ischemic or nonischemic cardiomyopathy who also have moderate to severe HF (Table 14-1), providing the basis for ICD therapy in these patients (Table 14-4).

Implantable Cardioverter Defibrillator Combined with Cardiac Resynchronization Therapy

Cardiac resynchronization therapy (CRT) with biventricular pacing improves survival in appropriately selected patients. CRT can be incorporated into a combination device with ICD capabilities with a further increase in survival.

The Comparison of Medical Therapy, Pacing, and Defibrillation in Heart Failure (COMPANION) trial randomly assigned patients with an LVEF ≤35%, NYHA class III or IV HF, and cardiac dyssynchrony (QRS >120 msec) to optimal medical therapy, biventricular pacing alone, or biventricular pacing in a device with ICD capabilities. Patients assigned to either of the CRT arms had improvements in clinical HF outcomes, whereas those assigned to the cardiac resynchronization therapy–implantable cardioverter defibrillator (CRT-ICD) arm also had improved overall survival. On the basis of these results, the physicians favor combined CRT-ICD devices in patients with severe systolic dysfunction, advanced HF, and evidence of dyssynchrony. There are some advanced HF patients for whom the palliative effects of CRT are desired but, because of poor quality of life and/or less aggressive goals of care, the ICD capabilities are not (Table 14-2). Biventricular pacing alone is a reasonable option in such patients.

Class IV Heart Failure without Dyssynchrony

The role of ICD therapy for primary prevention of SCD in patients with NYHA class IV HF without evidence of dyssynchrony (i.e., who are not CRT candidates) has not been definitively assessed. In general, such patients are not ICD candidates due to high nonarrhythmic mortality (i.e., "competing mortality"), poor quality of life, and less aggressive goals of care (Table 14-2). In selected patients with stable but advanced HF (i.e., "ambulatory class IV HF"), particularly young patients or those awaiting cardiac transplantation, ICD implantation may be reasonable. Such cases should be carefully evaluated on an individual basis, with detailed discussion between the patient and both EP and HF specialists.

TIMING OF IMPLANTATION

Patients present for consideration of ICD implantation at a variety of points along their clinical course, ranging from immediately following a large infarction to many years after an index event or diagnosis. The elapsed time since an MI or a diagnosis of cardiomyopathy impacts consideration of ICD therapy at both ends of this time span.

Early Implantation

ICD implantation is not recommended in the first weeks after an MI or for 9 months after the diagnosis of a nonischemic cardiomyopathy. The restriction early after an MI is, in some ways, counterintuitive. The risks of arrhythmic death are highest in the first days and weeks after an MI, as high as 2.5% in the first month in patients with severe LV dysfunction and HF. However, the Defibrillator in Acute Myocardial Infarction Trial (DINAMITE) specifically evaluated the role of ICD implantation early (6 to 40 days) after an MI, and found no survival benefit. Reasons for the lack of benefit are unclear, but may include recurrent ischemia causing early SCD, which would not be prevented by an ICD. In addition, many patients have improved LV function several weeks after their MI and such patients probably have relatively low long-term arrhythmic risks. Therefore, the failure to demonstrate benefit from early ICD placement likely reflects both early recurrent ischemia and an inability to identify appropriate candidates at this stage. The physicians currently defer ICD implantation for 4 weeks post-MI, at which time they reassess patients considered to be at increased arrhythmic risk. In selected cases, a wearable defibrillator vest may be a reasonable option until a determination is made regarding permanent device placement.

For patients with nonischemic cardiomyopathy and HF, it is recommended that ICD implantation be deferred for 9 months after the initial diagnosis. This period allows for the initiation of appropriate medical therapy, which may result in improved LV function and/or reduced HF symptoms. Patients who are enrolled in clinical trials or registries may have implantable cardioverter defibrillators (ICDs) implanted 3 to 9 months after the diagnosis of a nonischemic cardiomyopathy.

Late Implantation

On the other end of the spectrum, patients who are several years removed from an initial MI may appear to have low arrhythmic risk, particularly if they have been clinically stable for many years. Although it is true that arrhythmic risk declines in the first months after an MI, this decline eventually reaches a plateau and does not return to baseline, even after many years without an arrhythmic event. Illustrating this point, the control groups in the MUSTT and MADIT-2 were an average of 3 and 7 years removed from their initial MI, respectively. In such patients, ICD implantation resulted in substantial mortality benefit (Table 14-1). Therefore, despite many years of quiescence with a longstanding diagnosis, patients who meet established criteria for primary prevention ICD therapy should not be disqualified based on extended elapsed time from the index event.

SELECTED BIBLIOGRAPHY

Antiarrhythmics versus Implantable Defibrillators (AVID) Investigators. A comparison of antiarrhythmic-drug therapy with implantable defibrillators in patients resuscitated from near-fatal ventricular arrhythmias. *N Engl J Med*. 1997;337:1576.

Bardy GH, Lee KL, Mark DB, et al. Amiodarone or an implantable cardioverter-defibrillator for congestive heart failure. SCD-HeFT Investigators. *N Engl J Med*. 2005;352:225.

Bristow MR, Saxon LA, Boehmer J, et al. COMPANION Investigators. Cardiac-resynchronization therapy with or without an implantable defibrillator in advanced chronic heart failure. *N Engl J Med*. 2004;350:2140.

Buxton AE, Lee KL, Fisher JD, et al. Multicenter Unsustained Tachycardia Trial Investigators. A randomized study of the prevention of sudden death in patients with coronary artery disease. *N Engl J Med*. 1999;341:1882.

Connolly SJ, Gent M, Roberts RS, et al. Canadian Implantable Defibrillator Study (CIDS): A randomized trial of the implantable cardioverter defibrillator against amiodarone. *Circulation*. 2000;101:1297.

Josephson ME. *Clinical cardiac electrophysiology*, 4th ed. Philadelphia: Lippincott Williams & Wilkins; 2008.

Kuck KH, Cappato R, Siebels J, et al. The CASH Investigators. Randomized comparison of antiarrhythmic drug therapy with implantable defibrillators in patients resuscitated from cardiac arrest. The Cardiac Arrest Study Hamburg (CASH). *Circulation* 2000;102:748.

Lee DS, Green LD, Liu PP, et al. Effectiveness of implantable defibrillators for preventing arrhythmic events and death: A meta-analysis. *J Am Coll Cardiol*. 2003;41:1573; (Sec prev meta-analysis).

Moss AJ, Hall WJ, Cannom DS, et al. The Multicenter Automatic Defibrillator Implantation Trial Investigators. Improved survival with an implanted defibrillator in patients with coronary disase at high risk for ventricular arrhythmia. *N Engl J Med*. 1996;335:1933.

Moss AJ, Zareba W, Hall WJ, et al. MADIT II Investigators. Prophylactic implantation of a defibrillator in patients with myocardial infarction and reduced ejection fraction. *N Engl J Med*. 2002;346:877.

Zipes DP, Camm AJ, Borggrefe M, et al. ACCAHAESC 2006 guidelines for management of patients with ventricular arrhythmias and the prevention of sudden cardiac death-executive summary. A report of the American College of Cardiology, American Heart Association Task Force and the European Society of Cardiology Committee for Practice Guidelines (Writing committee to develop guidelines for management of patients with ventricular arrhythmias and the prevention of sudden cardiac death). *J Am Coll Cardiol*. 2006;48:1064.

Permanent Pacemakers

CLINICAL INDICATIONS

The clinical indications for permanent pacemaker (PPM) implantation are covered in detail in Chapter 11. A brief recapitulation is provided in the subsequent text.

Sinus Node Dysfunction

Sinus node dysfunction is the most common indication for pacemaker implantation, accounting for 40% to 60% of all implants. Symptomatic sinus node dysfunction (i.e., documented sinus bradycardia or sinus pauses with symptoms) as well as chronic chronotropic incompetence are a class I indication for PPM implantation. Less commonly, asymptomatic patients may require pacing for sinus node dysfunction. Pharmacologic therapy to treat sinus node dysfunction is limited and because many patients require medications that can suppress sinus node function (such as β-blockers, calcium channel blockers, or antiarrhythmia medications), pacemaker implantation may be required to treat sinus node dysfunction exacerbated by external (medication) causes. Often patients with sinus node dysfunction have accompanying supraventricular arrhythmias and the incidence of developing atrial fibrillation is 5% per year.

Pacing for Atrioventricular Block

Atrioventricular (AV) block is the second most common indication for pacemaker implantation. As detailed in Chapter 11, common causes include heightened vagal tone, medications, senile degeneration, infection, and infarction.

Pacing for Other Indications

Pacemaker implantation is occasionally utilized to treat other disorders. Neurocardiogenic syncope associated with bradycardia (particularly sinus arrest) documented spontaneously or during tilt table testing that is recurrent and unresponsive to medical treatment may benefit from PPM implantation although several large randomized trials have revealed conflicting results. Patients receiving a pacemaker for this indication may be treated with rapid pacing (e.g., at ~100 bpm) for a short period of time (i.e., 2 minutes) upon onset of vagal symptoms and may have fewer episodes of syncope (although, patients may still become highly symptomatic from a vasodepressor response).

Some patients undergo pacemaker implantation for ventricular resynchronization to treat heart failure. Candidates for this therapy are those patients with ischemic or nonischemic cardiomyopathy, reduced left ventricular ejection fraction (≤35%), heart failure symptoms despite optimal medical therapy, and left bundle branch block. These patients may have asynchronous activation of the septum and delayed activation of the left lateral wall resulting in a reduced stroke volume and often increased mitral regurgitation. Currently, the evidence for echocardiographic identifiers of interventricular dyssynchrony (dyssynchronous contraction of the right and left ventricles) is equivocal.

Randomized trials have demonstrated that some patients have improved clinical outcomes (quality of life, exercise capacity, maximum oxygen consumption, reduced heart failure hospitalizations, and improved survival) with biventricular pacing (simultaneous right and left ventricular pacing). Left ventricular pacing is performed by stimulating through an additional electrode that is placed transvenously through the coronary sinus to the epicardial LV (although occasionally the LV lead is placed on the epicardial surface of the heart through a surgical or thoracoscopic approach). Typically, the best place for left ventricular pacing is the posterolateral or lateral cardiac veins (see Chapter 1).

Dual chamber pacing is occasionally used for hypertrophic obstructive cardiomyopathy. Right ventricular pacing changes the septal activation sequence and therefore may induce dyssynchrony and decrease the outflow tract gradient. Results from clinical trials have found that the effects are at best modest—and in some cases may even be detrimental. Pacing may be beneficial to allow uptitration of β-blockers or calcium channel blockers for their lusitropic effect or to allow AV junctional ablation in the setting of poorly controlled atrial fibrillation.

Pacing may be beneficial in some patients with the long QT syndrome who present with bradycardia or pause-induced *torsade de pointes*.

PACEMAKER FEATURES

A pacemaker system consists of the pulse generator and lead(s) (see Fig. 15-1). The pulse generator consists of the device circuitry and battery whereas the pacemaker lead consists of the electrode, insulation, connector pin, and a fixation mechanism. The lead conducts the cardiac signals to the pulse generator in either a bipolar (two electrodes at the tip of the lead in the cardiac chamber) or unipolar (a single electrode at the tip of the lead with the pacemaker generator "can" functioning as the second electrode) configuration. Most modern implanted electrodes are bipolar because they are less prone to sensing noncardiac electrical signals. Several fixation mechanisms are available including passive fixation with tines, wings, or fins or active fixation using exposed or retractable screws (see Fig. 15-2). Passive fixation leads are anchored to the heart by entrapment to trabecular muscle whereas active fixation mechanisms allow the placement of the leads in any position of the heart.

Single-chamber pacemakers are most often utilized for patients with chronic atrial fibrillation (in whom sensing or pacing in the atrium is unnecessary). Although, single-chamber atrial pacing is still performed on some

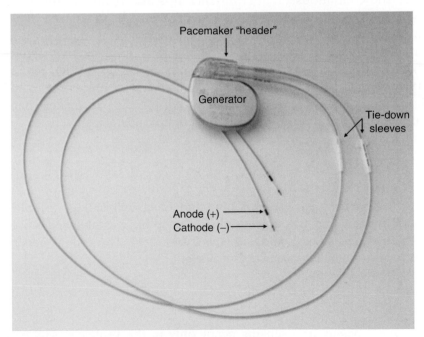

FIGURE 15-1. Pacemaker (battery and circuitry) and pacemaker leads.

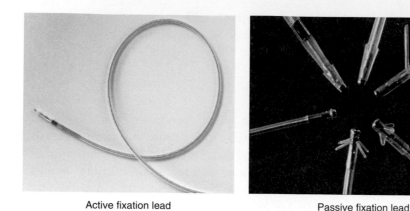

Active fixation lead   Passive fixation lead

FIGURE 15-2. Active and passive fixation pacing leads.

occasions, most patients with sinus node dysfunction receive dual-chamber pacemakers due to the common association of sinus node dysfunction with AV node dysfunction. In fact, patients with sinus node dysfunction but no evidence of AV nodal disease at the time of pacemaker implantation develop significant AV node disease at a rate of 0.6% to 2.7% per year. It is the authors' practice to implant dual rather than single-chamber pacemakers in most patients except in those with chronic atrial fibrillation.

Pacemaker batteries are expected to last for 6 to 12 years. The duration of battery life is related to the amount of pacing that occurs (single vs. dual chamber and continuous vs. intermittent). It is also related to the amount of energy needed to capture the respective chamber. All pacemakers have indicators signaling when the elective replacement time is reached. Common indicators include (a) a decrease in pacing rate upon magnet application, (b) change to a simpler pacing mode (from DDDR to VVIR), (c) reduced battery voltage, (d) increase in battery impedance, and (e) loss of programmability. If the pacemaker battery reaches end of life the pacemaker changes to the simplest pacing mode and may fail to communicate.

PACING MODES

The North American Society of Pacing and Electrophysiology (NASPE) and the British Pacing and Electrophysiology Group have established a five-letter code which is periodically updated (see Table 15-1). The code is generic and applies to all pacemaker makes and models.

VVI

In VVI mode, pacing and sensing occur only in the ventricle. Any paced or sensed event starts an internal timer—the expiration of the lower rate interval

TABLE 15-1 The Revised North American Society of Pacing and Electrophysiology/British Pacing and Electrophysiology Group (NASPE/BPEG) Generic Code for Antibradycardia, Adaptive-Rate, and Multisite Pacing

Position	I	II	III	IV	V
Category	Chamber(s) Paced	Chamber(s) Sensed	Response to Sensing	Rate Modulation	Multisite Pacing
	O = None	O = None	O = None	O = None	O = None
	A = Atrium	A = Atrium	T = Triggered	R = Rate modulation	A = Atrium
	V = Ventricle	V = Ventricle	I = Inhibited		V = Ventricle
	D = Dual (A + V)	D = Dual (A + V)	D = Dual (T + I)		D = Dual (A + V)

(LRI) without an intervening sensed event (i.e., ventricular beat) will cause the pacemaker to deliver a pacing impulse and reset the lower rate timer. A sensed event will also restart the lower rate timer and therefore will inhibit the pacemaker from delivering a paced beat. VVI pacing is most often used in patients with chronic atrial fibrillation.

AAI

AAI mode is identical to VVI mode, except that pacing and sensing occur in the atrium, not in the ventricle.

DDD

In DDD mode (see Fig. 15-3), pacing and sensing occur in both the atrium and ventricle. In addition, a sensed or paced beat in the atrium "triggers" pacing in the ventricle if intrinsic conduction does not occur spontaneously after a programmed delay.

Atrioventricular Interval

Most pacemaker timing intervals are based on the ventricle. A sensed or paced event in the ventricle will start the LRI timer. At the same time, a second timer for the VA interval is started. If no atrial event is sensed at the end of the VA interval a pacing impulse will be delivered in the atrium. An atrioventricular interval (AVI) is started at that time and a ventricular pacing spike will

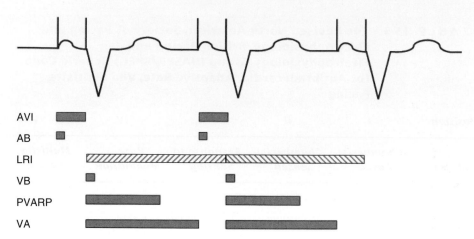

FIGURE 15-3. The timing intervals in a dual-chamber pacemaker are shown. AVI, atrioventricular interval; AB, atrial blanking period; LRI, lower rate interval; VB, ventricular blanking period; PVARP, postventricular atrial refractory period; VA, ventriculoatrial interval.

be delivered if no ventricular event is sensed. The sum of the VA interval and AVI is the LRI.

Postventricular Atrial Refractory Period

Two important programmable timers are started upon sensing or pacing events in the ventricle. The ventricular refractory period avoids T-wave oversensing. At the same time, the postventricular atrial refractory period (PVARP) timer is started. During that time no atrial sensing occurs in order to prevent sensing of retrogradely conducted P waves in the atrium, which may result in pacemaker-mediated tachycardia (PMTs) (see subsequent text). The upper tracking rate is limited by the sum of the PVARP and the AVI.

Cross Talk and Safety Pacing

Many pacemakers have the capability to shorten the AVI with increasing heart rates. Usually the sensed AVI is shorter than the paced AVI. After a paced atrial stimulus, the AVI is divided into two parts: A programmable blanking period starting with the atrial stimulus and followed by sensing in the ventricle during the remainder of the AVI. During the blanking period no sensing in the ventricles occurs in order to avoid sensing of the atrial stimulus for a ventricular event which would cause inhibition of ventricular pacing (cross talk inhibition). A sensed event in the ventricle during the second part of the AVI (possibly caused by a ventricular premature complex [VPC] or the atrial stimulus) will result in a ventricular safety pacing stimulus usually with an AVI of 100 msec (see Fig. 15-4). This ensures that no cross talk inhibition

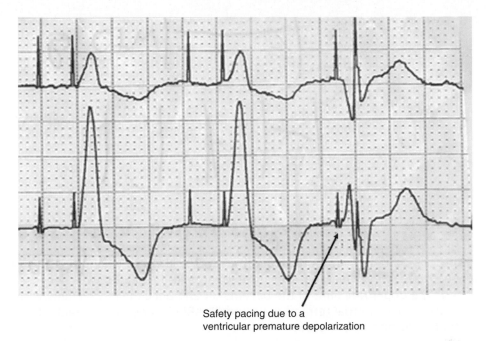

Safety pacing due to a
ventricular premature depolarization

FIGURE 15-4. Demonstration of safety pacing. In this case a ventricular premature depolarization. Safety pacing is characterized by the fixed AV interval of 100 msec. AV, atrioventricular.

occurs which could otherwise result in asystole in pacemaker-dependent patients.

Upper Rate Behavior and Pacemaker Wenckebach

DDD pacemakers have a programmable upper rate limit beyond which tracking of atrial events do not occur. If the atrial rate exceeds the upper limit in patients without AV conduction pacemaker Wenckebach or 2:1 AV conduction results (see Fig. 15-5). Initially in order not to violate the upper rate limit the pacemaker prolongs the AVI until a sensed atrial event falls into the PVARP and is therefore not tracked resulting in Wenckebach behavior. If the atrial rate increases further, the sensed atrial events fall into the atrial refractory period resulting in 2:1 conduction.

DDI

In this mode, sensing and pacing occur in both the atrium and ventricle but ventricular pacing is not triggered by sensed events in the atrium. Unlike the DDD mode, in DDI, a sensed atrial event does not start an AVI. Ventricular pacing will occur after atrial sensed events only at the lower rate limit (when no

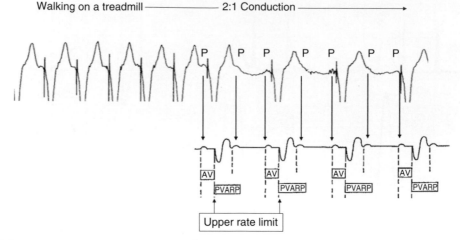

FIGURE 15-5. Demonstration of pacemaker Wenckebach phenomena. Sinus tachycardia occurs while walking on a treadmill. The sinus rate eventually exceeds the upper rate limit of the pacemaker and once the P wave falls within the postventricular atrial refractory period (PVARP) it is no longer tracked. This results in tracking of every other P wave and a 2:1 response. At slower sinus rates, the AV interval will gradually prolong and result in varying degrees of pacemaker Wenckebach cycles (e.g., 4:3 conduction).

intrinsic ventricular activity is sensed). Dual-chamber pacing will occur only when there is no sensed atrial activity or ventricular activity above the lower rate limit. This pacing mode is often used in patients with supraventricular arrhythmias to avoid ventricular tracking during paroxysmal episodes (e.g., paroxysmal atrial fibrillation). The mode switch feature (described in the subsequent text) allows many pacemakers to switch from DDD to DDI mode automatically once a supraventricular tachycardia is detected.

VDD

This is an uncommon pacing mode where sensing occurs in both the atrium and ventricle but there is only pacing in the ventricle. Atrial sensing will trigger ventricular pacing after a programmed AV delay as in DDD mode, but pacing will not occur in the atrium.

AOO and VOO

In AOO and VOO pacing modes (also known as *asynchronous pacing*), pacing occurs at a fixed programmed rate without regard to the underlying rhythm. This pacing mode is sometimes programmed to avoid inhibition of the pacemaker during surgical procedures or if oversensing is a problem in pacemaker-dependent patients.

ADDITIONAL FEATURES

Mode Switch

To avoid tracking of atrial arrhythmias and the resultant high-rate ventricular pacing, dual-chamber pacemakers can "mode switch" automatically to a non-tracking mode (i.e., DDI or VVI) if a supraventricular arrhythmia is detected above a programmable rate (e.g., 170 bpm). The device will automatically switch back to the tracking mode (DDD) if/when the arrhythmia terminates.

Strategies to Promote Intrinsic Conduction

Right ventricular pacing results in interventricular asynchrony and can lead to heart failure in a subset of patients. Therefore, conduction from the atria to the ventricles is preferable. This is sometimes difficult to maintain in patients with long PR intervals because with traditional pacing algorithms programming a long AV interval (to allow normal ventricular activation) may use up a lot of time in the AV timing cycle and result in a relatively low maximum tracking rate for the pacemaker (upper rate limit). Algorithms have been developed allowing pacemakers to favor native conduction in patients with intact AV conduction. The pacemaker stimulates the heart in AAI mode and monitors for native conduction to the ventricle. Should no native conduction occur the pacemaker switches to DDD pacing. After a certain time interval, the pacemaker tests for the native conduction again by gradually increasing the AVI. If conduction to the ventricle occurs it switches back to AAI pacing. One such algorithm is called *managed ventricular pacing* (MVP, Medtronic, Inc. Minnesota) and sometimes can mimic pacemaker dysfunction when a paced atrial beat is not followed by a ventricular beat (see Fig. 15-6).

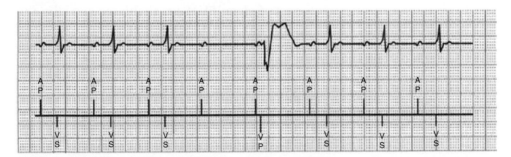

FIGURE 15-6. Managed ventricular pacing (MVP) mode: Atrial pacing captures the atrium with conduction to the ventricles through the atrioventricular (AV) conduction system. There is AV block after the fourth atrially paced beat (AP) which results in AV sequential pacing the following cycle to ensure capture of the ventricles.

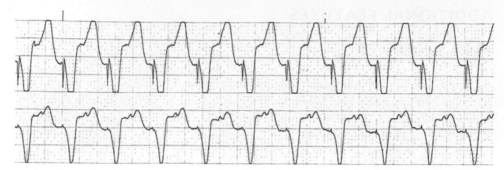

FIGURE 15-7. Pacemaker tachycardia. Note the retrogradely conducted P waves at the beginning of the T wave.

Rate Adaptive Pacing

Rate adaptive or rate responsive pacing allows the pacemaker to adjust the heart rate according to the physiologic demand. This feature is most useful for patients with sinus node dysfunction or atrial fibrillation with a slow ventricular rate. A variety of different sensors are utilized including activity sensors (which use either piezoelectric crystals or accelerometers) or minute ventilation sensors (which respond to respiratory rate as measured by transthoracic impedance). Less frequently, QT sensors (responsive to changes in autonomic status) or combined sensors (that utilize more than one of the aforementioned sensors) are employed.

Pacemaker-Mediated Tachycardia

Ventricular pacing with retrograde AV conduction may result in PMT. This can only occur if the pacing mode is DDD and if the retrograde conduction results in the atrial event occurring outside the programmed refractory period (postventricular atrial refractory period or PVARP). If this occurs, the retrograde atrial signal will be interpreted as a spontaneous P wave, resulting in tracking, ventricular pacing, and perpetuation of the cycle. Pacing at or near the upper rate limit of the pacemaker without physical activity should raise the suspicion for PMT in patients with dual-chamber pacemakers (see Fig. 15-7). Reprogramming the device to prolong the PVARP or switching to a nontracking mode will alleviate the problem.

PACEMAKER IMPLANTATION

The vast majority of pacemakers are implanted transvenously, although epicardial pacemaker lead placement is occasionally performed. The cephalic, axillary, or subclavian vein can be used for transvenous access (see Fig. 15-8).

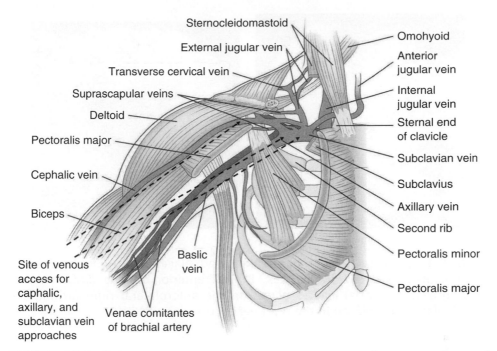

Sternocleidomastoid

External jugular vein

Transverse cervical vein

Suprascapular veins

Deltoid

Pectoralis major

Cephalic vein

Biceps

Site of venous access for caphalic, axillary, and subclavian vein approaches

Venae comitantes of brachial artery

Baslic vein

Omohyoid

Anterior jugular vein

Internal jugular vein

Sternal end of clavicle

Subclavian vein

Subclavius

Axillary vein

Second rib

Pectoralis minor

Pectoralis major

FIGURE 15-8. Relevant upper extremity venous anatomy for pacemaker and implantable cardioverter defibrillator (ICD) implantation. The most common sites of venous access include the cephalic, axillary, and subclavian veins.

Cephalic venous access carries the lowest risk of pneumothorax and compared with subclavian access, has a lower risk of subsequent lead fracture due to friction or compression by the ligament at the costoclavicular angle. Leads are passed through the venous system and secured in the atrium (usually the right atrial appendage) and ventricle (typically the right ventricular apex), respectively. Patients who have undergone cardiac surgery will often have the right atrial appendage removed and alternative right atrial sites are used. Figure 15-9 shows pacemaker lead positioning on chest roentgenogram.

After lead placement, electrical parameters are assessed to ensure adequate pacing threshold, sensing, and impedance. Pacing threshold is the minimum energy required to reliably capture the heart outside the refractory period. Figure 15-10 shows the strength-duration relationship. Any combination of pulse width duration and stimulation strength above the curve will result in capture of the stimulated chamber. Any increase in the pulse width duration beyond 0.5 to 0.6 msec has only minor effects on the voltage needed to capture the stimulated chamber. Conversely, any decrease of the pulse width below 0.5 msec results in considerable increase in the voltage needed to capture the stimulated chamber. Therefore, at a pulse width of 0.5 to 0.6 msec the most energy efficient stimulation combination is achieved (lowest voltage to capture).

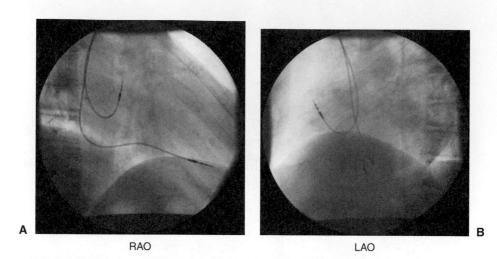

A   RAO

B   LAO

FIGURE 15-9. Dual-chamber pacemaker lead placement. **A:** Right anterior oblique (RAO) view at 30 degrees. **B:** Left anterior oblique (LAO) view at 60 degrees. The atrial lead is placed in the anterolateral right atrium, the ventricular lead is placed in the right ventricular apex.

Sensing refers to the ability of the device to "see" the cardiac signals. Sensitivity is a programmed value below which the device will ignore electrical signals. This allows the device to differentiate between true cardiac signals and external noise. The sensitivity can be thought of as a solid fence. Any intrinsic signal that is taller than the fence (i.e., greater amplitude than the programmed sensing amplitude) will be seen and will inhibit

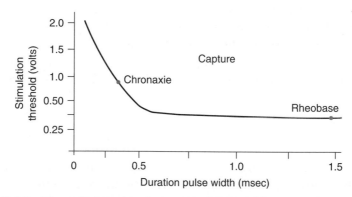

FIGURE 15-10. The relationship between the stimulation voltage (volts) and stimulation duration (msec) is shown. The rheobase is the minimal voltage at an infinitely long duration pulse that captures. The chronaxie is the pulse width at twice the rheobase voltage. Above a pulse width of 0.5 to 0.6 msec the voltage needed for capturing does not decrease significantly any further. Any combination of duration pulse width and voltage above the curve will result in capture.

the pacemaker. For example, if the sensing amplitude is set at 0.6 mV and the P wave sensed in the right atrium is 3 mV, the pacemaker will see the P wave and inhibit pacing. Conversely, any intrinsic signal which is smaller than the programmed sensing amplitude (obscured by the theoretic fence) will not be recognized and the pacemaker will deliver a paced beat (e.g., a sensed amplitude setting of 0.6 mV in the atrium may not recognize a fibrillatory wave of 0.3 mV and result in inappropriate atrial pacing during atrial fibrillation).

Lead impedance is assessed at implantation and routinely during follow-up. The lead impedance is a combination of the properties of the lead itself as well as the resistance at the interface of the electrode and the cardiac chamber. The lead impedance is inversely related to the amount of energy needed to capture the respective cardiac chamber at a fixed voltage (Ohm's law: Voltage = current × resistance). Tracking changes in the lead impedance is helpful to identify lead abnormalities (see the subsequent text).

Complications of pacemaker implantation are uncommon but can include infection, pneumothorax, hemothorax, bleeding, venous thrombosis, air embolism, lead dislodgement, cardiac perforation requiring drainage or surgery, neurovascular injury, or death.

ACUTE AND CHRONIC COMPLICATIONS

Infection

Infections are classified as acute and chronic in relation to the timing of device implantation. The most common pathogens include *Staphylococcus aureus* and *Staphylococcus epidermidis*. They can arise from the pocket and manifest as a localized pocket infection or they can spread through the circulation and result in an endovascular infection. Primary endovascular infections can secondarily infect indwelling pacemaker and implantable cardioverter defibrillator (ICD) leads and are very difficult to treat without lead extraction. Echocardiographic imaging is often performed to identify potentially infected material attached to the leads; however, these findings are nonspecific and their absence does not exclude lead involvement. Superficial erythema or a retained suture with small abscess formation can occur within days of the procedure and is usually curable with antibiotics. More commonly, infections present 3 or more months post device implantation and may be difficult to manage. If there is a breach of skin integrity over the device it must be considered infected and removed. If the skin is intact and there are no systemic signs of infection we advocate a trial of antibiotics under the guidance of an infectious disease consultant. If signs of infection recur despite antibiotics, the authors advocate complete extraction. Patients who are very debilitated from unrelated systemic illnesses or of advanced age can sometimes be managed with chronic suppressive antibiotics.

Pacemaker Syndrome

The pacemaker syndrome is a constellation of symptoms that may occur due to ventricular pacing and loss of AV synchrony. Specifically, atrial contraction against closed AV valves can trigger reflex mediated symptoms that may include fatigue, cough, decrease in exercise capacity, dizziness, syncope or presyncope, altered mental status, palpitations, and nausea. Hemodynamically, the syndrome is characterized by a decrease in stroke volume and hypotension. Sometimes jugular pulsation can be observed in patients. Of note the syndrome is not limited to the VVI pacing mode because AAI pacing with a long PR interval can have similar hemodynamic consequences.

Twiddler Syndrome

This syndrome (see Fig. 15-11) is caused by manual rotation of the pacemaker generator that results in twisting and retraction of the leads. Patients may do this while sleeping but even if awake are rarely aware of the action.

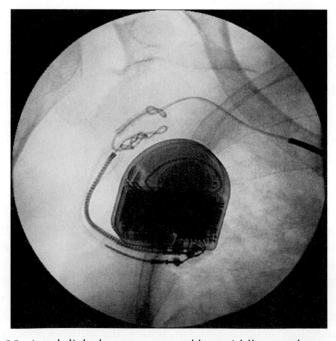

FIGURE 15-11. Lead dislodgement caused by twiddler syndrome in a patient.

PACEMAKER MALFUNCTION

Undersensing

Undersensing is the failure of the device to see an intrinsic cardiac electrical signal. It can be caused by multiple factors including inflammation, lead fracture, lead dislodgement, ischemia, electrolyte imbalances, arrhythmias, postcardioversion/defibrillation, and drug effects. Figure 15-12 shows an example of ventricular undersensing, although undersensing may occur in either cardiac chamber. Clinically, undersensing will result in a failure of the pacemaker to inhibit pacing and will result in inappropriate atrial and/or ventricular pacing. Rarely, this may lead to the initiation of tachycardia. Increasing the programmed sensitivity of the device may overcome this problem. Rarely, surgical lead revision is required.

Oversensing

Oversensing is the misinterpretation of electrical signals by the device and may lead to inappropriate inhibition of pacing, inappropriate triggered pacing

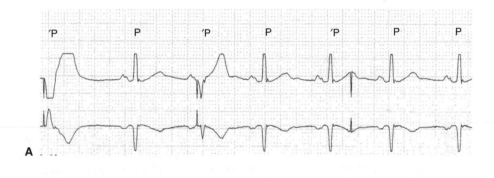

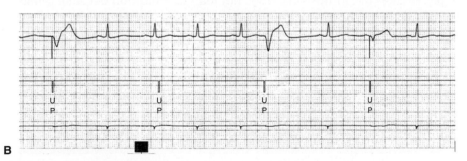

FIGURE 15-12. Undersensing of the ventricular lead. **A:** The telemetry of two-surface electrocardiographic (ECG) leads are shown with undersensing of the ventricular complexes resulting in inappropriate pacing. **B:** The intracardiac ECG and marker channels show ventricular undersensing.

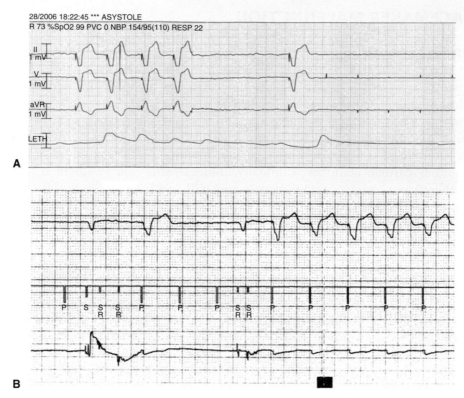

FIGURE 15-13. A pacemaker-dependent patient in chronic atrial fibrillation with a VVI pacemaker and lead fracture. **A:** The telemetry with three-surface electrocardiographic (ECG) leads and oximetry is shown. Four-paced ventricular complexes are followed by a period without pacing spikes or ventricular activity caused by ventricular oversensing. A fifth pacing spike is capturing the ventricle while the following pacing spikes fail to capture resulting in asystole. **B:** One-surface ECG, the ventricular marker channel, and the intracardiac ECG are shown. Pacing on the right and the first pacing spike (*P*) on the left result in capture of the ventricles. Noise in the intracardiac channel is recognized by the pacemaker but in this case does not lead to inhibition because it falls into the ventricular refractory period.

(i.e., atrial oversensing may lead to ventricular pacing), or both. Oversensing may be caused by myopotentials, cross talk (sensing of the paced output from one lead on the other lead), electromagnetic interference, insulation breaks, lead fractures, and inappropriate sensing of the P, R, or T wave. An example of oversensing caused by a lead fracture is shown in Figure 15-13.

Failure to Capture

An increase in the pacing threshold above the programmed parameters will result in a loss of capture. The electrocardiogram (ECG) will show pacing spikes which are not followed by a depolarization of the paced chamber. Lead failure, electrolyte disturbances, myocardial ischemia, myocardial infarction, drug therapy, and the healing process after lead implantation may cause the threshold to increase. Increased pacing thresholds may be transient. Device interrogation and chest x-ray should be obtained and are often helpful in making the diagnosis. Figure 15-13 shows an example of failure to capture.

No Output

In contrast to the failure to capture, no output conditions result in the absence of pacing spikes on the surface ECG tracing. All surface ECG leads should be assessed because the pacing spike in bipolar pacing can be very small and difficult to see. Output failure most commonly is caused by oversensing or battery depletion. Magnet application, which results in asynchronous pacing, may assist in making the diagnosis.

Large Impedance Change

Impedance should be checked at the time of lead placement and tracked with every device interrogation. Changes in the lead impedance over time which are >200 or 300 ohms should prompt concern for lead damage. Low lead impedances (i.e., <200 ohms) suggest an insulation breach, generally in the inner insulation in a bipolar coaxial lead. High lead impedances (i.e., >2,000 ohms) indicate an open circuit. This can occur with a lead fracture or a loose setscrew where the lead attaches to the header of the device.

PERIOPERATIVE PACEMAKER MANAGEMENT

Cardiologists are frequently consulted for patients undergoing surgery who have pacemakers and ICDs implanted. Electromagnetic interference encountered during surgery or diagnostic or therapeutic procedures in the hospital setting can have different pacemaker responses and potentially damage the device. Table 15-2 shows an overview of potential electromagnetic sources encountered in the operating or procedure rooms with electrocautery being the most common source.

Figure 15-14 suggests a flowchart for the perioperative management of patients undergoing pacemaker implantation. The pacemaker type, brand, and the pacemaker dependency should be determined preoperatively. If electrocautery is used in pacemaker-dependent patients the device should be programmed VOO or DOO or a magnet should be secured over the pacemaker during the procedure. To minimize the risk of damage to the pacemaker, the grounding pad should be positioned so that the pacemaker system is not in

TABLE 15-2	**Table Identifying Common Causes of Electromagnetic Interference**

Sources of electromagnetic interference

Electrocautery

Radiofrequency ablation

Lithotripsy

MRI

Electroconvulsive therapy

Radiation therapy

MRI, magnetic resonance imaging.

the field of current flow. Electrocauterization in close proximity to the pacemaker should be avoided and bipolar electrocautery should be encouraged. Continuous ECG monitoring is mandatory and an external defibrillator/pacer should easily be accessible.

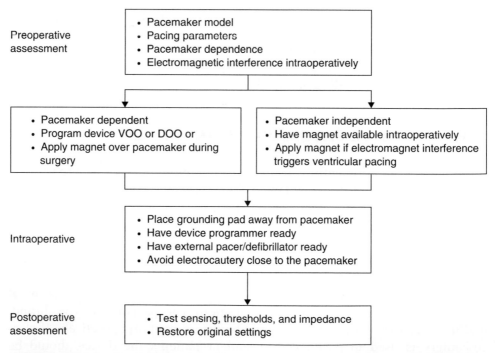

FIGURE 15-14. Our approach to the perioperative management of pacemaker patients.

SELECTED BIBLIOGRAPHY

Abraham WT, Fisher WG, Smith AL. Cardiac resynchronization in chronic heart failure. *N Engl J Med*. 2002;346:1845–1853.

American Society of Anesthesiologists Task Force. A Report by the American Society of Anesthesiologists Task Force on Perioperative Management of Patients with Cardiac Rhythm Management Devices. Practice Advisory for the Perioperative Management of Patients with Cardiac Rhythm Management Devices: Pacemakers and Implantable Cardioverter-Defibrillators. *Anesthesiology*. 2005;103:186–198.

Ammirati F, Colivicchi F, Santini M. Permanent cardiac pacing versus medical treatment for the prevention of recurrent vasovagal syncope a multicenter, randomized, controlled trial. *Circulation*. 2001;104:52–57.

Bernstein AD, Camm AJ, Fletcher RD, et al. The revised NASPE/BPEG generic pacemaker code for antibradyarrhythmia and adaptive rate and multiscale pacing. *Pacing Clin Electrophysiol*. 2002;25:260–264.

Bristow MR, Saxon LA, Boehmer J. Cardiac-resynchronization therapy with or without an implantable defibrillator in advanced chronic heart failure. *N Engl J Med*. 2004;350:2140–2150.

Cazeau S, Leclercq C, Lavergne T, et al. Effects of multisite biventricular pacing in patients with heart failure and intraventricular conduction delay. *N Engl J Med*. 2001;344:873–880.

Cleland JG, Daubert JC, Erdmann E, et al. The effect of cardiac resynchronization on morbidity and mortality in heart failure. *N Engl J Med*. 2005;352:1539–1549.

Connolly SJ, Sheldon R, Thorpe KE, et al. Pacemaker therapy for prevention of syncope in patients with recurrent severe vasovagal syncope. *JAMA*. 2003;289:2224–2229.

DAVID Trial Investigators. Dual-chamber pacing or ventricular backup pacing in patients with an implantable defibrillator. The dual chamber and VVI implantable defibrillator (DAVID) trial. *JAMA*. 2002;288:3115–3123.

Gregoratos G, Abrams J, Epstein AE, et al. ACC/AHA/NASPE 2002 guideline update for implantation of cardiac pacemakers and antiarrhythmia devices: Summary article: A report of the American College of Cardiology/American Heart Association Task Force on Practice Guidelines (ACC/AHA/NASPE Committee to Update the 1998 Pacemaker Guidelines). *Circulation*. 2002;106:2145–2161.

Kappenberger L, Linde C, Daubert C, et al. Pacing in hypertrophic obstructive cardiomyopathy. A randomized crossover study. *Eur Heart J*. 1997;18:1249–1256.

Clinical Management of Patients with Implantable Cardioverter Defibrillators

In the wake of numerous scientific studies demonstrating the clinical benefit of implantable cardioverter defibrillators (ICDs), millions of these devices have been implanted worldwide. A thorough understanding of basic ICD functions, ICD programming, and management of common ICD clinical scenarios is essential, not just for the electrophysiologist but for all health care providers who care for patients with ICDs.

INFORMED CONSENT

Patients must fully understand the indications for ICD implantation, the potential acute and long-term complications associated with ICD implantation, as well as issues related to device reliability and performance. It is worthwhile having a formal discussion of estimated risks for arrhythmic death based on patient characteristics (see Chapter 14). An equally important part of the discussion should address the fact that ICDs may prolong their life, but particularly in those with advanced heart failure this involves a shift in the mode of death from sudden cardiac arrest to intractable heart failure (see Table 16-1).

Longer-term issues include infection and/or erosion requiring device explant, device or lead malfunction, and inappropriate shock (~4% per year in sudden cardiac death in heart failure [SCD-HeFT]). In the SCD-HeFT cohort,

TABLE 16-1 Periprocedural Complications

Complication	Percentage Risk
Any complication	5–11
Mechanical complication with lead or pocket revision	4–7
Significant hematoma	2–3
Pneumothorax	1
Acute infection	0.4–1.4
Cardiac perforation/tamponade	0.3
Death	<1

14% of patients experienced a clinically significant complication due to the ICD over 5 years.

COMPONENTS OF THE IMPLANTABLE CARDIOVERTER DEFIBRILLATOR

The ICD consists of several components: sensing electrodes to provide both rate and arrhythmia sensing, defibrillation electrodes, and the pulse generator which consists of the battery, capacitor, and controlling circuitry.

Lead technology has evolved rapidly since the introduction of the first ICD systems. The earliest systems used standard pacemaker leads to pace and sense in combination with separate defibrillation leads that delivered therapeutic shocks. Current models combine these functions into a single lead. Some leads employ true bipolar sensing between the distal tip of the electrode and a ring electrode just proximal to the tip, whereas other leads use integrated bipolar sensing between the tip and the distal portion of the defibrillation coil. Integrated bipolar leads have a larger "antenna" over which they sense cardiac signals; as such there is greater potential for inappropriate oversensing of noise such as diaphragmatic myopotentials. At implant, the right ventricle (RV) sensing lead should have a local electrogram amplitude ("R wave") of at least 5 mV to ensure adequate sensing of lower amplitude fibrillatory waves during ventricular fibrillation (VF).

The defibrillation electrodes, once patches that were attached to the epicardial surface, are now coils that are an integrated part of the transvenous lead. One coil is in the distal portion of the lead and lies along the inferior wall of the RV. The shock vector is between the pulse generator, usually implanted in the pectoral site, and the RV coil. Many leads include a second coil in the section within the superior vena cava (SVC), which provides a broader tripolar

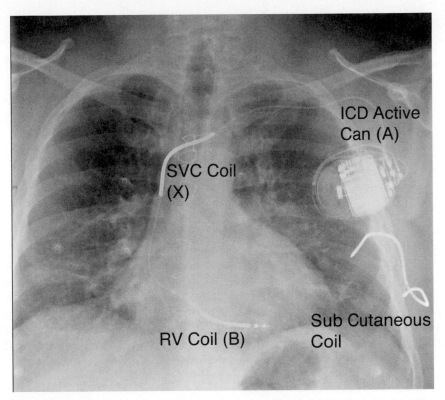

FIGURE 16-1. Chest x-ray demonstrating a standard dual coil implantable cardioverter defibrillator (ICD) lead with the proximal and distal coils labeled. There is a subcutaneous coil which originates in the pacemaker pocket and is tunneled subcutaneously along the lateral chest wall in a posterior orientation. In this case, the coil is not optimally positioned in the posterior orientation because it has migrated backward as often occurs. SVC, superior vena cava; RV, right ventricle.

shock vector with lower impedance, usually resulting in lower defibrillation thresholds (DFTs) (see Fig. 16-1).

The pulse generator consists of the metal housing that is an active part of the shock vector, internal circuitry, the battery which generally lasts for 5 to 7 years, and a high voltage capacitor for storing and delivering the charge.

DEVICE FEATURES

All ICDs perform pacing functions similar to pacemakers for treatment of bradyarrhythmias. In addition, ICDs are able to treat tachyarrhythmias through a number of different modalities: antitachycardia pacing (ATP), cardioversion, and defibrillation (see Figs. 16-2, 16-3, and 16-4). The sequence and manner in which these therapies are delivered is programmable and can be

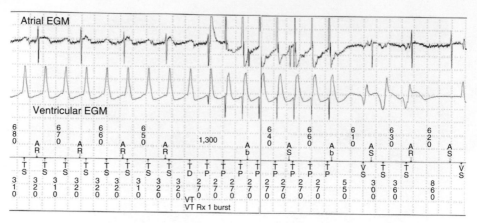

FIGURE 16-2. Implantable cardioverter defibrillator (ICD) electrograms from a dual chamber device demonstrating ventricular tachycardia at 320 msec. It is detected and antitachycardia pacing at 270 msec for 8 beats is delivered with successful termination of the ventricular tachycardia (VT). The atrial marker channel demonstrates (atrioventricular) AV dissociation. EGM, electrogram; AR, atrial even in refractory period; Ab, atrial far-field; AS, atrial sensed event; TS, ventricular tachycardia sensed event; TD, ventricular tachycardia detected; TP, antitachycardia pace; VS, ventricular sensed event. (Marker Channel Abbreviations for Medtronic [slightly different for other vendors].)

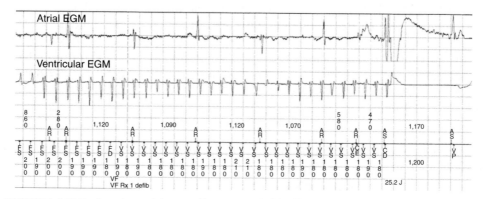

FIGURE 16-3. Implantable cardioverter defibrillator (ICD) electrograms from a dual chamber ICD demonstrating a rapid ventricular tachyarrhythmia (180 msec). The atrial channel shows atrial activity which is dissociated from the ventricular arrhythmia. The rapid rate of the tachycardia falls into a zone which is programmed to deliver a shock (25 J) and restores sinus rhythm. EGM, electrogram; AR, atrial even in refractory period; AS, atrial sensed event; FS, ventricular fibrillation sensed event; FD, ventricular fibrillation detected; VS, ventricular sensed event; CE, capacitor charged end; CD, charge delivered; VP, ventricular paced beat. (Marker Channel Abbreviations for Medtronic [slightly different for other vendors].)

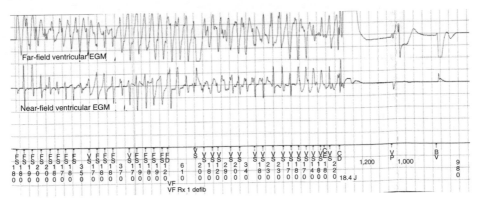

FIGURE 16-4. Implantable cardioverter defibrillator (ICD) electrograms from a dual chamber ICD. Ventricular fibrillation (VF) is sensed on the ventricular channel (near field) as well as the atrial channel (far field). EGM, electrogram; FS, ventricular fibrillation sensed event; VS, ventricular sensed event; FD, ventricular fibrillation detected; CE, capacitor charge end; CD, charge delivered; VP, ventricular paced beat; BV, biventricular paced beat. (Marker Channel Abbreviations for Medtronic [slightly different for other vendors].)

tailored to each patient depending on the specific clinical scenario. Such factors might include a known history of ventricular tachycardia (VT) with a specific tachycardia cycle length, or a high or low DFT.

ATP, when successful, allows the immediate delivery of therapy without the delay of capacitor charging as well as the avoidance of painful shocks. The ICD is usually programmed to deliver ATP as initial therapy in a tachycardia zone where one might expect VT to be readily discriminated from a supraventricular rhythm, but not so fast as to cause syncope. ATP is usually only effective in terminating VT due to reentry as it works by delivering multiple extra stimuli at a rate faster than the tachycardia cycle length (TCL). Once the extrastimuli enters the excitable gap of the reentrant circuit, it resets the circuit and terminates the circuit when the stimulus simultaneously blocks in the orthodromic direction and conducts antegradely in the circuit, colliding with the head of the preceding wavefront and abolishing the circuit. There are a variety of pacing algorithms used in ATP which are as follows:

- Burst pacing comprises a set of extrastimuli (usually 8 to 10) at a certain percentage of the TCL, usually between 81% to 94% of the arrhythmia cycle length. If one burst fails to convert the VT, subsequent bursts can be programmed to have shorter cycle lengths.

- Ramp pacing is similar except that the cycle length of each extrastimuli is decremented within each beat of the ATP cycle. This is a more aggressive pacing regimen that may terminate certain VTs but has increased risk of converting a regular tachycardia into polymorphic VT or VF.

TABLE 16-2 Typical Implantable Cardioverter Defibrillator (ICD) Therapy Programming

	VT Zone	VF Zone
Heart rate	170–200 bpm	>200 bpm
Cycle length	300–350 msec	<300 msec
Detection	18/24 intervals	18/24 intervals
Therapy 1	ATP (burst pacing)	35 J
Therapy 2	25 J	35 J
Therapy 3	35 J	35 J
Therapy 4	35 J	35 J
Therapy 5	35 J	35 J

VT, ventricular tachycardia; VF, ventricular fibrillation; ATP, antitachycardia pacing.

ATP can painlessly terminate VT in 70% to 75% of cases. However, ATP is not stand-alone therapy as it can be proarrhythmic in 30% of cases by accelerating the clinical VT into a faster VT or VF. Consequently, it is essential that high output shocks be programmed as subsequent therapy in case this should happen.

ICDs can deliver shocks with a programmable amount of energy. Lower-energy cardioverting shocks, usually 5 to 20 J, can be delivered more quickly because of the linear relationship between shock energy and charge time, but risk accelerating the tachycardia do not deliver enough energy to convert the rhythm. The highest output devices are currently able to deliver up to 35 to 40 J, which is sufficient energy to terminate most tachyarrhythmias (see Table 16-2). In the rare circumstance that a high-output device is tested and is not able to provide a safety margin of 10 J over the DFT, additional leads such as a subcutaneous lead along the lateral and posterior chest wall must be added to the system (Fig. 16-1).

Ventricular rate is the primary measure that determines the presence of ventricular arrhythmia; however, this alone can lead to inappropriate therapy for sinus tachycardia or supraventricular tachycardias (SVTs) with a ventricular response in the predetermined tachycardia zone. In order to minimize inappropriate therapies, ICDs have a number of methods to discriminate between VT and SVT (see Fig. 16-5). Sudden onset of the tachycardia, variability of the P-R interval, and stability of R-R intervals all favor VT. As well, many current models compare the morphology of the baseline electrogram with the ventricular electrogram during the tachycardia to discriminate between SVT and VT. This is most effective using a wide field electrogram such as from the RV-tip to the can. Abnormally rapid sensed activity in the atrial or ventricular

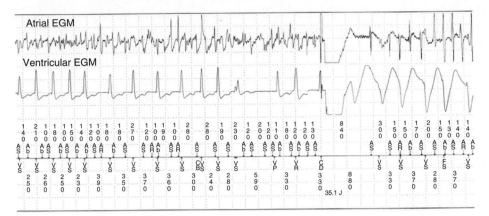

FIGURE 16-5. Implantable cardioverter defibrillator (ICD) electrograms from a dual chamber ICD demonstrating atrial fibrillation on the atrial channel resulting in a rapid ventricular response. The rapid ventricular rate is inappropriately interpreted as ventricular tachycardia and is treated with a 35-J shock. EGM, electrogram.

channel can represent damage to the lead such as lead fracture and can be misinterpreted by the device as VF resulting in device discharge (see Fig. 16-6).

Magnet Mode

Placing a magnet over an ICD will switch the device to "magnet mode" which will temporarily suspend all tachyarrhythmia monitoring. As discussed in

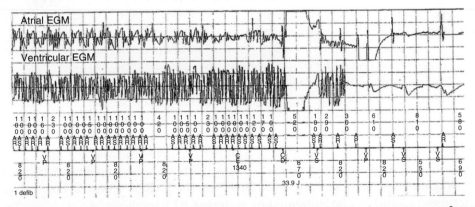

FIGURE 16-6. Implantable cardioverter defibrillator (ICD) electrograms from a dual-chamber ICD with fracture of both the atrial and ventricular leads due to likely crush injury at the costaclavicular junction. Noise is identified on both the atrial and ventricular channels by the very rapid (100 msec) activity. In this case the tachycardia is interpreted as ventricular fibrillation (VF) and a maximum output (34 J) shock is delivered. EGM, electrogram.

the subsequent text, this is a useful feature when there is suspicion that the patient is receiving inappropriate shocks or if they are going to be in a situation, such as surgery with electrocautery, where they may be at risk for oversensing environmental noise resulting in ICD discharge. It is important to realize that in contrast to pacemakers, which revert to asynchronous pacing in magnet mode, there is no change in the programmed pacing mode during magnet application to ICDs.

CLINICAL ISSUES

Periprocedural Considerations

ICD leads are inserted after vascular access is gained through either the cephalic, axillary, or subclavian vein, and the leads are attached to the myocardium through either active fixation using an integrated retractable screw or passive fixation with tines on the distal lead. The device is then placed subcutaneously in the pectoral space. ICDs are ideally placed on the left side so as to create the widest defibrillation field between the ICD can and RV and SVC coils. In the preprocedural setting, it is important to avoid factors that may compromise vascular access such as left subclavian catheters or long-standing left-sided peripheral IVs which may cause thrombosis. As well, other infectious risks such as indwelling urethral catheters should be minimized in the periprocedural setting.

Patients who will undergo ICD implantation are commonly anticoagulated for either atrial fibrillation or mechanical valves. Depending on the individual patient risk profile, it may be necessary to "bridge" them to the procedure with heparin after discontinuing warfarin. Most surgeons prefer the international normalized ratio (INR) to be <2 for ICD implantation, and if used, unfractionated heparin (UFH) or low molecular weight heparin should be discontinued sufficiently ahead of time (typically 4 and 24 hours preprocedure, respectively) to minimize the risk of bleeding (see Fig. 16-7).

Pocket hematoma is a source of morbidity and the risk is significantly increased in patients requiring anticoagulation. The importance of fastidious management of postprocedure anticoagulation cannot be overstated. Anticoagulation is usually resumed 6 hours after the procedure using UFH without a bolus and is titrated to a goal partial thromboplastin time (PTT) of 50 to 70 until the INR is therapeutic. The risk of hematoma appears to be most significant on postprocedure days 2 to 3 as the INR is elevated but not yet therapeutic, and can be mitigated by lowering PTT levels.

For any patient who may need a magnetic resonance imaging (MRI) in the future, for such issues as surveillance of malignancy or assessment of the central or peripheral nervous system, it is important to realize that this will be contraindicated once the ICD is implanted and any studies that are being considered should be performed before placement of the ICD.

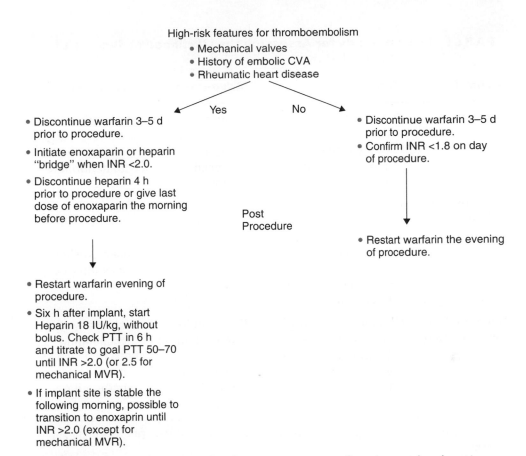

High-risk features for thromboembolism
- Mechanical valves
- History of embolic CVA
- Rheumatic heart disease

Yes / No

Yes branch:
- Discontinue warfarin 3–5 d prior to procedure.
- Initiate enoxaparin or heparin "bridge" when INR <2.0.
- Discontinue heparin 4 h prior to procedure or give last dose of enoxaparin the morning before procedure.

No branch:
- Discontinue warfarin 3–5 d prior to procedure.
- Confirm INR <1.8 on day of procedure.

Post Procedure

Yes branch (post):
- Restart warfarin evening of procedure.
- Six h after implant, start Heparin 18 IU/kg, without bolus. Check PTT in 6 h and titrate to goal PTT 50–70 until INR >2.0 (or 2.5 for mechanical MVR).
- If implant site is stable the following morning, possible to transition to enoxaprin until INR >2.0 (except for mechanical MVR).

No branch (post):
- Restart warfarin the evening of procedure.

FIGURE 16-7. An algorithm for the management of periprocedural anticoagulation. CVA, cerebrovascular accident; INR, international normalized ratio; PTT, partial thromboplastin time; MVR, mitral valve repair.

Defibrillation Threshold Testing

Testing the reliability of defibrillation by the ICD is usually performed at the time of device implantation. The DFT is the amount of energy required to restore sinus rhythm from VF with a 50% success rate. However, clinically, the term is often used to describe the energy level at which reliable defibrillation occurs. DFT testing is performed by inducing VF, using either a low-energy shock timed to the T wave or high-frequency ventricular stimulation, and assessing the amount of energy required to reliably defibrillate the patient. This is probabilistic in nature and there are a number of methods used to assess the DFT (see Table 16-3), which leads to some confusion and controversy on the subject. In addition to, there are many conditions that influence the DFT such as drugs, electrolytes, and ischemia that are variable; therefore, the ICD should be programmed to deliver therapy with a safety margin of at least 10 J over the DFT. Most patients will have a DFT of <15 at implant.

TABLE 16-3	Methods for Assessing the Likelihood of Successful Defibrillation		
Method	**Technique**	**Advantage**	**Disadvantage**
Verification	One or two successful defibrillations using 10 J less than maximum output of ICD	Minimal number of shocks Shorter procedure time	May significantly overestimate the energy needed to defibrillate
Step down to failure	Induce VF and repeatedly defibrillate with increasingly lower energy until failure to defibrillate. Lowest successful shock level is the DFT	May be more accurate in assessing DFT	May require multiple shocks Repeated shocks may alter DFT
Upper limit of vulnerability (ULV)	Critically timed shocks are delivered on the T wave at decreasing energy until fibrillation occurs	Only requires the patient to be in ventricular fibrillation once	Technically challenging Repeated shocks may shorten battery life

ICD, implantable cardioverter defibrillator; VF, ventricular fibrillation; DFT, defibrillation threshold.

Testing is done at initial implant, with generator changes, and in some patients electively during routine follow-up. Evaluation may be needed more frequently in certain patients such as those with recurrent shocks, known elevated DFT, significant clinical change such as myocardial infarction, and changes in drugs that affect the DFT such as addition of amiodarone. Special care should be taken if atrial fibrillation is present, due to the risk of stroke if the patient is cardioverted and has not been appropriately anticoagulated beforehand.

Management of the Patient with a High Defibrillation Threshold

Unless contraindicated, such as with atrial fibrillation without appropriate periprocedural anticoagulation, heart failure with severe volume overload, or recent cardiac arrest with significant neurologic impairment, a newly implanted ICD should be tested for adequate DFT (>10 J safety margin) at the time of implant. With the evolution of lead technology and higher output devices, inadequate safety margin is an increasingly uncommon situation; however, when present, it must be addressed. Simply reprogramming the polarity of the shock vector may result in a decreased DFT and is an uncomplicated way to achieve adequate DFT. The position of the lead is crucial to the DFT and one should be alert to the possibility of the SVC coil being too far into the right atrium. Some patients with high DFTs may require the addition of a subcutaneous coil positioned in the posterior chest wall. These third coils can be effective in lowering the DFT by broadening the shock vector to involve more myocardial mass and through lowering the impedance, which results in higher delivered current.

In the patient who is found to have an elevated DFT on routine testing, not associated with implant or generator change, the patient's medications and clinical status need to be carefully assessed for potential etiologies (see Table 16-4). All attempts should be made to correct the problem non-invasively before invasive measures to reconfigure the ICD system are performed.

Routine Follow-up

Routine follow-up of patients with ICDs involves evaluation every 3 to 6 months, either in clinic or through remote transtelephonic transmission. The patient's medications should be reviewed for changes that might impact device function, especially class I and III antiarrhythmic drugs which may alter pacing and DFTs. The examination should focus on the cardiovascular examination and the device site for signs of infection or impending erosion of the overlying skin. Patients should be encouraged to pay attention to the device site and call if changes occur such as erythema, warmth, swelling, or thinning of the skin over the device develop.

TABLE 16-4 Factors that Influence Defibrillation Threshold (DFT)	
Increase DFT	**Drugs:** amiodarone, carvedilol, disopyramide, diltiazem, mexilitine, verapamil
	Device: right-sided location of can, inactive can
	Leads: single coil (RV only), SVC coil positioned too distally, lead fracture
	Clinical: heart failure, pulmonary edema, acidosis, severely dilated LV
Variable or unclear effect on DFT	**Shock polarity:** direction of shock vector between coils and can
Lower DFT	**Drugs:** dofetilide, ibutilide, sotalol
	Leads: addition of a subcutaneous coil, dual coil rather than a single coil lead

RV, right ventricle; SVC, superior vena cava; LV, left ventricle.

Routine device interrogation entails assessment of the following parameters.

Battery Life

ICDs usually store enough energy for 5 to 7 years of surgery. Remaining life is generally monitored by following the battery voltage and is also influenced by the battery impedance and frequency of device activity. With battery depletion, the device will eventually enter the elective replacement interval (ERI). Times vary among manufacturers, but the ICD will usually function normally for weeks to months after entering the ERI. The device should be changed before entering the end of life (EOL) phase when ICD function will be unreliable and eventually cease.

Charge Time

A prolonged charge time indicates either battery depletion or defective capacitor function. The definition of normal charge times varies depending on manufacturer and model but is usually <12 seconds.

Sensing

Measurement of the sensed P and R waves is essential to assure normal device function both in baseline rhythm and tachyarrhythmia. Ideally, P wave electrograms are >2 mV and R waves are >5 mV. Insufficient R wave sensing puts the patient at risk for undersensing VF and catastrophic withholding of appropriate tachycardia therapy. It is also important to be alert to any abnormal ventricular sensing such as T wave oversensing that may lead to excessive R wave counting and inappropriate shock.

Pacing Threshold

Especially in patients who depend on pacemaker function, pacing thresholds need to be monitored and pacing outputs need to be adjusted to ensure reliable capture without excess use of battery draining output.

Lead Impedance

The pacing impedance should be monitored for decreased values that might suggest lead insulation failure or increased values suggestive of lead fracture. Overall trends, sudden changes, as well as manufacturer- and lead-specific values all need to be considered when deciding what is abnormal.

Monitored Events and Therapies

In the case of ICD shock, the patient is usually able to report the event; however, they are often unaware of other clinically significant episodes such as ATP termination, VT that is nonsustained or below the detection zone, or atrial fibrillation. On the basis of this data, one can reprogram the ICD for maximal effectiveness, for example, lowering the detection zone to incorporate slower VT.

Thoracic Impedances

Some newer ICDs are able to track transthoracic impedance which is a surrogate measure of pulmonary edema and worsening heart failure. Along with more traditional indicators of volume overload, this may prove helpful in guiding therapy.

Approach to the Implantable Cardioverter Defibrillator Discharge

When contacted about ICD discharge, the clinician is often in the position of triaging the patient remotely. For single isolated shocks without subsequent symptoms, the patient can be evaluated as an outpatient within 48 hours. Patients with more frequent shocks, or single shocks associated with symptoms such as syncope, chest pain, or new dyspnea should be evaluated urgently. Certain historical features can suggest an etiology for inappropriate discharge—strenuous activity may result in sinus tachycardia—shocks soon after implant suggest lead dislodgement or a loose setscrew; physical manipulation of the device or ipsilateral shoulder suggests lead noise. If an analyzer system is not immediately available in the setting of incessant shocks and suspected device malfunction, a magnet can be placed over the device to inhibit therapies. If the patient becomes unstable again, then arrhythmia should be suspected and the magnet should be removed to resume tachycardia therapies.

Alternatively, some patients with ICDs experience syncope or cardiac arrest without obvious ICD discharge. Interrogation of the ICD is essential in such situations and often helps clarify the etiology of the event. The interrogation should be directed toward identifying ICD therapies of which the patient was not aware, or tachycardias for which therapy was withheld because they were slower than the therapy zone. Indirect clues include low-amplitude R waves which may suggest undersensing of VF.

Electrical Storm

Electrical storm is typically defined as three or more appropriate ICD discharges in a 24-hour period and requires an urgent search for reversible etiologies such as ischemia, decompensated heart failure, electrolyte imbalance, or proarrhythmic effect of drugs. After the initial assessment, the patient should be treated with intravenous amiodarone and as much β-blockade as blood pressure and heart rate can tolerate. Sedation and intubation may be necessary both for patient comfort and to blunt the adrenergic drive that ICD discharge provokes, which may perpetuate recurrent tachycardia.

Perioperative Management

If properly managed, the patient with an ICD in place is at no higher surgical risk than the risk associated with his or her underlying medical condition. The major concern is the risk of electrocautery-induced noise leading to inhibition of pacing in the pacer-dependent patient, or inappropriate therapy for lead noise that is misinterpreted as VF. The risk can be minimized by using bipolar cautery, or with unipolar cautery, placing the grounding pad as far as possible from the ICD can, and by using short bursts of cautery. If the surgery is above the diaphragm or there is other concern of electrical interference, then either ICD therapies can be temporarily programmed off or a magnet can be placed over the ICD which will inhibit all tachycardia therapies. Unlike a pacemaker, the magnet will not force the device to pace asynchronously so it may be necessary to reprogram an ICD to an asynchronous pacing mode in the patient who is pacemaker dependent. With the earliest generation of ICDs, magnet application would reset the ICD but this is not a concern with contemporary ICDs. In all cases, when disabling ICD therapies (either by reprogramming

TABLE 16-5	**Perioperative Management of Implantable Cardioverter Defibrillators (ICDs)**
Preprocedure	Document the manufacturer of the device should a device programmer be needed to manage an urgent issue
	Determine the underlying rhythm; if the patient has an ICD and is pacemaker dependent, pacing should be reprogrammed to an asynchronous pacing mode
Interprocedure	For procedures at high risk for device oversensing, the device tachyarrhythmia therapies should be programmed off or a magnet should be placed over the device during the procedure, and removed immediately post procedure
	Patients should be continuously monitored on telemetry and have external pacing/defibrillation pads in place, attached to an external pacemaker/defibrillator, and should have monitoring throughout the procedure and while the magnet is in place over the device
Postprocedure	Device interrogation for: (a) patients undergoing chest surgery, or ipsilateral neck, upper abdominal surgery; (b) pacemaker dependent patients; (c) patients with evident device malfunction (such as asynchronous pacing in the absence of a magent); (d) ICD patients who had their device detection programmed *off* preoperatively

or by application of a magnet), the patient should be placed on continuous telemetry (see Table 16-5).

PRACTICAL PATIENT CONSIDERATIONS

Driving

Rules governing the issue of driving by patients with ICDs differ in various jurisdictions and it is important for physicians to be aware of the regulations in their area of practice. In the patient whose ICD is implanted for primary prevention, driving privileges need not be restricted after he or she has recovered from the implant procedure. For patients with prior syncope, resuscitated SCD, or appropriate ICD discharge for ventricular arrhythmia, most guidelines agree upon a minimum restriction of 6 months. The recommendation for all ICD patients is for a lifelong restriction from commercial driving.

Other Electronic and Magnetic Devices

ICDs are adequately shielded enough that patents need not worry about electromagnetic interference (EMI) from common household appliances such as microwave ovens. Most metal detectors will detect ICDs when patients pass through security. There is no evidence that the field generated by these devices can alter ICD function; however, it is advisable for the patient to proceed directly through the detector without stopping inside. Many of the handheld metal detectors/wands can alter ICD function and should not be held in place directly over the ICD. Many electronic surveillance systems employed in stores use systems that may generate EMI but patients are safe as long as they walk directly through such systems without touching them. Digital cellular telephones and portable music players are safe to use except when placed directly over an ICD, such as in a shirt pocket, as there are case reports of this causing EMI.

Magnetic Resonance Imaging

There are multiple reasons for concern in performing MRI on patients with ICDs. Least concerning of these is the magnet mode temporarily inhibiting tachycardia therapy. Other concerns include induction of rapid pacing by the magnetic field and pulsed radiofrequency, damage to the battery through magnetic torque, and generation of an ablative current through the ICD leads. Modern ICDs have improved EMI protection and use less ferromagnetic material and there are now small reports suggesting the it may be safe to perform MRIs on patients with ICDs in very controlled circumstances. However, in general, MRI should still be considered contraindicated in patients with ICDs.

Electroconvusive Therapy and Implantable Cardioverter Defibrillators

There are reports of safe and successful use of electroconvusive therapy (ECT) in patients who have an ICD implanted. The tachycardia therapies should be disabled before ECT because of the risk of ECT-induced seizures causing oversensing of myopotentials by the ICD lead, which can be misinterpreted as VF and result in inappropriate shocks.

Other Medical Devices

Devices such as neurostimulators for treatment of patients with Parkinson disease and transcutaneous electrical nerve stimulation (TENS) devices run the theoretic risk of interfering with the sensing function of ICD or pacemaker due to delivery of electrical stimulation. However, these devices are considered compatible, especially with newer stimulators that use bipolar stimulation current and with modern cardiac devices that use bipolar sensing. If a patient has an older unipolar sensing system in the ICD or pacemaker, the device should be examined carefully and sensitivity reduced to avoid oversensing far-field signals from the stimulator.

Philosophic Issues

Discontinuation of Implantable Cardioverter Defibrillators

Occasionally a patient will wish to discontinue ICD therapy (e.g., not replace a depleted generator, or turn off the device). If the patient understands the risks of living without a functioning device it may reasonable to remove or not replace the ICD generator. Removal of the leads, if chronic, adds significant morbidity to the procedure.

In patients with ICDs who develop terminal illness with limited life expectancy, it is reasonable to disable tachycardia therapies.

SELECTED BIBLIOGRAPHY

Alter P, Waldhans S, Plachta E, et al. Complications of implantable cardioverter defibrillator therapy in 440 consecutive patients. *Pacing Clin Electrophysiol.* 2005;28:926–932.

Ellenbogen K, Kay GN, Wilkoff BL, et al. *Clinical cardiac pacing, defibrillation, and resynchronization therapy*, 3rd ed. Philadelphia: WB Saunders; 2007.

Goldschlager N, Epstein A, Friedman P, et al. Environmental and drug effects on patients with pacemakers and implantable cardioverter/defibrillators: A practical guide to patient treatment. *Arch Intern Med.* 2001;161:649–655.

Reynolds MR, Cohen DJ, Kugelmass AD, et al. The frequency and incremental cost of major complications among medicare beneficiaries receiving implantable cardioverter-defibrillators. *J Am Coll Cardiol*. 2006;47:2493–2497.

Stevenson WG, Chaitman BR, Ellenbogen KA, et al. Clinical assessment and management of patients with implanted cardioverter-defibrillators presenting to nonelectrophysiologists. *Circulation*. 2004;110:3866–3869.

Zimetbaum P. A 59-year-old man considering implantation of a cardiac defibrillator. *JAMA*. 2007;297:1909–1916.

CHAPTER 17

Noninvasive Diagnostic Testing

THE ELECTROCARDIOGRAM

The 12-lead electrocardiogram (ECG) provides an enormous amount of useful information for the prediction of arrhythmia risk.

QRS Interval

Prolongation in the QRS interval with an intraventricular conduction delay (IVCD) or left bundle branch block (LBBB) pattern has consistently been correlated with an increase in total and arrhythmic mortality in patients with underlying cardiomyopathy. Right bundle branch block (RBBB) does not appear to be associated with a worse prognosis.

QT Interval

The QT interval is the ECG representation of cardiac repolarization. Prolongation in the QT interval in association with the development of polymorphic ventricular tachycardia is called *torsades de pointes* (*TDP*). QT prolongation with TDP can be a congenital abnormality or can be acquired.

Measurement of the QT Interval

The QT interval is measured from the onset of the Q wave to the termination of the T wave. The end of the T wave is defined as the point at which the T wave crosses the baseline. If the baseline is difficult to assess, a line can be drawn from the preceding TP interval to the next TP interval. The lead with the most distinct T wave and clear termination should be chosen. Lead II or V_2 are the most commonly utilized leads.

The U wave is a small positive or negative deflection which follows the QT interval (see Fig. 17-1). It is generally not included in the measurement of the QT interval unless it is >50% of the T-wave amplitude.

The QT interval normally decreases with increasing heart rates and lengthens with slower heart rates. A failure to shorten the QT interval during increased heart rates is a response consistent with long QT syndrome. The QT interval can vary up to 100 msec over the course of the day, felt largely due to autonomic tone. It is longer in the night compared with the morning and daytime hours.

There are many methods to measure the corrected QT interval. Three commonly used methods are as follows:

$$\text{Bazett formula: } QTc = QT \text{ interval}/RR^{1/2}$$

$$\text{Fredericia formula: } QTc = QT/RR^{1/3}$$

$$\text{Framingham formula: } QTc = QT + 0.154 \, (1 \, RR)$$

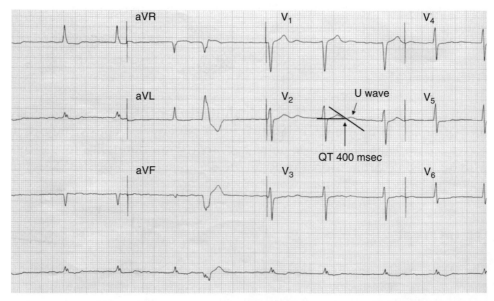

FIGURE 17-1. Demonstration of QT interval measurement in the presence of a positive U wave.

The most widely used formula to determine the QT interval corrected for heart rate is the Bazett formula. This formula is limited by overcorrection at high heart rates and undercorrection at low rates.

Normal QT Values

Normal QT interval ranges are similar in males and females until late adolescence. During adulthood, females have a slightly higher normal range than men.

	Childhood (through adolescence)	Adulthood
Males	up to 0.44–0.046	<0.43
Females	up to 0.44–0.046	<0.45

Special Circumstances

Atrial Fibrillation

There is no standard method for assessing the QT interval during atrial fibrillation (AF). Options include averaging ten consecutive QT intervals or the longest and shortest QT interval on an ECG.

Bundle Branch Block

The prolongation in the QRS interval may lead to prolonged QT intervals which are not solely due to abnormal repolarization. A typical correction normalizes the QRS to 100 or 110 msec—therefore, if the QRS is 160 msec, 50 msec is subtracted from the QT interval.

AMBULATORY ARRHYTHMIA MONITORING

Ambulatory arrhythmia monitoring is used most often for the identification of symptomatic arrhythmias to determine the cause of palpitations, the documentation of asymptomatic arrhythmias including the determination of the cause of syncope, the identification of nonsustained ventricular tachycardia (NSVT) for sudden death risk assessment, or the cause of stroke such as AF (see Table 17-1). These devices are also useful for the assessment of heart rate during chronic arrhythmias such as AF.

Holter monitors are large devices which are generally worn for 48 hours. They record continuously and save all data for the entirety of the monitoring period. Patients can keep a diary of their symptoms to correlate with the arrhythmias identified with scanning of the 48-hour monitoring period. These

TABLE 17-1	Ambulatory Monitoring Arrhythmia Devices and Common Indications	
Device	**Description**	**Indication**
Holter	24–48 h of continuous monitoring	AF rate control AF identification Identification of NSVT in patients at risk for sudden death Identification of sinus node dysfunction
Event recorder	Continuous or postevent monitoring Generally used for 14–30 d	Palpitations Daily asymptomatic transmission to evaluate for AAD toxicity
MCOT	Continuous monitoring devices with wireless download of information Generally used for 14–30 d	AF rate control AF identification Syncope
Reveal	Insertable recorder 18 mo	Syncope

AF, atrial fibrillation; NSVT, nonsustained ventricular tachycardia; AAD, antiarryhthmic drugs; MCOT, mobile continuous outpatient telemetry.

devices are ideal for monitoring the heart rate in chronic AF or documenting chronotropic competence. They are less helpful for the diagnosis of palpitations or syncope given the short duration of monitoring.

Event recorders refer to devices which are activated by the patient during a symptomatic event. Continuous loop recorders use three electrodes attached through leads to a beeper-sized device. The heart rhythm is continuously monitored but data is only saved when the patient activates the device. The duration of recording before and after the activation is programmable. Newer continuous looping event recorders also have automatic triggers for rapid and slow heart rates. Postevent recorders are not connected to the patient continuously but are applied at the time of a symptomatic event. These devices have the disadvantage of having to be applied at the time of the event, risking the possibility of missing a transient event. They have the advantage of being small (credit card–sized, or wristwatch type) and not requiring sticky electrodes that sometimes cause skin rash. Both types of event recorders are generally worn for 2 to 4 weeks and events are transmitted transtelephonically.

Mobile continuous outpatient telemetry (MCOT) devices record continuously with periodic automatic downloading of information over a wireless network. Reports are available on the Internet, which display rate histograms as well as tachyarrhythmias and bradyarrhythmias. These devices combine the advantages of comprehensive monitoring with the portability of event recorders.

Implantable (insertable) loop recorders are now available. The Reveal is a small device (roughly the size of a pacemaker) that is subcutaneously implanted in the chest. It can be programmed to save up to 40 minutes of events which are automatically triggered as well as triggered by the patient. The battery lasts up to 18 months and information is downloaded in the same way pacemaker diagnostic information is obtained. Information can also be transtelephonically telemetered. These devices are used primarily for infrequent episodes of syncope.

HEAD-UP TILT TESTING

This test is most commonly employed for the diagnosis of neurocardiogenic syncope.

Tilt table testing is a procedure in which patients are placed on a table and secured with a strap across their midsection. The patient remains supine for at least 5 minutes following which the table is tilted with the head up to an angle of 60 to 80 degrees. Passive tilting involves a 20- to 45-minute period of tilt without the administration of drugs. Tilt table testing can also be performed in conjunction with the administration of medications designed to provoke a neurocardiogenic reflex (e.g., isoproterenol, adenosine).

A common protocol is a two-stage test with an initial passive phase which if negative is followed up after a 5-minute period of lying flat, with a second active phase using isoproterenol. The dose of isoproterenol is titrated to a target heart rate of 20% above the resting heart rate. The most common abnormal responses to tilt table testing include the following (see Fig. 17-2):

1. Neurocardiogenic response characterized by an abrupt drop in blood pressure with varying degrees of bradycardia

2. Dysautonomic response characterized by a gradual but significant drop in blood pressure with a flat or increasing pulse

3. Postural orthostatic tachycardia syndrome (POTS) response characterized by a slight drop in blood pressure with a significant and prolonged increase in heart rate

Other drugs used to augment the sensitivity of tilt testing include sublingual nitroglycerine and adenosine. The reproducibility tilt table testing is limited (~70%); therefore it is difficult to assess the efficacy of therapy with this study. A positive study is defined by the loss of consciousness but clinicians may terminate the study before a complete syncopal reaction.

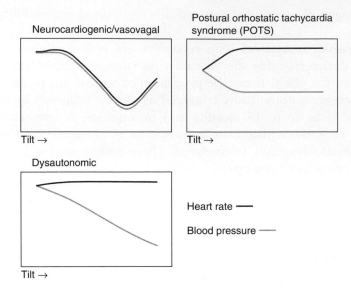

FIGURE 17-2. The most common abnormal responses to tilt table testing.

OTHER NONINVASIVE TESTS

The Signal-Averaged Electrocardiography

Signal-averaged electrocardiography (SAECG) is a method of identifying late potentials in the QRS complex. Late potentials represent areas of slowed conduction or delayed activation due to scar, edema, fibrosis, or local inflammation. These areas identified by the SAECG may represent the substrate for reentrant arrhythmias. The technique involves the signal processing of 2 to 400 ventricular beats to generate a single, high-resolution QRS complex. Criteria for an abnormal or positive SAECG include a total duration of the filtered QRS of >114 msec, root mean square (RMS) voltage of the terminal portion of the QRS of <40 mV, or low-amplitude (<40 mV) signals which persist for >38 msec at the end of the QRS (see Fig. 17-3). The SAECG, particularly if positive based on a prolonged filtered QRS has been shown to be predictive of arrhythmic death and total mortality in studies of patients with reduced left ventricular (LV) function (<40%) due to myocardial infarction (MI). The value of this test in patients with more preserved LV function is less well validated.

T Wave Alternans

T wave alternans (TWA) refers to the variations in T wave morphology that occur in a beat-to-beat and alternating pattern. The exact mechanism underlying TWA is unknown but the overarching theory is that alternans represents temporal and spatial variations in repolarization. These large spatial gradients of repolarization can result in unidirectional block, reentry, and an increased

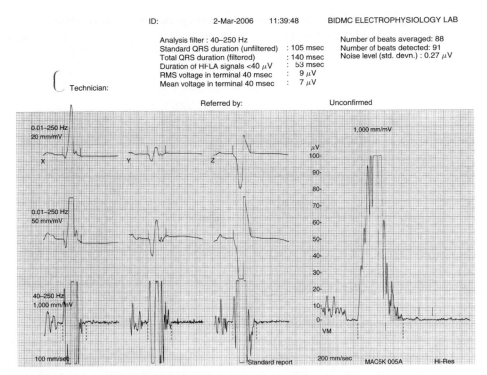

ID: 2-Mar-2006   11:39:48   BIDMC ELECTROPHYSIOLOGY LAB

Analysis filter : 40–250 Hz   Number of beats averaged: 88
Standard QRS duration (unfiltered)   : 105 msec   Number of beats detected: 91
Total QRS duration (filtered)   : 140 msec   Noise level (std. devn.) : 0.27 µV
Duration of HFLA signals <40 µV   : 53 msec
RMS voltage in terminal 40 msec   : 9 µV
Mean voltage in terminal 40 msec   : 7 µV

FIGURE 17-3. Criteria for an abnormal or positive signal-averaged electrocardiography (SAECG) include a total duration of the filtered QRS of >114 msec, root mean square (RMS) voltage of the terminal portion of the QRS of <40 mV, or low amplitude (<40 mV) signals which persist for >38 msec at the end of the QRS. HFLA, high frequency low amplitude.

likelihood of ventricular arrhythmias. Alternation of the T wave can rarely be seen on the 12-lead ECG. Computer spectral analysis allows the identification of microvolt TWA.

The standard technique for recording TWA involves graded exercise with a requirement of a stable regular heart rate target of at least 110 bpm. Chronotropic incompetence (e.g., β-blockade) and AF are two contraindications to TWA testing. At present one third of patients will have an indeterminate test. TWA has been tested primarily in the post-MI, low ejection fraction (EF) population. The results suggest a poor positive predictive value (10%) with a good negative predictive value (99%). The coming years will see the analysis of a number of well-done clinical trials which should more clearly elucidate the role of TWA in risk prediction.

Heart Rate Variability

Heart rate variability (HRV) is the natural fluctuation in heart rate due to the effects of parasympathetic and to a lesser extent, sympathetic input to the sinus node. Autonomic balance has important influences on many aspects of electrophysiology (afterpotentials, refractory periods, automaticity, and fibrillation thresholds) and HRV has been studied as a measure of susceptibility to ventricular arrhythmias. The two main categories of HRV are time domain measures and frequency domain measures. Time domain measures (e.g., standard deviation of RR intervals, RMS of successive RR intervals) are measures of the variation of RR intervals over time. Frequency domain measures (high-frequency measures reflect vagal influence, low frequency reflect vagal and sympathetic influence) compute power spectral density. Low values of HRV are considered abnormal.

The balance of data supports the ability of HRV to identify patients with LV dysfunction and a significant all cause or total mortality. It has been less successful at identifying those patients with a high risk of arrhythmic death who would most benefit from implantable cardioverter defibrillator (ICD) implantation.

Baroreceptor Sensitivity

Baroreceptor sensitivity (BRS) assesses the baroreceptor response to increased blood pressure (generated by an infusion of an α-adrenergic drug). The slope of the regression line of increased blood pressure to heart rate slowing gives an index of vagal tone. The baroreceptor response is normally reduced with age and hypertension. Recently, impaired BRS (<3.1 to 6.1 msec per mm Hg) has been correlated with increased mortality in patients post MI, independent of EF.

Heart Rate Turbulence

Heart rate turbulence (HRT) is another test of autonomic function. This study measures the initial increase in heart rate that occurs after the blood pressure drop associated with an ectopic beat followed by the decrease in heart rate as the blood pressure rises to normal. Lower levels of HRT are associated with a more impaired autonomic response and worse prognosis.

SELECTED BIBLIOGRAPHY

Bazett JC. An analysis of time relation of electrocardiograms. *Heart*. 1920;7:353–367.

De Ferrari G, Sanzo A, Bertoletti A, et al. Baroreflex sensitivity predicts long-term cardiovascular mortality after myocardial infarction even in patients with preserved left ventricular function. *J Am Coll Cardiol*. 2007;50:2285–2290.

Exner D, Kavanagh K, Slawnych M, et al. Noninvasive risk assessment early after a myocardial Infarction. *J Am Coll Cardiol*. 2007;50:2275–2284.

Fredericia LS. Dir systolendaeur in elecktrokardiogram bei normalen menchen und bei Herzkranken. *Acta med Scand*. 1920;53:469–486.

Josephson ME. *Clinical cardiac electrophysiology*, 4th ed. Philadelphia: Lippincott Williams & Wilkins; 2008.

Narayan S. T-wave alternans and the susceptibility to ventricular arrhythmias. *J Am Coll Cardiol*. 2006;47:269–281.

Zimetbaum P, Buxton A, Batsford W, et al. Electrocardiographic prectors of arrhythmic death and total mortality in the Multicenter Unsustained Tachycardia Trial. *Circulation*. 2004;110:766–769.

Antiarrhythmic Drugs

Antiarrhythmic drugs are widely used in clinical electrophysiology to both prevent and terminate arrhythmias. The drugs can also be used to slow arrhythmias to make them hemodynamically tolerated (e.g., atrial fibrillation) or facilitate pacing-mediated termination (e.g., ventricular tachycardia [VT]). Their safe and effective use requires a thorough understanding of their indications and toxicities. Reentry is the predominant mechanism of arrhythmias treated with antiarrhythmic drugs. Although the mechanism by which drugs stop automatic or triggered rhythms and reentrant rhythms involving the atrioventicular (AV) node is understood, it is unclear how drugs terminate reentrant arrhythmias confined to the atrial or ventricular myocardium.

Prevention of a reentrant arrhythmia in the atrium or ventricle is most likely to occur by prolongation of refractoriness without affecting conduction or by abolishing conduction—a more difficult task. Antiarrhythmic drugs are classified according to the predominant ion current they block (Vaughn-Williams classification) (see Table 18-1). There are many limitations to this classification, not least of which is the recognition that many antiarrhythmic drugs block multiple ion currents. In general, blockade of sodium channels depresses the rate of rise of the action potential (V_{max}) and blockade of potassium channels prolongs repolarization.

Class 1 antiarrhythmic drugs primarily block sodium channels which result in a decrease in the rate of rise of phase 0 of the action potential. Class 1 drugs are further divided into class 1A, 1B, and 1 C subclasses which

---

TABLE 18-1   Vaughan-Williams Classification

Type 1 Na channel blockers
  A Intermediate rate of binding and dissociation
  Rapid binding and dissociation
  C Slowest binding and dissociation
Type 2 β-Blockers
Type 3 Potassium channel blockers
Type 4 Calcium channel blocker

---

are distinguished by different rates of drug binding and dissociation from the sodium channel receptor. For example, during tachycardia less time is available for drug dissociation from the sodium receptor. This results in a greater number of blocked channels (see Table 18-2). If more sodium channels are blocked there will be a decrease in conduction velocity with prolongation in depolarization and resultant QRS prolongation. The slower a drug dissociates from a receptor the more drug will be bound at rapid heart rates (i.e., use dependence).

Class 1A sodium channel blocking drugs include quinidine, procainamide, and disopyramide. These drugs predominantly block potassium channels (Ikr) at slow rates and normal concentrations and sodium channels at faster rates and higher concentrations. This pattern of potassium channel blockade at slow rates is called *reverse use dependence*. This group is distinguished by an intermediate rate of binding and dissociation from the sodium channel.

Class 1B antiarrhythmic drugs include lidocaine and mexilitine. They have rapid binding and dissociation kinetics. They are particularly effective on His-Purkinje fibers with less binding to atrial tissues. Atrial tissues have a shorter action potential duration which accounts for the lesser effect of type 1B agents on atrial tissue compared with ventricular tissue. Binding of type 1B agents to the sodium channel is greater in the inactivated state and in the presence cellular acidosis as occurs during myocardial ischemia.

Class 1C drugs have the slowest binding and dissociation kinetics. Slower dissociation kinetics result in a greater amount of bound drug at rapid heart rates which facilitates the termination of rapid arrhythmias (tachycardias). These drugs slow cardiac conduction to the greatest extent of the class 1 agents.

Class 2 drugs are the β-blockers.

Class 3 drugs prolong refractoriness by prolonging the action potential duration. Most block potassium channels but some also allow persistence of the inward sodium current (e.g., ibutilide). The potassium channel blocking drugs predominantly block Ikr and thereby result in prolongation of repolarization with an increase in refractoriness and action potential duration.

Class 4 drugs are calcium channel blocking drugs. The calcium channel blockers of predominant interest to arrhythmia management are the nondihydropyridine compounds (diltiazem and verapamil).

TABLE 18-2 Electrophysiologic Manifestations of Antiarrhythmic Drugs

Antiarrhythmic Drug	Channel(s) Blocked	Electrophysiologic Effects	ECG Manifestations	DFT
Quinidine	INa Ik Ito ACH Alpha	↑ HV, ↑ A and V RP	May ↑ sinus rate ↑ QT (not dose related) ↑ QRS high dose	
Procainamide	INa Ikr (related to amount of NAPA)	↑ HV, ↑ A and V RP	↑ QT (not dose related) ↑ QRS high dose	Varies NAPA ↓
Disopyramide	INa Ik ACH	↑ HV, ↑ A and V RP	May ↑ sinus rate ↑ QT (not dose related) ↑ QRS high dose	↑
Lidocaine (IV) Mexilitine (PO)	INa particularly in ischemic tissue	↓ or ↑ HV, ↔ A and V RP	None	↑
Propafenone	INa BB	↑ HV, ↑ A and V RP	May ↓ sinus rate ↑ PR, ↑ QRS	Varies
Flecainide	INa	↑ HV, ↑ A and V RP ↑ Pacing threshold	May ↓ sinus rate ↑ PR, ↑ QRS	↑
BB	I$_f$ pacing current		↓ Sinus rate	↔
Sotalol	Ik, Beta	↑ AH, ↑ A and V RP	↓ Sinus rate, may ↑ PR, ↑ QT (dose related)	↓

(continued)

TABLE 18-2 *Continued*

Antiarrhythmic Drug	Channel(s) Blocked	Electrophysiologic Effects	ECG Manifestations	DFT
Dofetilide	Ik	↑ A and V RP	↑ QT (dose related)	↓
Ibutilide (IV)	Ik INa agonist	↑ AH, ↑ A RP	↑ QT (dose related)	NA
Amiodarone	Ik INa, ICa, Beta, alpha, ACH	↑ AH, ↑ A and V RP	↓ Sinus rate, ↑ PR, ↑ QRS, ↑ QT	↑
CCB (non dihydropyridone)	ICa	↑ AH, ↔ A and V RP	↓ Sinus rate, ↑ PR	↑
Adenosine	Ik channel opener	↑ AH, ↓ A and V RP	↓ Sinus rate, AVN delay or block, ↓ atrial and ventricular refractoriness	↔
Digoxin	Na/K pump inhibition Parasympathetic agonist Sympathetic inhibition	↑ AH, ↔ A and V RP	↓ Sinus rate AVN delay or block	↔

ECG, electrocardiogram; DFT, defibrillation threshold; NAPA, *N*-acetylprocainamide; ACH, acetylcholine; AVN, atrioventricle node.

Digoxin blocks the Na/K pump resulting in an increase in intracellular sodium. This results in increased activity of the Na/Ca exchanger and increased intracellular calcium. Digoxin also is a vagomimetic agent, which accounts for its modest AV and sinus nodal–slowing effects.

PRINCIPLES OF ANTIARRHYTHMIC DRUG TOXICITY

The major toxicity of drugs which prolong the QT interval (potassium channel blockers) is *torsades de pointes* (TDP). This arrhythmia is a form of polymorphic VT associated with QT prolongation. It often occurs as salvos of nonsustained polymorphic VT which may result in ventricular fibrillation. An important factor which predisposes to TDP is bradycardia, particularly with a pause following conversion of atrial fibrillation to sinus rhythm. Other risk factors for TDP include hypokalemia, female gender, congenital long QT syndrome, and congestive heart failure (see Table 18-3). Importantly, TDP is not a dose-related phenomena when associated with class 1A drugs. Conversely it is dose related with class 3 agents.

Management of TDP includes intravenous magnesium sulfate (2 g IV bolus with 2 to 4 g repeated if necessary). The potassium should be repleted to levels above 4.0 mEg/L. In addition, an increase in the heart rate will shorten the QT interval and reduce the likelihood of ongoing polymorphic VT. This is best accomplished with isoproterenol and or pacing. It is the authors' preference to pace the atrium rather than the ventricle at rates of >90 bpm if AV conduction is normal. Atrial pacing through a catheter in the coronary sinus or right atrial appendage requires fluoroscopic guidance. If atrial pacing is not possible, ventricular pacing is also effective.

Very wide-complex VT can be a complication of sodium channel blockers, particularly type 1C agents. This occurs most often in association with prior structural heart disease (e.g., myocardial infarction), which in combination with strong sodium channel blockade can facilitate the development of reentrant VT.

Another important toxicity of antiarrhythmic drugs is the conversion of atrial fibrillation to atrial flutter with accelerated conduction. This is particularly common with class 1C drugs which organize atrial fibrillation into atrial flutter in up to 15% of instances. The atrial cycle length of flutter in these cases is often slower than the typical 300 bpm and can conduct through the AV node in a 1:1 manner. This arrhythmia is recognized by a wide QRS complex and impaired myocardial contractility, which may be associated with hemodynamic collapse (see Fig. 18-1). It is the authors' practice to use an AV nodal blocking drug with type 1C drugs to prevent 1:1 conduction of atrial flutter.

Digoxin is an important source of drug toxicity. It often occurs in the setting of renal insufficiency or hypokalemia (see Table 18-4). Proarrhythmia is manifest as a wide array of abnormalities including sinus bradycardia or

TABLE 18-3 Cardiovascular and Noncardiovascular Toxicities of Antiarrhythmic Drugs

Antiarrhythmic Drug	Metabolism/ Dose	Noncardiovascaular Toxicity	Cardiovascular Toxicity	Special Considerations: Oral Loading/ Monitoring and Pregnancy
Quinidine	Hepatic CYP 3A4 (70%), renal (30%) Dose: sulfate—600 t.i.d. Gluconate—324 to 648 q8h Dose reduce for renal failure	Thrombocytopenia Cinchonism Pruritus, rash	QRS prolongation with toxic doses, *torsades de pointes* (not dose related)	Load in sinus rhythm Pregnancy: C though decades of experience Enters breast milk
Procainamide	Mostly hepatic—rapid acetylators produce more NAPA, NAPA is renally cleared PO dose: 50 mg/kg/24 h. IV dose: 1 g over 25 min, then 20–60 μg/kg/min infusion Reduce dose for renal dysfunction or low cardiac output	Rash, fever, arthralgias, drug-induced lupus particularly in slow acetylators (α histone abs) Agranulocytosis	QRS prolongation with toxic doses *Torsades de pointes* (not dose related) IV formulation: hypotension, QRS and QT prolongation	Load in sinus rhythm Pregnancy: C, less experience than with quinidine Enters breast milk
Disopyramide	Renal, hepatic (CYP 3A4) Dose: 100–400 q 8–12 h. Maximum dose 800 mg/24 h Reduce dose for renal or hepatic dysfunction	Anticholinergic (contraindicated for narrow-angle glaucoma): dry mouth, urinary retention, constipation, blurry vision	CHF exacerbation, torsades de pointes	Load in sinus rhythm Pregnancy: C, case reports of initiation of preterm labor Enters breast milk

Lidocaine	Hepatic CYP 3A4 IV 75 mg loading dose followed by 50 mg boluses every 5 min for a total of 225 mg. Infusion of 2 mg/min. Reduce load and infusion for hepatic dysfunction or severe CHF	Dizziness, confusion. drowsiness, seizures, paresthesias, muscle twitching	Conduction abnormalities Sinus arrest	Pregnancy: C
Mexilitine	Hepatic CYP 2D6	Ataxia, tremor, GI complaints, rarely seizures	Bradycardia	Pregnancy: C, enters breast milk
Propafenone	Hepatic: 150–300 q8h or SR 225–425 b.i.d.	Metallic taste, dizziness, SIADH	Atrial flutter with 1:1 conduction Ventricular tachycardia May unmask Brugada Contraindicated with coronary disease	Safe to load during atrial fibrillation Safe to load in ambulatory setting Prenancy: C, enters breast milk

(continued)

TABLE 18-3 *Continued*

Antiarrhythmic Drug	Metabolism/ Dose	Noncardiovascaular Toxicity	Cardiovascular Toxicity	Special considerations: Oral loading/ Monitoring and Pregnancy
Flecainide	Renal/hepatic CYP 2D6 50–100 mg b.i.d., maximum dose 300–400 mg/d	Dizziness, headache, visual blurring	Atrial flutter with 1:1 conduction Ventricular tachycardia May unmask Brugada Contraindicated with coronary disease	Safe to load during atrial fibrillation Safe to load in ambulatory setting Pregnancy: C, a fair amount of data for its safety
BB	Hepatic/renal Only renal (atenolol, nadolol)	Fatigue, depression, bronchospasm, impotence	Sinus bradycardia, AVN conduction disease	Pregnancy: risk of intrauterine growth retardation, fetal hypoglycemia, and bradycardia, particularly during first and third trimester
Sotalol	Renal: 80–120 mg b.i.d., maximum dose 240 mg b.i.d.	Bronchospasm	Bradycardia, *torsades de pointes*	Load in sinus rhythm Pregnancy: B, enters breast milk

| Dofetilide | Renal, hepatic CYP 3A4
CrCL >60 (500 μg b.i.d., CrCl 40–60 (250 μg b.i.d.), CrCl 20–39 (125 μg b.i.d.) | None | *Torsades de pointes* | Mandatory in hospital drug initiation
Check creatinine two three times a year
Pregnancy: C, not recommended if breast feeding |
| Amiodarone | Hepatic
T1/2 50 d:
PO load 10 g over 7–10 d, then 400 mg for 3 wk, then 200 a day for atrial fibrillation
Maintenance dose of 400 mg/d for VT
Dose reduce load for bradycardia or QT prolongation
IV: 150–300 mg bolus, then 1 mg/min infusion for 6 h followed by 0.5 mg/min thereafter | Pulmonary (acute hypersensitivity pneumonitis, chronic interstitial infiltrates), hepatitis
Thyroid (hypo or hyperthyroidism)
Photosensitivity, blue gray discoloration with chronic high dose, nausea, ataxia, tremor, alopecia
Avoid if identified thyroid nodule | Sinus bradycardia
Rarely *torsades de pointes* | Safe to load during atrial fibrillation and in ambulatory setting
LFTs two to three times a year, TFTs twice yearly, PFTs and CXR at initiation and CXR yearly thereafter
Pregnancy: D, risk of thyroid abnormalities in fetus |

287

(*continued*)

TABLE 18-3 *Continued*

Antiarrhythmic Drug	Metabolism/ Dose	Noncardiovascaular Toxicity	Cardiovascular Toxicity	Special considerations: Oral loading/ Monitoring and Pregnancy
Dronedarone	Hepatic: reduce renal creatinine clearance without changing renal function 400 mg b.i.d.	Gastrointestinal (diarrhea, nausea), small increase in creatinine without a change in renal function	Sinus bradycardia, possibly *torsades de pointes*	No significant considerations
Ibutilide (IV)	Hepatic CYP 3A4 1 mg IV over 10 min, repeat after 10 min if necessary	Nausea	*Torsades de pointes*	Must monitor for 4 h following drug initiation
CCB (nondihy-dropyridine)	Hepatic Inhibit CYP 3A4	Constipation, rash, peripheral edema	Sinus bradycardia, AVN conduction disease	Levels increased with liver and renal disease
Adenosine	Erythrocyte/endothelial cell. 6 mg IV push followed if necessary by 12 mg after 1–2 min	Nausea, headache, flushing, chest pain, bronchospasm (contraindicated if asthma)	AV nodal block, decrease in atrial and ventricular refractoriness can cause development of atrial fibrillation and ventricular ectopy	Pregnancy: C, verapamil and diltiazem widely used as first-line therapy for SVT during pregancy

| Digoxin | Renal, hepatic, GI, 0.125–375 mg/d | Anorexia, nausea, fatigue, confusion, altered vision with green/yellow halos | Bradycardia, accelerated atrial and juncitonal tachycardia with AV nodal block, bidirectional ventricular tachycardia | Pregnancy: C, many decades of experience Can use with breast feeding |

Pregnancy categorization

A = controlled trials demonstrate safety

B = no risk demonstrated in humans

C = risk has not been adequately assessed

D = positive evidence of risk

NAPA, *N*-acetylprocainamide; CHF, cognestive heart failure; GI, gastrointestinal; SR, slow release; SIADH, syndrome of inappropriate antidiuretic hormone secretion; AVN, atrioventricular node; VT, ventricular tachycardia; TFT, thyroid function test; PFT, pulmonary function test; CXR, chest x-ray; AV, atrioventricular; SVT, supraventricular tachycardia.

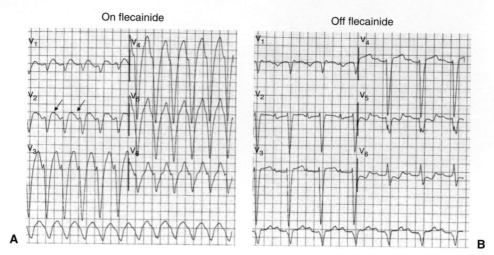

FIGURE 18-1. Demonstration of QRS widening associated with a rapid rate in a patient on flecainide **(A)** compared with baseline in the same patient at a slower heart rate off of flecainide.

arrest, nonparoxysmal atrial tachycardia with block, accelerated junctional rhythm with block (see Fig. 18-2), fascicular rhythms, and bidirectional VT (see Fig. 18-3).

ANTIARRHYTHMIC DRUG INITIATION AND MONITORING

In general, drugs which prolong the QTc interval should be discontinued for QT intervals in excess of 500 msec. If there is an underlying bundle branch block the maximum QT interval is 550 msec. Amiodarone is an exception to this rule given the very low incidence of TDP associated with this medication. The authors use a QTc of ≥550 msec as a limit beyond which amiodarone is discontinued.

Drugs which prolong the QRS duration (sodium channel blocking agents) should be discontinued or dose reduced if the QRS duration exceeds 25% of the starting interval. In the case of type 1 C drugs which possess use dependence, the degree of QRS prolongation is best assessed with a stress test.

SPECIAL DRUGS USED IN THE ELECTROPHYSIOLOGY LABORATORY

Adenosine is a short-acting antiarrhythmic drug which does not fit into standard classifications. Adenosine receptors exist throughout the body (brain,

TABLE 18-4 Selected Drug Interactions

Antiarrhythmic Drug	Selected Drug Interactions
Quinidine	↑ Digoxin and amiodarone concentrations Quinidine inhibits CYP 2D6 and may increase drugs metabolized by this enzyme e.g., ↑ effect of tricyclic antidepressants, haloperidol (Haldol), some β-blockers, fluoxetine, narcotics Quinidine metabolism is inhibited by cimetidine Quinidine metabolism is increased by phenobarbital, phenytoin, and rifampicin
Procainamide	Procainamide clearance is reduced by trimethoprim, cimetidine, and ranitidine
Disopyramide	None
Lidocaine	Levels may be increased by drugs which inhibit CYP 3A4
Mexilitine	Levels increased by amiodarone, quinidine, fluoxetine, haloperidol (Haldol), paroxetine, and cimetidine
Propafenone	May decrease the metabolism of warfarin Increase digoxin levels
Flecainide	May increase digoxin levels Flecainide levels are increased by amiodarone, haloperidol (Haldol), quinidine, cimetidine, and fluoxetine
BB	Minimal except for carvedilol and metoprolol whose levels may be increased by amiodarone, propafenone, quinidine, fluoxetine, haloperidol (Haldol), paroxetine, and cimetidine
Sotalol	No significant interactions
Dofetilide	Contraindicated with verapamil, ketoconazole, cimetidine, megestrol, prochlorperozine, and trimethoprim; hydrochlorthiazide increases dofetilide levels; must discontinue amiodarone at least 3 mo before dofetilide initiation
Ibutilide	None
Amiodarone	Inhibits CYP 450 enzymes—increases concentrations of warfarin, digoxin, cyclosporine, alprazolam, carbemazepine, HMG-CoA inhibitors, phenytoin, and quinidine

(continued)

TABLE 18-4 *Continued*

Antiarrhythmic Drug	Selected Drug Interactions
CCB (nondihydropyridone)	Inhibits CYP 3A4 will increase levels of alprazolam, carbamazepine, dihydropyridine, cyclosporine, HMG-CoA inhibitors; verapamil (but not diltiazem) increases digoxin levels
Adenosine	Methylxanthines compete for adenosine receptors with adenosine; dipyridamole decreases the metabolism of adenosine
Digoxin	Levels of or sensitivity to digoxin increased by hypokalemia, cyclosporine, spironolactone, quinidine, verapamil, amiodarone, propafenone, renal failure, rifampin, hypoxia, decreased muscle mass. Hypercalcemia also increases sensitivity to digoxin and calcium repletion should be avoided in the setting of digoxin toxicity Levels of or sensitivity to digoxin decreased by malabsorption, hyperkalemia, and hypocalcemia

BB, β-Blockers; CCB, calcium channel blocker; HMG-CoA, 3-hydroxy-3-methyl-glutaryl coenzyme A.

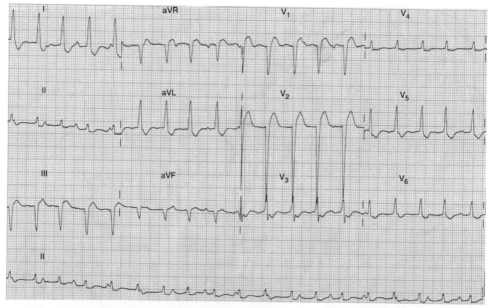

FIGURE 18-2. Digoxin toxicity manifested as an accelerated junctional rhythm with atrioventricular (AV) dissociation.

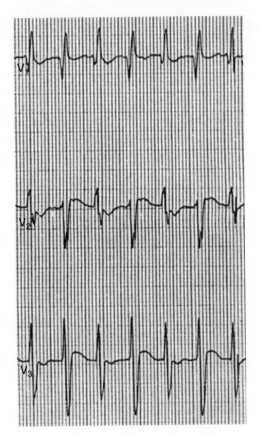

FIGURE 18-3. Digoxin toxicity manifested as bidirectional ventricular tachycardia.

lungs, heart, kidney, blood vessels, etc.) and the A1 receptor is the most cardiac selective subtype. Activation of the adenosine channel opens the adenosine-sensitive potassium channel and slows AV nodal conduction through hyperpolarization of AV nodal cells. Adenosine also indirectly diminishes calcium channel opening (see Table 18-5).

Atropine—(1 to 3 mg) muscarinic blocker—results in 25% to 50% increase in sinus rate.

Isoproterenol (1 to 3 μg per minute)—at least 25% increase in sinus rate.

Autonomic blockade: blockade of sympathetic and parasympathetic systems is achieved by 0.04 mg per kg of atropine and 0.2 mg per kg of propranolol.

TABLE 18-5 Specific Clinical Utility	
Antiarrhythmic Drug	**Specific Clinical Utility**
Quinidine	SVT: inhibits retrograde fast pathway in AVNRT Inhibits accessory pathway conduction VT: particularly in the presence of an ICD ? Brugada, idiopathic VF due to block of Ito
Procainamide	IV: AF termination and VT termination. PO: AF, SVT, VT
Disopyramide	AF treatment in HCM (particularly, if ICD in place)
Lidocaine	VT associated with ischemia or VT felt to be due to triggered mechanism
Mexilitine	Adjunctive therapy to other antiarrhythmic drugs (e.g., sotalol) for management of VT
Propafenone	SVT including AF, idiopathic VT
Flecainide	SVT including AF, idiopathic VT
BB	SVT, rate control of AF, and atrial flutter, catecholaminergic VT
Sotalol	SVT including AF, VT with and without structural heart disease
Dofetilide	AF, VT
Ibutilide	Termination of atrial flutter and atrial fibrillation
Amiodarone	AF, SVT, and VT
CCB (nondihydropyridone)	SVT, rate control of AF and atrial flutter, idiopathic LV septal VT
Adenosine	SVT termination
Digoxin	AF rate control, SVT, weak inotrope

SVT, supraventricular tachycardia; AVNRT, atrioventricular nodal reentry tachycardia; VT, ventricular tachycardia; ICD, implantable cardioverter defibrillator; VF, ventricular fibrillation; AF, atrial fibrillation; HCM, hypertrophic cardiomyopathy; LV, left ventricle.

SELECTED BIBLIOGRAPHY

Crijns HJ, Van Gelder IC, Lie KI. Supraventricular tachycardia mimicking ventricular tachycardia during flecainide treatment. *Am J Cardiol*. 1988;62:1303–1306.

Josephson ME. *Clinical cardiac electrophysiology*, 4th ed. Philadelphia: Lippincott Williams & Wilkins; 2008.

Roden D, Woosley R, Primm K. Incidence and clinical features of the quinidine associated long QT syndrome: Implications for patient care. *Am Heart J*. 1986;111: 1088–1093.

Task Force of the Working Group on Arrhythmias of the European Society of Cardiology. The Sicilian gambit. A new approach to the classification of antiarrhythmic drugs based on their actions on arrhythmogenic mechanisms. *Circulation*. 1991;84:1831.

Zimetbaum P. Amiodarone for atrial fibrillation. *N Engl J Med*. 2007;356:935–941.

Index

A

AAI pacing, 235
Ablation, 80
    AVNRT, 114–115
    of concealed posteroseptal accessory
        pathways, 115
Action potential, 13–15
    atrial myocytes, 14–15
    of atrioventricular node, 13–14
    calcium-dependent nodal, 14
    His-Purkinje system, 14–15
    ion channels and phases, 16
    selected alterations and influence on
        electrocardiogram, 15
    of sinus node, 13–14
    sodium-dependent, 14
    ventricular myocytes, 14–15
Adenosine, 292
Amiodarone, 58, 67, 291
Anatomy, clinical electrophysiology, 1–12
    atrioventricular node, 7
    fluoroscopic anatomy, 10–12
    His-Purkinje system, 8–9
    left atrium, 5–7
    left ventricle, 9–10
    ligament of marshall, 7
    right atrium, 1–5
    right ventricle, 9

Anterior wall myocardial infarction, 154–155
Antiarrhythmic drugs, 279–294
    atrial fibrillation, initiation for, 69
    electrophysiologic manifestations,
        281–282
    electrophysiology laboratory, special drugs
        used in, 290–294
        clinical utility, 294
    initiation, 290
    monitoring, 290
    toxicity, principles of, 283–289
        cardiovascular and noncardiovascular
            toxicities, 284–289
    Vaughan-Williams classification, 280
Antidromic tachycardias, 88
AOO pacing, 238
Aortic leaflet, 9
Arrhythmia, 19–20
    clinical presentation, 20
    mechanism of, 21
Arrhythmogenic right ventricular
        cardiomyopathy (ARVC), 203
Arrhythmogenic right ventricular dysplasia
        (ARVD), 159–160, 203–207
    diagnosis, 204–205
    management, 205–207
    tetralogy of Fallot, 159
Ashman phenomenon, 51

Asynchronous pacing, 238
Athlete's heart, 209
Atrial conduction, 41
Atrial fibrillation, 55–71
 management and consultation, 71
 natural history and subtypes, 56–62
  age, 57
  alcohol and, 59
  autonomically triggered, 57
  cardiovascular surgery, associated with, 58
  familial, 59
  hyperthyroidism, associated with, 57
  ischemia/infarction as a trigger, 58
  post MAZE or percutaneous AF ablation procedure, 58
  specific electrocardiographic patterns, 59
  symptoms and hemodynamic consequences, 61
  tachybrady syndrome, 60
  with reduced ventricular function at presentation, 62
  workup of new-onset, 61
 nomenclature, 56
 stroke risk, 62–71
  antiarrhythmic medications, 67
  cardioversion, 63–67
  choice of antiarrhythmic agents, 68–69
  nonpharmacologic therapy, 69–70
  principles of rate control, 70–71
  rhythm versus rate control, 63
Atrial flutter, 73–83
 clinical characteristics, 73–77
  diagnosis of isthmus-dependent, 75
  ECG characteristics, 74
 electrocardiographic clues to the diagnosis, 77–78
 electrophysiology laboratory, evaluation in the, 78–81
 management of, 81–83
  clinical pearls, 82
Atrial pacing, 35
Atrial premature depolarizations, 113
Atrial tachycardia, 88
 atrial activation sequence and atrioventricular relationship, 108
 effect of atrial and ventricular stimulation, 109
 effect of BBB, 108
 initiation, 107
 pharmacologic and physiologic maneuvers, 109

requirement of atria and ventricles, 109
 treatment, 115–116
Atrioventricular block, 232
Atrioventricular nodal echo beat, 38
Atrioventricular nodal reentrant tachycardia (AVNRT), 85
 atrial activation sequence and atrioventricular relationship, 98
 effect of atrial and ventricular stimulation, 100–101
 effect of BBB, 99
 initiation, 98
 pharmacologic and physiologic maneuvers, 101–102
 requirement of atria and ventricles, 99–100
 treatment, 114–115
Atrioventricular node function, 7, 43–44
Atrioventricular reentrant tachycardia (AVRT), 86–88
 atrial activation sequence and atrioventricular relationship, 103–104
 effect of atrial and ventricular stimulation, 105–106
 effect of BBB, 104
 initiation, 102
 pharmacologic and physiologic maneuvers, 107
 requirement of atria and ventricles, 104–105
Atrioventricular Wenckebach cycle length, 43
Atropine, 67, 293
Automatic ventricular tachycardia, 141

B
Bachmann bundle, 1
 location of, 3
Baroreceptor sensitivity, 276
Bazett formula, 270
Bezold Jarsch reflex, 167
Bifascicular block, 172
Bisoprolol, 177
β-Blockers, 57, 199
Bradbury-Eggleston syndrome, 183
Bradyarrhythmias, 183
Bradycardias, 163–177
 atrioventricular conduction disease, 165–169
  associated with myocardial infarction, 167–169
  congenital atrioventricular block, 166
  heart block associated with trauma, 167

infection, 165–166
  neurodegenerative disorders, 166
  paroxysmal atrio ventricular block,
    167
  clinical syndrome, 163–165
  diagnosis, 169–173
    electrocardiogram clues, 171–173
    electrophysiology laboratory evaluation,
      173
    symptoms/signs, 169–171
  treatment, 173–177
Brugada syndrome, 200–203
  diagnosis, 201
  management, 201–203
Bundle Branch Block (BBB)
  QT interval, 271
  ventriculoatrial interval, effect on, 99, 104,
    108
Bundle branch reentry
  beats, 37
  ventricular tachycardia, 158
Burst pacing, 255

C

Cardiac conduction system, 2
Cardioversion, 63–67
  anticoagulation pericardioversion, 65
  complications, 67
  methods of, 65–67
Catecholaminergic polymorphic ventricular
    tachycardia (CPVT), 211–212
  clinical course and management, 211–212
  diagnosis, 211
Cellular electrophysiology, 13–17
  action potential, *See* Action potential
  depolarization and the QRS interval,
    15–16
  repolarization and the QT interval,
    16–17
CHADS2 risk assessment score, 62–63
Class IV heart failure, 228
Concealed conduction, 46
Concentric retrograde activation, 31–32
Congenital atrioventricular block, 166
Cross talk, 236
Cycle length, 31

D

DDD pacing, 235
DDI pacing, 237
Decremental conduction, 35
Defibrillation threshold testing, 259–261
Delayed after depolarizations, 19

Differential pacing, 113
  basal right ventricular versus right
    ventricular apical pacing, 113
  Para-Hisian pacing, 113
Digoxin, 57, 283, 292
Diltiazem, 280
Disopyramide, 68, 280, 291
Dofetilide, 58, 68, 291
Dual atrioventricular nodal pathways, 44
Duchenne and Beckers muscular dystrophy,
    166

E

Early after depolarizations, 19
Eccentric conduction, 31
Eccentric retrograde conduction, 32
Echo beat, 22
Effective refractory period, 33
Electrical cardioversion, 66
Electrical storm, 263
Electrocardiogram (ECG), 269–271
  QRS interval, 269
  QT interval, 269–271
    measurement of, 270
    normal values, 271
    special circumstances, 271
  site of block determination, 173
Electroconvulsive therapy, 266
Electrophysiology, 25–38
  abnormal intervals, 30–31
    retrograde atrial activation, 31
  atrial pacing, response to, 35
  normal intervals, 27–30
  pacing techniques, 31–35
    refractory periods, *See* Refractory
      periods
  ventricular pacing, response to, 35–38
    repetitive ventricular responses, 37–38
Emery Dreifuss syndrome, 166
Endocarditis, 165
Entrainment, 23
  mapping, 152
  of ventricular tachycardia, 24
Epsilon wave, 204
Erb dystrophy, 167
Excitable gap, 22

F

Familial atrial fibrillation, 59
Fascicular ventricular tachycardia, 156
Fasciculoventricular pathways, 128
Fixed rate pacing, 32
Flecainide, 66, 68, 291

Framingham formula, 270
Fredericia formula, 270
Functional refractory period, 33

G
Gap phenomenon, 47–48

H
Head-up tilt testing, 273
Heart rate turbulence, 276
Heart rate variability, 275–276
His-Purkinje system, 8, 14–15
　cycle length, abrupt changes in, 35
Holter monitors, 271

I
Ibutilide, 280, 291
Implantable cardioverter defibrillator
　components, 252–253
　features, 253–258
　　magnet mode, 257–258
　indications, 219–229
　　general principles, 219–222
　　primary prevention, 224–228
　　secondary prevention, 223–224
　　timing of implantation, 228–229
　patient, clinical management of, 251–266
　　defibrillation threshold testing, 259–261
　　discharge, 263
　　driving, 265
　　electronic and magnetic devices,
　　　265–266
　　informed consent, 251
　　perioperative management, 264–265
　　periprocedural considerations, 258–259
　　philosophic issues, 266
　periprocedural complications, 252
　routine device interrogation
　　battery life, 262
　　charge time, 262
　　lead impedance, 262
　　monitored events and therapies,
　　　262–263
　　pacing threshold, 262
　　sensing, 262
　　thoracic impedances, 263
Infarction, 58
Inferior myocardial infarction, 155
Infranodal block, 172
Infranodal conduction, 47
Inspiration, 41
Ion channelopathies, 194
Ischemia, 58

Isoproterenol, 293
Isthmus ablation, 81
Isthmus-dependent atrial flutter,
　diagnosis, 75
　intracardiac recordings, 80

J
Jervell and Lange-Nielsen (JLN) syndrome,
　194

K
Kearns-Sayre syndrome, 167

L
Left anterior oblique (LAO), 10–11
　fluoroscopic projection of catheter
　　placement, 10
Left atrium, 5–7
　epicardial exposure, 7
Left ventricle, 9
Left ventricular systolic dysfunction
　heart failure, 227
　prior myocardial infarction, 225–227
LeNegre disease, 165
Lev disease, 165
Lidocaine, 280, 291
Ligament of Marshall, 7
Limb girdle muscular dystrophy, 166
Limbus, 4
Long QT syndrome, 194–199
　acute management, 199
　causes, 195
　clinical syndrome, 195–196
　diagnosis, 196–198
　management, 199
Lown-Ganong-Levine syndrome, 130

M
Magnetic resonance imaging, 265
Mahaim fibers, 130
Managed ventricular pacing (MVP) mode,
　239
Mexiletine, 199, 280, 291
Midodrine, 190
Mitral annular ventricular tachycardia, 156
Mode switch, 239
Myocardial diseases, 194
Myocardial infarction, 225
Myotonic dystrophy, 166

N
Neurocardiogenic syncope, 232
Noninvasive diagnostic testing, 269–276

ambulatory arrhythmia monitoring,
271–273
baroreceptor sensitivity, 276
ECG, 269–271
head-up tilt testing, 273
heart rate turbulence, 276
heart rate variability, 275–276
signal-averaged electrocardiography, 274
T wave alternans, 274–275
Non–isthmus-dependent flutter, 74
electrocardiogram, 75

O
Orthostasis, 183–184
Overdrive acceleration, 20
Oversensing, 245–246

P
P waves, 90–91
Pacemaker syndrome, 244
Pacemaker-mediated tachycardia, 240
Pacemakers, permanent, 231–248
acute and chronic complications, 243–244
infections, 243
pacemaker syndrome, 244
Twiddler syndrome, 244
additional features, 239–240
intrinsic conduction promotion, 239
mode switch, 239
pacemaker-mediated tachycardia, 240
rate adaptive pacing, 240
clinical indications, 231–232
atrioventricular block, 232
other indications, 232
sinus node dysfunction, 231
features, 233–238
AAI pacing, 235
active fixation pacing leads, 234
AOO pacing, 238
atrioventricular interval, 235
cross talk and safety pacing, 236
DDD pacing, 235
DDI pacing, 237–238
modes, 234
passive fixation pacing leads, 234
postventricular atrial refractory period,
236
upper rate behavior and pacemaker
Wenckebach, 237
VDD pacing, 238
VOO pacing, 238
VVI pacing, 234–235
implantation, 240–243

malfunction, 245–247
failure to capture, 246–247
large impedance change, 247
no output, 247
oversensing, 245–246
undersensing, 245
perioperative management, 247–248
Pacing rate, 31
Para-Hisian pacing, 113
Paroxysmal atrio ventricular block, 167
Pericardioversion anticoagulation, 65
guidelines for, 66
Permanent pacemakers, *See* Pacemakers,
permanent
Pindolol, 177
Postural orthostatic tachycardia syndrome
(POTS), 184, 273
Principles, clinical electrophysiology,
41–54
aberration forms, 50–53
acceleration-dependent block,
51–52
associated with premature beats,
50–51
deceleration-dependent block, 52
retrograde invasion, 52–53
atrioventricular node function, 43–44
dual atrioventricular nodal pathways,
44–49
concealed conduction, 46
gap phenomenon, 47
infranodal conduction, 47–49
supernormal conduction, 47
mechanisms of aberration, 49–50
aberration/transient bundle branch
block, 49–50
atrial premature complex, 49
ventricular premature complex, 49
normalization of aberration, 53–54
sinus node and atrial conduction,
41–43
influences on sinus node function, 43
sinoatrial conduction time, 42
sinus node recovery time, 42
PR interval, 95
Pre-excitation index, 111
Procainamide, 30, 280, 291
Propafenone, 66, 68, 291
Propranolol, 293

Q
QRS alternans, 96
QRS interval, 15–16, 269

QT interval, 16–17, 269
Quinidine, 280, 291

R
Ramp pacing, 255
Rate adaptive pacing, 240
Reentry, 22, 139
Reflex syncope, 179
Refractory periods
    cycle length, abrupt changes in, 35
    effect of heart rate, 33–35
    effective, 33
    functional, 33
    relative, 33
Relative refractory period, 33
Right anterior oblique (RAO), 10
    coronary sinus venogram, 6
    fluoroscopic projection of catheter
        placement, 11
Right atrium, 1–5
Right ventricle, 9
Right ventricular outflow tract (RVOT), 9
Romano-Ward syndrome, 194
RP interval, 95

S
Schwartz score, 196
Short QT syndrome, 200
Shy-Drager syndrome, 183
Sinoatrial conduction time, 42
Sinus arrhythmia, 41
Sinus cycle length, 42
Sinus node
    and atrial conduction, 41–43
    dysfunction, 163–164, 231
    recovery time, 42
Sodium channel blocking drugs, 280
Sotalol, 58, 68, 291
Staphylococcus aureus, 243
Staphylococcus epidermidis, 243
Stroke, 62–71
    antiarrhythmic medications, 67
    cardioversion, 63–67
    choice of antiarrhythmic agents, 68–69
    nonpharmacologic therapy, 69–70
    principles of rate control, 70–71
    rhythm versus rate control, 63
Sudden cardiac death (SCD), 193
Sudden death syndromes, 193–216
    arrhythmogenic right ventricular
        dysplasia, 203–207
    athletes, special considerations in,
        213–216

12-element American Heart Association
    (AHA) recommendations, 216
Brugada syndrome, 200–203
general diagnostic approach, 212–213
hypertrophic cardiomyopathy, 207–211
    CPVT, *See* Catecholaminergic
        polymorphic ventricular tachycardia
        (CPVT)
    diagnosis, 208–209
    genes linked to, 208
    management, 210
    risk stratification, 210
long QT syndrome, *See* Long QT
    syndrome
short QT syndrome, 200
Supernormal conduction, 47
Supraventricular crest, 9
Supraventricular tachycardia, 85–116
    atrial tachycardia, *See* Atrial tachycardia
    atrioventricular reentrant tachycardia, *See*
        Atrioventricular reentrant
        tachycardia (AVRT)
    AVNRT, *See* Atrioventricular nodal
        reentrant tachycardia (AVNRT)
    clinical presentation, 89–90
        demographics, 89
        symptoms and circumstances, 90
    diagnosis, 90–97
        atrioventricular block, 96
        bundle branch block, 96
        electrocardiography, 90–96
        vagal maneuvers, 97
        ventricular premature depolarizations,
            96
    electrophysiologic evaluation, 97
    pacing maneuvers, 110–113
        atrial premature depolarizations, 113
        differential pacing, 113
        His-atrial and ventriculoatrial intervals,
            111–112
        response to ventricular pacing, 111
    treatment, 113–116
        of atrial tachycardia, 115–116
        AVNRT ablation, 114–115
        concealed posteroseptal accessory
            pathways, ablation of, 115
    ventricular tachycardia, differentiation
        from, 142–146
Syncope, 179–191
    clinical history, 184–186
    in athlete, 186
    during pregnancy, 185

motor movements from epilepsy,
distinguishing with, 186
symptoms and circumstances,
184–185
diagnostic evaluation, 187–189
ambulatory monitoring, 187
exercise testing, 187–188
tilt table testing, 189
differential diagnosis, 179–184
arrhythmic, 182–183
cardiovascular or pulmonary
obstruction, 181–182
neuropsychiatric, 183
orthostasis, 183–184
reflex syncope, 179–181
electrophysiology study, 189
management, 189–191
driving restrictions, 190–191

T
T wave alternans, 274
Tachybrady syndrome, 60
Tachycardias, mechanism of, 19–24
abnormal automaticity, 22
reentry, 22–24
triggered activity, 19–22
influence of electrophysiologic study
and drugs, 21
response to electrophysiologic study,
20–21
response to premature stimuli, 22
Tendon of Todoro, 3
Tetralogy of Fallot, 159
Thromboembolic prophylaxis, 64
Tilt table testing, 189
Todd paralysis, 186
Torsades de pointes (TDP), 269
management of, 283
Transient ischemic attack, 62
Triangle of dysplasia, 204
Triangle of Koch, 3–4
Tricuspid valve, 3
Triggered activity, 19
Triggered ventricular tachycardia,
140–141
Twiddler syndrome, 244

U
Undersensing, 245

V
Vasovagal syncope, 179
Vaughan-Williams classification, 280

VDD pacing, 238
Ventricular echo beat, 38
Ventricular pacing, 35–38
in atrial tachycardia, 101
Ventricular premature beats, 130
Ventricular premature depolarizations,
111
Ventricular refractoriness, 35
Ventricular tachycardia, 137–161
arrhythmogenic right ventricular
dysplasia, 159–160
differential diagnosis, 138, 160–161
differentiation from supraventricular
tachycardia with aberration,
142–146
evaluation and therapy, electrophysiology
laboratory role in, 146–148
diagnosis, 147
mechanism, 147–148
localizing the site of origin, 149–154
electrocardiogram localization,
149–151
mapping techniques, 151–154
mechanisms, 139–140
automatic, 141
reentry, 139–140
triggered, 140–141
specific clinical patterns, 154–159
anterior wall myocardial infarction,
154–155
bundle branch reentrant, 158–159
fascicular, 156
idiopathic verapamil-sensitive,
157–158
inferior myocardial infarction,
155
intrafascicular reentry, 159
left ventricular outflow tract,
156
mitral annular, 156
right ventricular outflow tract,
155
substrate, 141–142
Verapamil, 280
VOO pacing, 238
VVI pacing, 234–235

W
Warfarin, 83
Wenckebach phenomena, 237–238
Wolff-Parkinson-White syndrome,
119–134
clinical evaluation, 120–126

Wolff-Parkinson-White syndrome (*contd.*)
    asymptomatic patients, 121–123
    electrocardiographic interpretation,
        123–126
    symptomatic patients, 123
  definition, 119
  electrophysiologic study, 126–133

ablation strategies, 132–133
accessory pathway, characterizing the,
    127–128
induction and evaluation of tachycardia,
    129–130
tachycardias involving preexcitation
    variants, 130–132

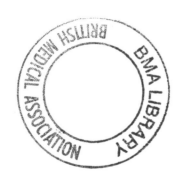